Medical Care
in Down Syndrome

PEDIATRIC HABILITATION

Series Editor

ALFRED L. SCHERZER
Cornell University Medical Center
New York, New York

Medical Care in Down Syndrome

A Preventative Medicine Approach

Paul T. Rogers
Mt. Washington Pediatric Hospital
Baltimore, Maryland, USA

Mary Coleman
Georgetown University School of Medicine
Washington, D.C., USA

With a special chapter on education by
Sue Buckley
Portsmouth Polytechnic
Portsmouth, England

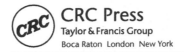

CRC Press
Taylor & Francis Group
Boca Raton London New York

CRC Press is an imprint of the
Taylor & Francis Group, an **informa** business

CRC Press
Taylor & Francis Group
6000 Broken Sound Parkway NW, Suite 300
Boca Raton, FL 33487-2742

First issued in paperback 2019

© 2008 by Taylor & Francis Group, LLC
CRC Press is an imprint of Taylor & Francis Group, an Informa business

No claim to original U.S. Government works

ISBN-13: 978-0-8247-8684-7 (hbk)
ISBN-13: 978-0-367-40278-5 (pbk)

A CIP record for this book is available from the British Library.

Library of Congress Cataloging-in-Publication Data available on application

**Visit the Taylor & Francis Web site at
http://www.taylorandfrancis.com**

**and the CRC Press Web site at
http://www.crcpress.com**

To the children and parents, who have been a continual source of inspiration and renewal

To our spouses, for their generous patience

To my father, who continually finds enjoyment, awe, and fulfillment in caring for children after nearly 40 years of pediatric practice—PTR

Preface

This book was written to provide contemporary information on the medical aspects of Down syndrome and preventive medical management. Contemporary information is needed because the increased knowledge about Down syndrome and its management often are not reported by popular reference books. For example, a contemporary pediatric textbook uses the archaic term "Mongolism" in the index and a current genetics reference book discusses institutionalization of young infants with Down syndrome. Care of young infants has changed dramatically in the last generation. Institutionalization is an obsolete practice; most state institutions in the United States do not accept young infants. Instead, community placement options such as foster care and adoption have gained prominence. In addition, community services often are available to help families care for their child.

Another reason for writing this book was to provide information about the preventive medical management of persons with Down syndrome. The preventive approach identifies early the medical problems that are common in Down syndrome and corrects them before they interrupt developing skills.

Our goal is to provide updated information to the physician to help all children and adults reach their highest potential. To facilitate access to this material, part of the book is organized developmentally, according to age. Chapter 1 briefly presents background information about the history, genetics, and epidemiology of Down syndrome. The second chapter discusses child development in Down syndrome and its implication for education. Chapters 3 to 7 detail medical management at different age periods: the neonatal period, the first year, the young child, the adolescent, and, finally, the adult. In Chapters 8 through 18, a detailed review of the medical literature is provided, including chapters on obesity and dental care. The final chapters discuss topics such as controversial therapies, legal and financial issues, and the future of research in Down syndrome.

This book will assist any practicing physician who has the following responsibilities: (1) recognition, diagnosis, and initial management of the newborn with Down syndrome; (2) managing medical problems of persons from early childhood through adulthood (from the practical problem of teaching an infant with Down syndrome how to suck to the most esoteric problem of diagnosing keratoconus of the eye in an adult); and (3) educating the family about their child's special needs and providing continuing support. This book will also benefit parents, teachers, intervention specialists, and others who have a special interest in the person with Down syndrome. In summary, the volume will help those who endeavor to maximize the developmental skills of persons with Down syndrome.

This book can be very useful to the busy clinician. Chapters 3 to 7 contain a checklist of clinical management suggestions. For example, if you are about to enter the examination room to see a 2-year-old child with Down syndrome, Chapter 5 can be consulted for a summary of medical management suggestions for a child of that age.

The book also serves as a reference source for the medical literature and can be used by professional and parent organizations that help individuals with Down syndrome.

We wish to thank the following individuals who contributed their thoughtful suggestions or their own work to the preparation of this book: Mark Jacobstein, M.D., Julie Korenberg, M.D., Roberta Kripko, M.D., John Kuehn, M.D., Greg Laforme, M.D., Professor Jerome Lejeune, Valerie Lindgren, M.D., R. A. Rogers, Ph.D., W. B. Rogers, M.D., Nancy Roizen, M.D., Alfred Scherzer, M.D., William Sherilla, M.D., Carolyn Thomas, Ph.D., James Vaughan of the University of Chicago Medical Library, Johanna Vogelsang, the artist, John Vollman, M.D., John Waterson, M.D., David C. Ward, M.D. and Ira Weiss, Ph.D. We also wish to thank the Medical Illustration Department of Johns Hopkins University, the National Down Syndrome Society, and the National Down Syndrome Congress. Special thanks go to the individuals with Down syndrome—and their parents—who allowed their photographs to be used in this book.

Paul T. Rogers
Mary Coleman

Contents

Medical Care
in Down Syndrome

I

INTRODUCING DOWN SYNDROME

1

Introduction

A holiday was coming; Jason was in an exuberant mood. The assignment was to write a poem using the letters of the name of Martin Luther King, Jr. The seventh grade boy wrote:

Martin was his name
Amazing dream
Reverend who preached love
Turned the people's ideas
Important to know black people
Nice to know

Loved everyone
Unhappy about hatred
Thought about world changing
Happy to help people
Excited because he changed the laws
Rights for all people

Kind to everyone
Ideas to make life better
Nobel prize winner
Good to everyone

Justice for all
Remember him.

This poem was the pride of the seventh-grade learning disability class. It was written by a 12-year-old boy with trisomy 21.

The extraordinary progress of many children with Down syndrome surprises many health care professionals. Many hold a very outdated picture of children with Down syndrome—that they all test in the severe mental retardation range, burden the family, require institutionalization, and die in early adulthood. In addition, there used to be the view that medical problems, such as cardiac disease, strabismus, and obesity, are part of the syndrome and need no correction.

In reality, in the 1990s, the developmental outcome of children with Down syndrome has greatly improved because of early learning programs, physician and parent updated education about the syndrome, and appropriate medical management. These children need more, not less, love and limits; they need more, not less, medical care; and they need more, not less, opportunities in life.

The goal of this book is to provide medical information to the physician to help all children and adults with Down syndrome to reach their highest potential. Many treatable problems with these children have been neglected in the past. It has happened that the patients were written off as unable to learn when, in fact, they often could not hear well because of chronic otitis media (a treatable condition) and often could not see well because of refractive errors (another treatable condition). In addition, the children sometimes lost part of the educational gains they may have made despite all obstacles caused by the effect of the childhood onset of hypothyroidism (also a treatable condition) on their brains.

The underlying problems with brain function are many (see Chapter 13), and no amount of medical intervention can correct all of the brain dysfunction at this time. However, like any other child, each child with Down syndrome is a unique result of genetic and environmental factors—a special and unique individual who must be evaluated and judged as an individual (Fig. 1.1). Although all the patients share extra chromosomal material of the twenty-first chromosome, this effect is expressed slightly differently in each child. There are three modifying effects.

One major modifying effect is the remainder of the genotype that modifies and balances the trisomy effects on the phenotype. This effect should not be underestimated in the individual evaluation of a child with Down syndrome.

A second modifying effect is the physical and emotional environment surrounding this child. It became especially clear when these children were abandoned to institutions (usually on the advice of the family's physician) that living away from one's family in an institution had an effect on the expression of the phenotype. To take just one example, there now appears to be a difference

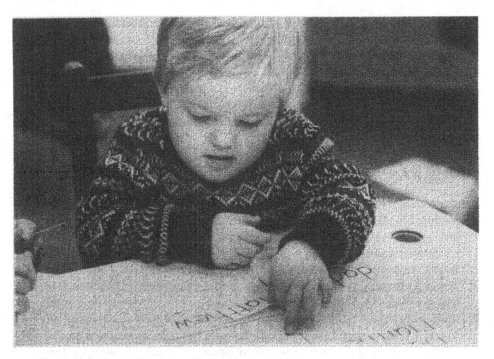

Figure 1.1 Boy with trisomy 21 learning to read.

in the age of onset of puberty in children raised at home compared to those raised in institutions (see Chapter 12).

Finally, a third modifying factor is the unevenness of appropriate medical care. If a researcher is studying brain function in a population of children with Down syndrome who have failed to be regularly tested for thyroid disease, the results of such a study will be determined by the medical condition of the children. This would not be a study of the effect of the extra twenty-first chromosomal material on these children; it would be a study of the effect of the extra chromosome plus the effect of thyroid disease in some unknown percentage of the particular population. In contemporary science, where attempts are being made to correlate the genotype with the phenotype using the tools of molecular biology and where sophisticated studies of brain function are now being proposed, it is important not to lose sight of factors that can have a major effect on the expression of the phenotype.

Intelligence and personality in a child with Down syndrome are affected by dedicated parents just as they are in non-Down syndrome children. Many studies in the medical literature report on children whose health care, there is reason to believe, has not met modern standards for individuals with Down syndrome. The validity of such studies needs careful scrutiny. Future studies of adequately nurtured and educated and medically cared-for children will lead to sounder concepts of the specific effects of the extra chromosome.

A look at the long, tortuous history of children born with Down syndrome has led to this realization of the limitations of our knowledge about this patient group.

HISTORY OF DOWN SYNDROME

The earliest evidence of Down syndrome may be found in works of art produced by the Olmec people who lived in Central America between 1500 BC and AD 300 (Fig. 1.2). Archaeologists uncovered numerous figurines that represent a young child with a round and puffy face and slanted eyes, well-marked epicanthic folds, a short nose with a broad bridge, and an obese body. The head shape was brachycephalic with a flattened occiput. The Olmec had adopted the most powerful animal that shared their habitat, the jaguar, as their main totem. These figurines are called "were-jaguar" babies by archaeologists. There is some archaeological evidence to suggest these sculptures represent babies whom the Olmec believe were the offspring of a mating between a jaguar deity and a human woman. A contemporary interpretation is that the figurines actually represent infants with Down syndrome born to the Olmecs [1].

Locating other representations of persons with Down syndrome in art is difficult until nearly the twentieth century [2]. Possible reasons for this underrepresentation in art include the smaller populations and the high infant mortality rate in the Middle Ages [3]. There have been suggestions that these infants were sometimes used by painters as models in the fourteenth, fifteenth, and sixteenth centuries in Europe because they could be unusually quiet babies that held still longer than other infants, but definite identification of the syndrome in these paintings remains controversial [4]. Today, Down syndrome children are seen so often and are so clinically apparent that it is almost hard to believe that the syndrome was identified as a distinct clinical entity only in 1866. Attempts to explain the existence of these children before that included all kinds of wild theories, such as the one that suggested that babies with Down syndrome were "changelings," that is, babies that elves used to replace normal babies [5]. According to northern European legend, elves replaced the normal baby with the "changeling" so that the special baby could have human care and milk.

When John Langdon Down published the first clinical description of individ-

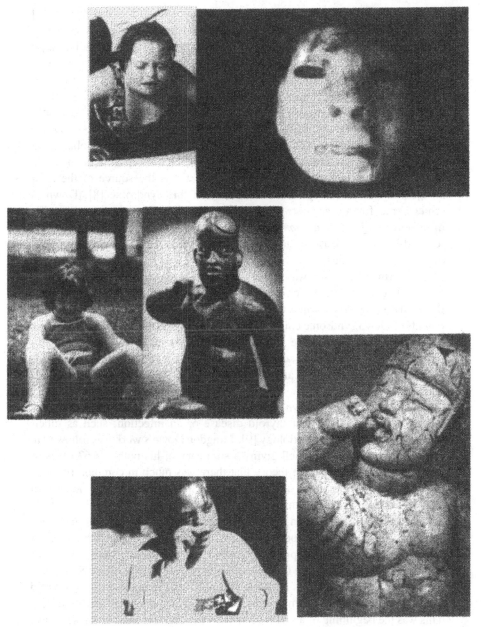

Figure 1.2 Were-jaguar figurines from Olmec culture and corresponding child with Down syndrome.

uals with Down syndrome in 1866, he earned a place in medical history [6] (Fig. 1.3). While superintendent of the Earlswood Asylum for Idiots in Surrey, England, he described retarded individuals with epicanthic folds, large tongues, and small noses who were distinct from retarded patients with cretinism. He adopted his classification system for individuals with mental retardation from a dissertation by Blumenbach who described the divisions of the human race as Caucasians, Malay (Native American), Ethiopians (African), and Mongolians [7]. Although his clinical description of persons with Down syndrome was accurate, his theory that they resembled the Mongolians and represented an arrest in ethnic development was later interpreted as an ethnic slight. This theory was discarded long ago but was the source of the term *mongoloid* that was adopted for persons with this syndrome [8]. Down is remembered for his accurate description of this patient group and for his mistaken use of the term *mongoloid*. He also should be remembered for his forward-looking endeavors such as training persons with Down syndrome to improve their abilities.

The term *mongolism* was never used in Russia where Mongol people actually live; in Russia, the children were called *Down's*. The term came under fire in the early 1960s when Chinese and Japanese investigators, as well as parents of Down syndrome children in the West, found the term offensive. The Mongolian delegation to the World Health Organization (WHO) informally requested the term not be used [7]. The term was dropped by *Lancet* in 1964, WHO publications in 1965, and *Index Medicus* in 1975 [7]. The term now is considered archaic.

The specific cause of Down syndrome was not known, but historically many investigators speculated that thyroid disease or an infection, such as tuberculosis or syphilis, was the etiology [9]. Langdon Down's work was followed in 1876 by an article by Mitchell giving a summary of his notes on 62 cases of mongolism [10]. He held the theory that there was much in common between the condition of mongolism and that of cretinism (infant hypothyroidism). In 1886, Shuttleworth decided that these were "unfinished children" [11]. In 1890, Wilmarth examined the brain of five children. He was surprised that the brains were of what he called "good size for imbecile brains," yet he advanced the theory that imperfect development or absence of certain cell groups in the pons and medulla was responsible for the condition [12]. In 1896, Telford Smith also noting certain resemblances between cretinism and mongolism gave thyroid treatments and reported an improvement in physical and mental condition [13]. This was the beginning of a series of investigators up to recent times who have recommended thyroid therapy for all children with Down syndrome (see Chapter 18 for the work of Benda who advocated giving thyroid therapy to all children with Down syndrome as late as 1969).

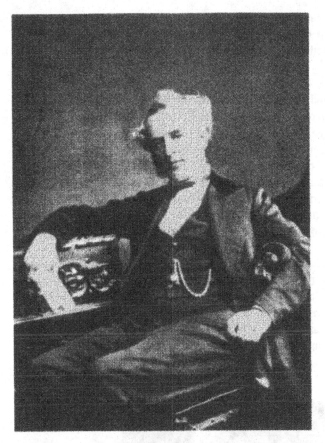

Figure 1.3   Dr. John Langdon Down.

Down's great contribution was that he was one of the pioneer practitioners who alerted his fellow physicians as early as 1866 that there are distinctive types of mental retardation and that the syndrome that he described was a clinical entity different from cretinism. Both Down syndrome and cretinism share some physical characteristics (see Chapter 12) that led to the original confusion and the century-long attempt to treat children with Down syndrome by thyroid therapy even after they were differentiated from cretins. Today, advanced laboratory testing allows us to identify one subgroup of individuals with Down syndrome who do also have thyroid disease. Thyroid treatment is, of course, contraindicated in the many euthyroid individuals with Down syndrome. (The fact that there is a subgroup of individuals with Down syndrome who also have thyroid disease continues to intrigue present-day investigators—current hypotheses question the relationship of thyroid problems in some adults with Down syndrome both to Alzheimer's disease [14] and zinc deficiency [15].)

The actual etiology underlying all cases of Down syndrome is a chromosomal aberration. Nondisjunction of the chromosomes was first suggested by Waardenburg, a Dutch ophthalmologist, in 1932 [16]. In 1934, Adrian Bleyer in the United States suggested the possibility of a chromosomal trisomy causing the syndrome [17]. In 1959, an extra chromosome was reported almost simultaneously by Jerome Lejeune et al. (Fig. 1.4) in France [18] and Patricia Jacobs et al. in England [19]. In 1960, Polani et al. discovered that some persons with Down syndrome have translocations [20]; in 1961, Clarke et al. described the first patients with mosaicism [21]. It is now known that one portion of the extra chromosome in triplicate is responsible for the phenotype of Down syndrome.

The discovery of a chromosomal aberration in Down syndrome ended a dismal period in the history of the syndrome and ushered in a new era of interest and research. Perhaps this first period, 1866–1958 (see Table 1.1), reached its greatest depth of mistreatment of children and adults with Down syndrome in the 1930s when the Nazi party of Germany began experimenting with euthanasia (or extermination) of persons with a mental disability, including Down

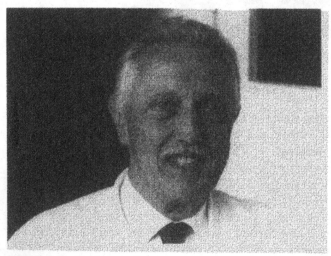

Figure 1.4 Dr. Jerome Lejeune.

Table 1.1 History of Down Syndrome

Period	Years	Historical event	Concomitant events
I.	1866–1958	Clinical delineation of Down syndrome from other forms of mental retardation	Parent bonding increasingly disrupted as younger and younger infants are placed into institutions
			Unsuccessful attempt to reverse mental retardation with various medical therapies
			Patients often denied minimal medical care
II.	1959–1972	Discovery of chromosomal aberration in patients with Down syndrome	Often further regression in humane and medical care and parent bonding due to accuracy of diagnosis in the newborn period
			Increased medical and educational research stimulated by chromosomal finding
III.	1973–present	Development of infant learning and other educational programs	Marked improvement in development of most patients receiving adequate educational and medical therapies
		Children and adults with Down syndrome begin to receive appropriate medical care	Beginning of mainstreaming in school
		Public acceptance increases	Beginning of vocations in competitive jobs

syndrome. Racism, embodied by the eugenics movement, contaminated much of Western society, and one of its secondary results was to isolate the "feeble-minded" in large depersonalized institutions [22].

The second period (1959–1972) in the history of Down syndrome was opened by the discovery of the presence of extra chromosomal material in the tissues of persons with Down syndrome [18,19]. One immediate effect was an increased admission to institutions of very young infants because with chromosome testing available, a physician could be quite sure of the diagnosis before parent bonding to the infant was developed. Many chromosomal laboratories sprang up, and a large number of different distinct chromosomal entities were discovered very rapidly [23].

However, the value of institutionalizing infants with Down syndrome was beginning to be questioned, partly as the result of the long waiting lists at institutions. Studies, such as those by Stedman and Eichorn (1964), were describing the negative impact of institutionalization on Down syndrome children [24]. In addition to the lack of a significant continuing caregiver whom a human child needs for emotional reasons, it was realized that the lack of stimulation in an institutional environment appeared to be lowering cognitive functioning even further. In medicine, it was a time of coming to recognize the emotional needs of the hospitalized child and to understand the importance of a multidisciplinary perspective for disabled children of all kinds. A new subspeciality of medicine, developmental pediatrics, was created to train physicians for the specialized needs of retarded children. (One of the authors of this book, Dr. Paul Rogers, is such a specialist.)

In the field of education, early education for mentally handicapped children was being developed during this period. Basic research on infants and young children increased, stimulated by new ideas such as those of Piaget [25]. In the United States, this interest was furthered by a climate of concern for underprivileged children in general, as the "Head Start" programs indicate. The Bureau of the Education of the Handicapped took a leadership role in first pilot and, then, fully funded programs for infants with Down syndrome [22].

The third period (1973 to the present) of Down syndrome history in the United States was opened with a landmark 1972 court decision (the PARC case) that declared that every child, regardless of mental ability, had a right to a free, appropriate public program of education. The following year (1973) in the United States, a national organization—the Down Syndrome Congress—was established by parents of Down syndrome children and professionals. Quietly, but dramatically, the movement to make it possible for families to care for their children at home was developing. In 1975, the Education for All Handicapped Children Act (PL. 94–142) was passed by the U.S. Congress. This was the most important of a group of laws that protect the educational rights of Down syndrome children to this day [22].

The rise of the community care movement was associated with a significant decrease in the number of persons in institutions and an increase in the number and quality of community programs for infants and young children. Today, many institutions will not accept newborn infants with Down syndrome; if it is not possible to stay with their family, they are placed in foster care or adopted. The first educational programs for home-reared children, originally called early intervention programs, not only educated parents about their child's special needs but began a systematic infant education protocol. For older children, federal laws such as PL 94–142 guaranteed a least restrictive, appropriate education for handicapped children of all ages.

Exactly what form of infant and childhood education is most useful to children with Down syndrome is still a topic under discussion (see Chapter 2 for a discussion of this topic). There is a consensus that early infant and family education is important. Adults with Down syndrome also have been helped by legislation in the United States. The Rehabilitation Act of 1973 (PL 93–112) has prescribed far-reaching civil rights protections that have led to enhanced opportunities for living and working in the community [22].

As the newborns with Down syndrome started to come home to their families rather than institutions, the medical profession began to take a more active interest in the medical care of this patient group. In addition to the researchers in chromosome laboratories, clinicians began to include these children in their populations receiving modern cardiac care, gastrointestinal surgery, auditory evaluations, and so on. Advances in the treatment of congenital cardiac disease, surgically repairable gastrointestinal lesions, and infectious disease has increased the life expectancy of persons with Down syndrome [26]. In 1978, this medical literature was brought together into one newsletter that reviewed the literature and highlighted the special medical needs of children and adults with Down syndrome [27]. In 1981, a special protocol or checklist presenting specific medical management suggestions was developed and initially updated every 2 years [28]. "The Down's Syndrome Preventive Medicine Checklist" was created for the use of clinics springing up throughout the world and especially designed for the competent, modern medical care of individuals with Down syndrome. A number of clinics throughout the world currently use the checklist to care for persons with Down syndrome. Chapters 3–7 of this volume present the medical information on which the preventive medicine program is based and provide the latest checklist currently being used in the clinics. The checklist currently is updated by the consensus of the clinic directors at regular intervals.

During the 1980s, further progress was made not only in clinical care but also in educational and vocational opportunities. Down syndrome adults work in a great variety of competitive jobs from creating "fast food" to starring in television series. During this decade, the study of the chromosomes has grown increasingly sophisticated with the development of gene assignments to the twenty-first and other chromosomes.

CHROMOSOME STUDIES

Threadlike structures, later called chromosomes, were observed for the first time in the nuclei of plant cells by K. Naegeli, a Swiss botanist in 1842. Naegeli called these structures transient cytoblasts. The term *chromosome* was coined by W. Waldeyer in 1898, and in 1902, Sutton identified the chromosomes as carriers of the genetic information in a cell [23]. The hypothesis that chromosome abnormalities could produce human pathology such as Down syndrome was proven almost simultaneously by Jerome Lejeune et al. in France [18] and Patricia Jacobs et al. in England [19].

Down syndrome results from a mistake, called nondisjunction, when chromosomes divide. The creation of the egg or sperm occurs when a cell with 46 chromosomes divides in half to create two germ cells—each with 23 chromosomes. In normal disjunction, the process of separation called meiosis, which takes two steps, results in equal cell division each time. Each egg and each sperm has 23 chromosomes. At fertilization, the union of the egg and sperm results in a zygote (a potential infant) with the full component of 46 chromosomes in 23 pairs.

In nondisjunction, the cell with 46 chromosomes fails to divide properly. One germ cell has 24 chromosomes, another only 22 chromosomes. At fertilization, the germ cell with only 22 chromosomes when combined to another germ cell produces a zygote of 45 chromosomes that is rarely viable. The germ cell with 24 chromosomes combines with a normal germ cell of 23 chromosomes, and a zygote is created with a total of 47 chromosomes (Fig. 1.5). This zygote with 47 chromosomes is more likely to survive.

By analyzing a specific marker called a DNA polymorphism in children with Down syndrome and their parents, researchers are developing techniques where they can identify the stage at which the chromosome division went wrong. Preliminary results suggest that error occurs in nearly 75% of the cases in the first stage of meiosis on formation of the mother's egg (when she herself is still a fetus) [29]. In the other 25% of the cases, the error probably occurs in stage 2 of meiosis during ovulation. This kind of analysis can be used to help genetic counseling in families that already have a child with Down syndrome.

Most patients with Down syndrome have an entire extra chromosome in their cells. Because the extra chromosome makes for three twenty-first chromosomes (a pair plus one extra), the chromosomal karyotype of these patients is called trisomy 21. *Tri* is the Greek word for "three." About 90% (89.3–93.9%) of Down syndrome individuals have a total of 47 cells instead of the usual 46, with a karyotype of trisomy 21 [30]. So trisomy 21 is, by far, the most usual karyotype found when one checks blood, skin, bone marrow, or other tissues of a Down syndrome individual.

Another small group of patients have a mixture of two types of cells in their bodies—trisomy 21 with 47 chromosomes and the normal cell pattern of 46 chromosomes. These patients are labeled chromosome mosaics. The frequency of this patient group is difficult to establish because theoretically it is impos-

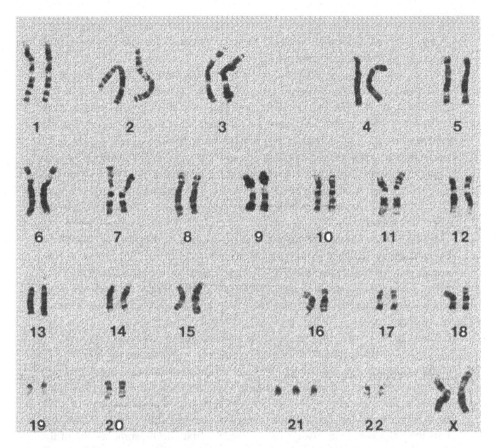

Figure 1.5 Chromosomal karyotype of a baby girl with trisomy 21. From the laboratory of Dr. Valerie Lindgren, University of Chicago.

sible to rule out the presence of a second cell line in a tissue studied from an individual. Therefore, each laboratory sets its own arbitrary limit to distinguish pure trisomy from mosaicism by the number of cells counted in each particular patient.

There are three types of mosaicism. The most common form, thought to occur in about 3% of affected persons, is *cellular mosaicism*. This is usually established by studying lymphocytes from the blood or fibroblast cells from the skin. Two types of cells are found in the tissue under study—one cell line has trisomy 21 (47 chromosomes), and the other cell line has a normal karyotype

(46 chromosomes). The cell lines are not found in permanently fixed percentages in any one individual because there is evidence for changes over time toward an increase of the normal cell line.

A second type of mosaicism is *tissue mosaicism*. In this rare type of mosaicism, one tissue will show trisomy 21, whereas another tissue will have a normal karyotype. For example, the lymphocytes in the blood might show trisomy 21, whereas the fibroblasts of the skin have a normal karyotype. In another rare form of mosaicism, *chimerism*, a fusion of two products of conception occurs at the time of conception to form a single individual. It is as if potential twins turned into one person. Each original zygote could have had separate chromosomal information, such as one having trisomy 21 and the other having a normal karyotype, which is expressed in two different cell lines in the single individual.

While on the subject of mosaicism, it should be noted that up to 10% of the normal parents of Down syndrome children may be mosaics themselves. The parents may be undetected clinically because they have good intelligence and little, if any, stigmata of Down syndrome. [30]. When there is no other explanation for familial Down syndrome, a search for parental mosaicism may be indicated [31a].

Sometimes breaks in two separate chromosomes may be followed by unification of the fragment of one chromosome with the wrong fragment of another chromosome. This rearrangement of chromosomes is a *translocation*. The most frequent translocations in Down syndrome are centric fusions (also known as Robertsonian translocations) where the two short arms of both chromosomes and the center (centromere) of one of them are lost. Translocations in Down syndrome always have a twenty-first chromosome as one of the two translocated chromosomes. The second involved chromosome is usually either another twenty-first chromosome or a fourteenth chromosome, although other chromosomes can sometimes be seen.

Translocations can be inherited, so a check of the parents for genetic counseling is indicated. If the child has normal siblings and a double 21q:21q translocation, the parents usually are not carriers. The frequency with which carrier translocation parents have Down syndrome offspring varies with the type of translocation but is usually less than the percentage theoretically predicted probably because of the loss of Down syndrome fetuses early in pregnancy.

In addition to these three main groups of chromosomal errors found in persons with Down syndrome, there also are very rare chromosome types occasionally reported. Ring chromosomes, isochromosomes, and double aneuploidy have been reported.

It is recommended that every individual with Down syndrome have a chromosomal karyotype performed. This is usually done by cell cultures and metaphase chromosome spreads (Fig. 1.5). Another technique, hybridization in situ, is also now commercially available in the United States [31b]. With chromosome 21 DNA specific probes, a digital image processing of single cells is illustrated (Fig. 1.6). Currently used for diagnosis of neonatal cells, amniotic fluid samples, and chorionic villus samples, this technique may eventually become applicable to fetal cells found in the maternal blood.

The individuals with translocation sometimes do not exhibit all the clinical features of Down syndrome, having only a partial trisomy 21 [32]. The molecular genetic methodology has made it possible to begin the correlation of the phenotypic components of Down syndrome with imbalance in specific regions of the twenty-first chromosome. By studying these rare translocation/partial trisomy 21 cases, it is now possible to begin these correlations. Such

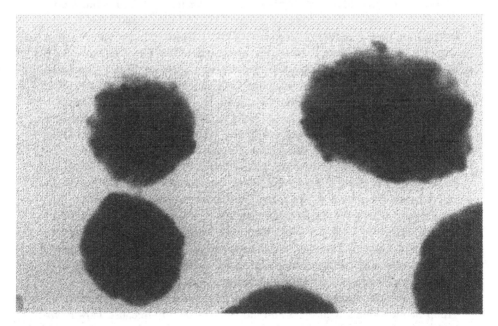

Figure 1.6 DNA probe showing three, rather than two, fluorescent signals, which is another way of diagnosing the presence of trisomy 21. From the laboratory of Dr. David Ward, Yale University.

phenotypic mapping eventually should make it possible to discover exactly which genes are responsible for which aspects of the phenotype of Down syndrome.

The initial studies suggested that the distal region of chromosome 21 was responsible for the recognizable features of Down syndrome [33]. In Fig. 1.7, a phenotypic map has been constructed from 17 well-defined cases of chromosome 21 duplications published since 1973 [34]. Observations such as these have led to the suggestion that a small region of chromosome 21 band q22 may contain a cluster of genes that may independently contribute to the development of the brain, heart, gastrointestinal tract, and immune system. This cluster of genes may also contribute to some dysmorphic features; epicanthic folds, Brushfield spots, and the gap between the first and second toes are a few examples of phenotypic features now being studied in the mapping system. This map indicates only the minimal regions involved in producing a particular clinical feature and will be refined as other cases are studied. It is already clear that genes in other regions contribute to the Down syndrome phenotype.

Advances in the field of human gene mapping have allowed for the creation of a detailed molecular map of chromosome 21 emerging from studies conducted by a number of investigative groups [35]. In Fig. 1.8 and Table 1.2, the information now available is correlated. Table 1.2 also indicates genes (DNA sequences) that are known to be expressed but whose function is unknown. It is of interest that the region defined for congenital cardiac disease comprises about 9 million base pairs and includes the genes ETS2 oncogene, the ETS2 related gene, ERG, and CBS [36].

Of note, although any of the genes included in a given region may contribute to a feature, the genes now defined in any region likely represent less than 10% of all genes located in that region of chromosome 21. Nevertheless, it is tempting to speculate on the potential relationship between the gene and phenotype. It is possible that abnormalities in the expression of CRYA1 (the major structural protein of the ocular lens) may predispose to cataracts. It is possible that IFN A/BR, the interferon receptors or CD18, may be related to the immune defects [37]. It is possible that ETS2, the oncogene, may be related to one of the leukemias found more frequently in patients with Down syndrome [38]. Does the amyloid beta protein precursor gene play a role in the frequency of Alzheimer's disease in adults with Down syndrome [39]?

These questions and many more are leading to new approaches to help this group of individuals with extra chromosomal material. Because Down syndrome is the most common chromosomal abnormality seen in newborns, this kind of molecular genetic information being teased out of the twenty-first chromosome may be a paradigm for studies of many less frequent chromosomal aberrations.

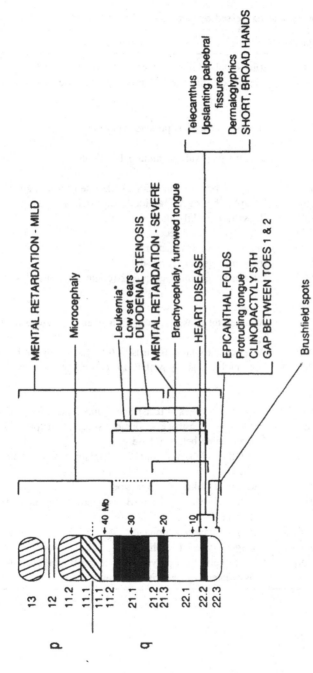

Figure 1.7 Down Syndrome phenotypic map—cytogenetic: 1973–1989. (Courtesy of J. Korenberg, Ph.D.)

Table 1.2 Genes and Expressed Sequences on Chromosome 21

DNAs	Genes	Expression
	RNR4	Ribosomal 4 (cluster of genes for ribosomal RNA)
	AD1	Alzheimer's disease 1 (familial; by genetic linkage)
D21S13		
D21S95		
	APP	Amyloid beta (A4) precursor protein
D21S93		
	SOD1	Cu-Zu superoxide dismutase 1, soluble
D21S58		
	PAIS	Phosphoribosylglycinamide synthetase (purine biosynthesis)
	PGFT	Phosphoribosylglycinamide formyl transferase
	PRGS	Phosphoribosylglycinamide synthetase
	IFNAR	Interferon, alpha; receptor
	IFNBR	Interferon, beta; receptor
	IFNGT1	Interferon, gamma; transducer 1
	IFNGR2	Interferon, gamma; receptor 2 (confers antiviral resistance)
D21S17		
D21S55		
	ERG	Avian etythroblastosis virus E26 (v-ets) oncogene related
D21S57		
	ETS 2	Avian erythroblastosis virus E26 (v-ets) oncogene homolog 2
	HMG 14	High mobility group protein 14 (chromatin-associated protein)
D21S3		
D21S15		
	MX1, 2	Myxovirus influenza resistance 1 and 2, homologs of murine
	BCEI	Breast cancer, estrogen-inducible sequence, expressed in
	CBS	Cystathionine beta synthase
	CRYA1	Crystallin, alpha polypeptide 1 (major protein of the ocular lens)
	PFKL	Phosphofructokinase, liver type
	CD18	Antigen CD18 (p95) (LFA-1B), lymphocyte function–associated antigen 1
	COL6A1	Collagen, type VI, alpha 1
	COL6A2	Collagen, type VI, alpha 2
	S100B	S100 protein, beta polypeptide (neural); glial specific protein associated with neurite outgrowth

EPIDEMIOLOGY

The incidence of births of babies with Down syndrome appears to be changing. In the 1976 textbook *Down's Anomaly*, 32 studies from the previous 25 years were analyzed, and an incidence of the order of 1 in 700 births was reported with "the results of various investigators in good agreement" [40]. Ten years later, industrialized countries were reporting a decline in the incidence of infants at birth with Down syndrome [41]. In 1985, the United States reported an incidence of 1 in every 1250 births [42], whereas England and Wales reported a similar figure of 1 in every 1265 births [43].

An example of this phenomenon is seen in the 1990 report from the Alsace region of northeastern France [44]. Although this study reports a conception incidence of 1 in 854 pregnancies, the actual live birth incidence was 1 in 1041. Stillbirths (3.6%) and induced abortions (14.4%) made the difference. In France, prenatal diagnosis is offered to every pregnant woman more than 38 years old. This study was conducted from 1979 to 1987, which included the data of the Chernobyl accident in May 1986, and was part of a collaborative study undertaken in 19 birth defects registries in Europe that sought to determine the impact of this radiological contamination. This collaborative study, which analyzed frequency rates by month of conception, did not indicate any immediate increases in birth defects right after the Chernobyl accident [45].

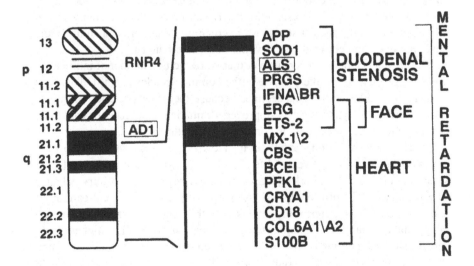

Figure 1.8 Chromosome 21 expressed genes.

The incidence figures for births always have varied from country to country when detailed epidemiological studies were done. Kuwait has one of the highest consanguineous marriage rates in the world—about 50% of all marriages. A study by Alfi et al. reported a fourfold increase in the incidence of Down syndrome within consanguineous marriages in Kuwait after controlling for maternal age and gravidity [46].

In Denmark, the age of the birth-giving mothers is older in studies conducted during the 1980s than in those in the 1960s [47]. This phenomenon could result in increases in the number of births because there is a close relationship between the frequency of births and advanced maternal age [48–50] (Table 1.3). this relationship between maternal age and frequency of births has long been established. Changes in maternal age patterns can affect the incidence statistics [51].

Therefore, it was somewhat of a surprise when evidence surfaced of paternal origin in some cases of Down syndrome. According to cytogenetic techniques, the paternal origin was thought to be between 12% and 20%, but DNA polymorphic analysis shows that a figure of 5% is more likely for the paternal origin of nondisjunction [29,52].

Screening during gestation for Down syndrome is now done by amniocentesis and chorionic villus sampling. The development of a battery of screening tests by sampling the blood of the mother are now being developed but are yet to be fully reliable [53]. Also under consideration are techniques screening the early embryo during the first trimester. (Ultrasound techniques for identification described in second trimester fetuses have the disadvantage of being late in the pregnancy.) One such first trimester screening technique is a study of the deviating development of the embryonic heart rate pattern [54].

The prevalence of Down syndrome, that is, the actual number of individuals alive at a given time, is likely to rise in the coming decades [26,55]. This is so even as the incidence of births declines because the life expectancy of infants born with Down syndrome has improved dramatically in recent years. The number one killer, infections, is coming under better control.

In 1953, Oster reported that 53% of the Down syndrome infants in a hospital series died during the first year of life [56]. In contrast, recent studies of Down syndrome infants in Denmark and Japan have shown estimates of survival rates of more than 92% until the age of 1 year [57,58]. Better medical care at all levels, especially in preterm tiny infants, and the aggressive intervention with congenital anomalies are factors in these improved statistics. The highest death rate for Down syndrome infants occurs between the ages of 28 days and 1 year, where in one recent Danish study it was still 30 times greater than the death probability in the Danish population of normal infants of the same age interval

Table 1.3 Rates of Down Syndrome per 1000 Live Births by Single-Year Maternal Age Intervals

Maternal age in years	Massachusetts study[a]	New York study[b]	Swedish study[c]
20	0.57	0.52	0.64
21	0.60	0.69	0.67
22	0.64	0.65	0.71
23	0.67	0.71	0.75
24	0.70	0.77	0.79
25	0.74	0.83	0.83
26	0.77	0.89	0.87
27	0.80	0.95	0.92
28	0.84	1.01	0.97
29	0.87	1.07	1.02
30	0.90	1.13	1.08
31	0.93	1.21	1.14
32	1.15	1.38	1.25
33	1.55	1.69	1.47
34	1.98	2.15	1.92
35	2.53	2.74	2.51
36	3.22	3.49	3.28
37	4.11	4.45	4.28
38	5.24	5.66	5.60
39	6.68	7.21	7.32
40	8.52	9.19	9.57
41	10.86	11.71	12.51
42	13.85	14.91	16.36
43	17.66	19.00	21.39
44	22.51	24.20	27.96
45	28.71	30.84	36.55
46	36.61	39.28	47.79
47	46.68	50.04	62.47
48	59.52	63.75	81.67
49	75.89	81.21	106.76

[a]Ref. 48.
[b]Ref. 49.
[c]Ref. 50.
Source: Reprinted with permission of Ware Press, Cambridge, Mass.

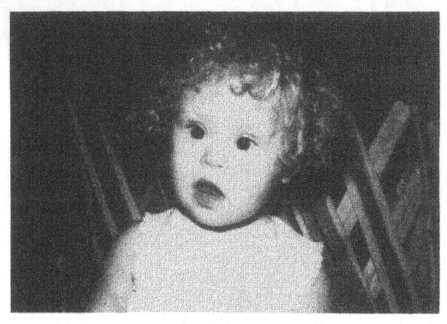

Figure 1.9   Child with Down syndrome.

[47]. A major factor affecting the probability of survival in young children is the presence of congenital cardiac disease.

Recently, a prevalence study of Down syndrome by 5-year age groups was performed in a province in northeast Italy (Belluno) [59]. Until 40 years of age, the prevalence was remarkably stable between 1:1100 and 1:1550. After 40 years of age, the rates began to rise to 1:2800 from 40 to 44 years of age, 1:3250 from 45 to 49 years of age, and 1:19,750 at greater than 50 years of age. This study also recorded the frequency of complicating disorders in this population; the study showed a relatively high incidence of ocular pathology, infectious diseases, autoimmune diseases, and anxiety or depressive disorders. Starting with Chapter 3, the medical care needed by such individuals will be the focus of this book.

The health and emotional well being of individuals with Down syndrome has implications in today's societies. In the industrial nations, there already is unemployment among nonhandicapped persons. In the twenty-first century, high technology is changing the vocational opportunities for everyone. The young adults with Down syndrome need maximum opportunity to maintain their cognitive gains of early childhood and their health and strength as adults.

It is a high priority that these children and adults get appropriate medical care designed to enhance the quality of their lives. Because each person with Down syndrome is unique, only the physician in full command of the history, physical examination, and laboratory results can decide what is needed for that individual. The preventive medical checklists (at the end of Chapters 3–7) suggest questions that might help the physician anticipate and head off potential medical problems.

REFERENCES

1. Milton G, Gonzales R. Jaguar cults—Down's syndrome—were-jaguar. Expedition 1974;16:33–37.
2. Mirkinson AE. Is Down's syndrome a modern disease? (Letter to the editor). Lancet 1968;ii:103.
3. Richards BW. Is Down's syndrome a modern disease? (Letter to the editor). Lancet 1968;ii:353–354.
4. Volpe EP. Is Down syndrome a modern disease? Perspect Biol Med 1986;29:423–436.
5. Levin. Changelings. S Afr Med J 1971;45(16):444–447.
6. Down JLH. Observations of an ethnic classification of idiots. Clinical Lectures and Reports by the Medical and Surgical Staff of the London Hospital 1866;3:259–262.
7. Howard-Jones N. On the diagnostic term "Down's Disease." Med Hist 1979;23:102–104.
8. Gould SJ. Dr. Down's syndrome. MD April 1983;55–61.
9. Brousseau K, Brainerd HG (rev.) Mongolism: A study of the physical and mental characteristics of mongolian imbeciles. Baltimore, MD: Williams & Wilkins, 1928.
10. Mitchell A. J Ment Sci 1876;xxii:174.
11. Shuttleworth GE. Clinical lecture on idiocy and imbecility. Br Med J 1886; i:183.
12. Wilmarth SW. Report on the examination of one hundred brains of feeble-minded children. Alienist and Neurologist October 1890.
13. Smith T. Thyroid treatment of cretinism and imbecility in children. Br Med J 1896; ii:1429.
14. Percy ME, Dalton AJ, Markovic VD, McLachlan DRC, Jera E, Humnel JT, Rusk ACM, Somerville MJ, Andrew DF, Walfish PG. Autoimmune thyroiditis associated with "subclinical" hypothyroidism in adults with Down syndrome: A comparison of patients with and without manifestations of Alzheimer's disease. Am J Med Genet 1990;36:148–154.
15. Nupditano G, Polka G, Lio S, Bucci I, DeRemigs P, Stuppiai L, Monoco F. Zinc deficiency a cause of some clinic hypothyroidism in Down syndrome? Ann Genet 1990;33:9–15.
16. Waardenburg PJ. Das menschliche Auge und seine Erbanlagen. The Hague, Netherlands: Martinus Nijhoff, 1932.

17. Bleyer A. Indications that mongoloid imbecility is a gametic mutation of the degenerative type. Am J Dis Child 1934;47:342.

18. Lejeune J, Gautier M, Turpin R. Etude des chromosomes somatiques de neuf enfants mongoliens. CR Acad Sci 1959;248:1721–1722.

19. Jacobs PA, Baikie AG, Court-Brown WM, Strong JA. The somatic chromosomes in mongolism. Lancet 1959;i:710.

20. Polani PE, Briggs JH, Ford CE, Clarke CM, Berg JM. A mongol girl with 46 chromosomes. Lancet 1960;i:721.

21. Clarke CM, Edwards JH, Smallpiece V. 21 trisomy/normal mosaicism in an intelligent child with mongoloid characteristics. Lancet 1961;i:1028–1030.

22. Rynders JE. History of Down syndrome. In: Pueschel SM, Tingey C, Rynders JE, Crocker AC, Crutcher DM, eds. New Perspectives on Down Syndrome. Baltimore, MD: Paul H Brooks, 1987:1–20.

23. Zellweger H, Simpson J. Chromosomes of Man. London: William Heinemann Medical Books, 1977.

24. Stedman D, Eichorn A. A comparison of the growth and development of institutionalized and home-reared mongoloids during infancy and early childhood. Am J Med Def 1964;391–401.

25. Spiker D. Early intervention. In: Cicchetti D, Beeghly M, eds. Children with Down Syndrome: A Developmental Perspective. Cambridge: Cambridge University Press, 1990:424–448.

26. Declining mortality from Down syndrome—No cause for complacency. Lancet 1990; i:888–889. Editorial.

27. Coleman M, ed. Down's Syndrome: Papers and Abstracts for Professionals. Washington DC: Children's Brain Research Clinic, 1978;1:1–4.

28. Coleman M. Down's syndrome preventive medicine checklist. In: Coleman, ed. Down's Syndrome: Papers and Abstracts for Professionals 1981;4:1–2.

29. Antonarakis SE and the Down Syndrome Collaborative Group. Parental origin of the extra chromosome in trisomy 21 as indicated by analysis of DNA polymorphisms. N Engl J Med 1991;324:872–876.

30. Thuline HC, Pueschel SM. Cytogenetics in Down syndrome. In: Pueschel SM, Rynders JE, eds. Down Syndrome: Advances in Biomedicine and the Behavioral Sciences. Cambridge, Mass: Ware Press, 1982:133–167.

31a. Timson J, Harris R, Gadd RL, Ferguson-Smith ME, Ferguson-Smith MA. Down's syndrome due to maternal mosaicism and the value of antenatal diagnosis. Lancet 1971;i:549–550.

31b. Lichter P, Jarch A, Cremer T, Ward DC. Detection of Down syndrome by in situ hybridization with chromosome 21 specific DNA probes. In: Patterson D, Epstein CJ, eds. Molecular Genetics of Chromosome 21 and Down Syndrome. New York: Wiley-Liss, 1990:69–78.

32. Jenkins EC, Duncan CJ, Wright CE, Giordano FM, Wilbur L, Wisniewski KE, Sjilower SL, French JH, Jones C, Brown WT. Atypical Down syndrome and partial trisomy 21. Clin Genet 1983;24:97–102.

33. Niebuhr E. Down's syndrome: The possibility of a pathogenetic segment on chromosome 21. Hum Genet 1974;21:99–101.
34. Korenberg J. Unpublished, 1991.
35. Patterson D, Epstein CJ, eds. Molecular Genetics of Chromosome 21 and Down Syndrome. New York: Wiley-Liss, 1990.
36. Korenberg JR, Kojis TI, Bradley C, Distech C. Down syndrome and band 21q22.2: Molecular definition of the phenotype. Am J Hum Genet 1989;45:A71.
37. Jones C, Morse H, Jung V, Rashidbaigi A, Langer J, Pestka S. The interferon receptor and inducer genes and chromosome 21. In: Patterson D, Epstein CJ, eds. Molecular Genetics of Chromosome 21 and Down Syndrome. New York: Wiley-Liss, 1990:131–136.
38. Papas TS, Watson DK, Sacchi N, Fujiwara S, Seth AK, Fisher RJ, Bhat NK, Mavrothalassitis G, Koizumi S, Jorcyk CL, Schweinfest CW, Kottaridis SD, Ascione R. ETS family of genes in leukemia and Down syndrome. Am J Med Genet 1990;(suppl 7):251–261.
39. Tanzi RE. The Alzheimer disease-associated amyloid beta protein precursor gene and familial Alzheimer disease. In: Patterson D, Epstein CJ, eds. Molecular Genetics of Chromosome 21 and Down Syndrome. New York: Wiley-Liss, 1990: 187–200.
40. Smith GF, Berg JM. Down's Anomaly. Edinburgh: Churchill Livingstone, 1976: 234–250.
41. Janerich DT, Bracken MB. Epidemiology of trisomy 21: A review and theoretical analysis. J Chronic Dis 1986;39:1079–1093.
42. Centers for Disease Control. Congenital malformation surveillance report: January 1981–December 1983. September 1985.
43. Office of Population and Censuses and Surveys. Congenital malformations, 1984. OPCS Monitor MB3 85/2.
44. Stoll C, Alembik Y, Dott B, Roth M-P. Epidemiology of Down syndrome in 118,265 consecutive births. Am J Med Genet 1990;(suppl 7):79–83.
45. De Wals P, Bertrand F, De La Mata I, Lechat M. Chromosomal anomalies and Chernobyl. Int J Epidemiol 1988;17:230–231.
46. Alfi OS, Chang R, Azen SP. Evidence for genetic control of nondisjunction in man. Am J Hum Genet 1980;32:477–483.
47. Mikkelsen M, Poulsen H, Nielsen KG. Incidence, survival and mortality in Down syndrome in Denmark. Am J Med Genet 1990;(suppl 7):75–78.
48. Hook EB, Fabia JJ. Frequency of Down syndrome by single-year maternal age interval: Results of a Massachusetts study. Teratology 1978;17:223–228.
49. Hook EB, Chambers GM. Estimated rates of Down's syndrome in live-births by one-year maternal age intervals for mothers aged 20 to 49 in a New York state study—implications of the "risk" figures for genetic counseling and cost-benefit analysis of prenatal diagnosis programs. In: Bergsma D, Lowry RB, Trimble BK, Feingold M, eds. Numerical Taxonomy on Birth Defects and Polygenic Disorders. Birth Defects Original Series 1977;13:124–141.

50. Hook EB, Linnsajo A. Down's syndrome in live births by single-year maternal age intervals in a Swedish study: Comparison with results from New York state. Am J Hum Genet 1978;30:19–27.
51. Baird PA, Sadovnick AD. Maternal age-specific rates for Down syndrome: Changes over time. Am J Med Genet 1988;29:917–927.
52. Petersen MB, et al. Use of short sequence repeat DNA polymorphisms after DCR amplification to detect the parental origin of the additional chromosome 21 in Down syndrome. Am J Hum Genet 1991;48:65–71.
53. Smithells D. Biochemical screening for chromosome disorders. Dev Med Child Neurol 1990;32:172–178.
54. Schats R, Jansen CAM, Wladimiroff JW. Abnormal embryonic heart rate pattern in early pregnancy associated with Down's syndrome. Hum Reprod 1990;5: 877–879.
55. McGrother CW, Marshall B. Recent trends in incidence, morbidity and survival in Down's syndrome. J Ment Defic Res 1990;34:49–57.
56. Oster J. Mongolism: A clinicogenealogical investigation comprising 526 mongols living in Seeland and neighboring islands in Denmark. Kobenhaven: Danish Science Press, 1953.
57. Masaki M, Higurashi M, Iijima K, Ishikawa N, Tanaka F, Fujii T, Kuroki Y, Matsui I, Iinuma K, Matsuo N, Takeshita K, Hashimoto S. Mortality and survival for Down syndrome in Japan. Am J Hum Genet 1981;33:629–639.
58. Dupont A, Vaeth M, Videbech P. Mortality and life expectancy of Down's syndrome in Denmark. J Ment Defic Res 1986;30:111–120.
59. Bacchichetti C, Lenzini E, Pegoraro R. Down syndrome in the Belluno district (Veneto region, northeast Italy): Age distribution and morbidity. Am J Med Genet 1990;(suppl 7):84–86.

2

The Development of the Child with Down Syndrome: Implications for Effective Education

INTRODUCTION

For parents, one of the most pressing questions on hearing that their child has Down syndrome is "What will he or she be able to do, as a 5 year old, as a teenager, as an adult? Will he or she ever be able to read and write, be able to leave home, be able to work?" In summary, "What kind of development can we expect?"

The next question may well be "What can we do to improve our child's development?" and by the age of 3 years, the most pressing question may be "What sort of education should we choose, special school or mainstream school? Where will he or she do best?"

These are the questions to be addressed in this chapter, which presents a review of the current state of knowledge to enable practitioners to give informed answers to parents and to plan effective early intervention and education services (Fig. 2.1).

Our understanding of the development of children with Down syndrome has progressed significantly in the last decade. There has been a great deal of research into all areas of psychological development, and psychologists are beginning to describe in detail some of the subtle ways in which Down syndrome affects the processes of development causing delay in the early years [1]. Much of this information has practical implications and should enable us to

This chapter was prepared by Sue Buckley.

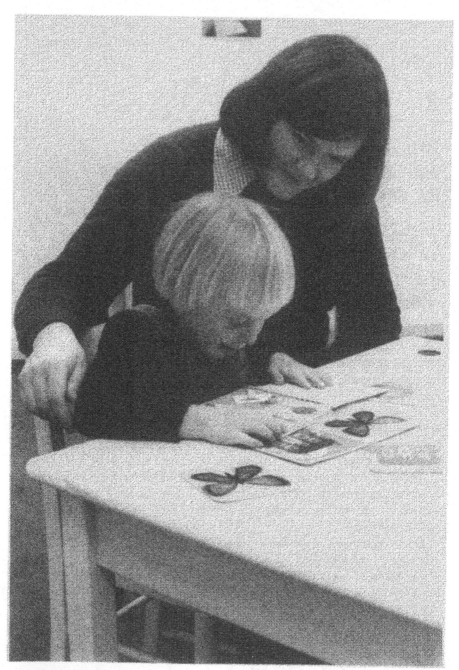

Figure 2.1 Early learning program.

design more effective remedial programs targeted at the children's specific learning difficulties.

It has been a decade of great optimism and progress. Many children with Down syndrome are now making faster progress than they did 25 years ago as a result of advances in medical care, education, remedial services, and more positive attitudes toward disability in the community [2,3]. Sufficient numbers of children have now progressed through early intervention programs and through mainstream school for some critical evaluation of outcomes to be possible [3–5].

During the same period, researchers have also been concerned with the needs of families, beginning to identify the coping strategies that enable most families to adjust [6] and the particular characteristics that may increase the vulnerability of the family [7]. It is increasingly being acknowledged that any intervention offered by service providers must recognize the need of the family system as a whole and not simply focus on the child [8]. This is especially important in the early years. Parents have a right to be presented with accurate information about the positive and negative effects of any sort of intervention that they are offered and to be encouraged to make informed choices, aware of the implications of those choices for all members of the family.

The answer to the first question, "What kind of development can we expect?" will be considered in three stages: infancy, the early school years, and teenage years drawing on the studies available at present. The answer to the second question, "What can we do to improve our child's development" will be preceded by considering what is known about the reasons for delayed progress, "Why these delays?" Finally, the planning and delivery of services will be considered in the light of research into both the child and family needs.

Before beginning to discuss the early development of the infant with Down syndrome, it may be useful to consider the current understanding of development in ordinary children and the processes that affect it to provide a framework in which to discuss the processes of development in Down syndrome.

THE DYNAMIC PROCESS OF DEVELOPMENT

Developmental psychology is a young science. In-depth study of the processes and pathways of development in the past 20 years has begun to lead to a greater understanding of some aspects of ordinary development. Two important principles have emerged: first, the process of development is a transactional one [9], depending on complex interactions between the child and the environment at each stage; second, the infant is very active in initiating and controlling this interaction with his or her world. The development and functional organization of the brain after birth is an ongoing process affected by the child's experiences and activities as well as his or her genes [10,11]. Ordinary development is a dynamic, interactive process that can be disrupted in many ways.

At each step from birth onward, the infant's developmental progress is dependent on the quality of these interactions and experiences and on his or her capacity to understand and learn from them. To begin to understand the development of a child with a disability, it is necessary to look at each step of development and identify the ways in which the normal interactive process has been altered, thereby changing or delaying the child's progress.

The interactive processes may be altered by biological limitations or delays, by differences in the infant's responsiveness to his or her environment in terms of initiating interactions or understanding and learning from them, by differences in the behavior of those interacting with the child because of his or her disability, and by differences in the range of social and educational experiences offered.

To understand the reasons for the developmental delay in Down syndrome, it will be necessary to look at the evidence for differences at each of these levels, the biological/physical, the psychological (the infant as interactor, initiator, and learner), the interpersonal (parent-child and peer interaction), and the wider social and educational environment.

The way in which Down syndrome affects physical development is the focus of the rest of this book so it will only be referred to briefly in this chapter where it is relevant to the child's progress in a particular area.

Our knowledge of the effects of Down syndrome on psychological development is mostly on outcomes. Until the last decade, studies simply described the age at which milestones may be reached, identifying that progress was likely to be slower than normal but not exploring the possible reasons for these delays. In what ways does Down syndrome alter the pathways and processes that lead to the development we describe as ordinary? Only when we can begin to answer that question will we be in a position to develop optimally effective remedial strategies. Some of the research of the past decade to be considered later in the chapter is asking questions about processes rather than outcomes and reporting findings with positive remedial implications.

MEASURING DEVELOPMENT IN TERMS OF IQ

It has been accepted since the condition was first described that an inevitable consequence of Down syndrome is delay in all areas of development leading to a permanent state of moderate to severe mental retardation. In most published studies, children with Down syndrome achieve scores from about 20 to 85 IQ (intelligence quotient) points on intelligence tests [12]. This means that the most able Down syndrome children are achieving scores within the lower end of the normal range of development (i.e., IQ range 70–130, mean 100), whereas the low-scoring Down syndrome children must be seen to be very delayed.

In these studies, development was measured solely in terms of IQ. Although this allows some sort of crude comparison with ordinary development, it gives little useful information about the individuals' progress in achieving the skills and abilities that matter in everyday life. Any practically useful discussion of development needs to consider the child's progress in terms of behaviors that have relevance for parents, such as the age at which the child may walk, dress unaided, learn to read, use the telephone, cook a meal, or get a job. Development in the rest of this chapter will therefore be discussed in terms of the acquisition of meaningful knowledge and functional skills. However, before going on to do this, there are some issues that have arisen in relation to IQ measures that need some consideration to dispel some common misunderstandings.

Factors Affecting Outcomes of IQ Scores

Studies since the turn of the century have indicated that even on crude IQ measures the developmental outcomes for this group were improving [13,14], indicating that they were not solely determined by biological limitations but could be influenced by environmental factors.

A number of investigators have considered the question of broad influences on IQ scores and therefore on development for this group. When IQ is the measure used, evidence for the usual effect of social class and parental education on the children's development has been inconclusive, with some studies reporting such a link and others not finding it. However, there has been general agreement in the past that there is a significant sex difference, with girls doing better than boys on IQ measures (for a comprehensive review of IQ studies up to 1985, see Carr [12]).

Recent studies that have used measures of everyday living skills across a variety of areas of development, rather than IQ scores, have shown that the development of young people with Down syndrome is as sensitive to the quality of their environment and responds to the same factors in the same way as in ordinary youngsters [14–16]. In the most comprehensive study of teenage development available [15], the teenagers with Down syndrome showed the same advantages of family position, social class, and quality of school. This study did not find any sex difference in overall levels of functioning either. The teenage boys as a group were more delayed in terms of language development only. On a measure of everyday skills taking account of all areas of functioning, there was no difference between the boys and girls. In fact, the boys were ahead in independence skills and more likely to be out and about in the community as a consequence.

Interpreting the Decline in IQ

Another issue that has been frequently discussed but is often misinterpreted in terms of its significance for the children's progress is the decline in IQ scores with age. The fact that the IQ scores do decline has been shown by many studies [12] and is a consequence of the way IQ scores are computed. At each age, the child is being compared with ordinary children. If his or her rate of progress is not as fast as that of the ordinary child, then he or she will inevitably get lower IQ scores each year despite actually making progress in all areas of development.

Reliability and Validity of IQ

A number of investigators have questioned the value of IQQ (or norm-referenced) tests as meaningful measures of development for children with disabilities. None of the major tests used has been standardized for use with delayed populations, and as Wishart points out [17], they are versions of tests developed up to 50 years ago. Commonly used infant scales such as the Bayley are little more than measures of physical abilities and coordinations, particularly in the first years of life; few have even face validity now as measures of cognitive function. The predictive validity of such infant tests is low; average correlation with later intelligence, even just two years later, is only .14 [18]. The tests usually attempt to measure both mental and motor abilities (or verbal and performance IQ on tests for older children), and the final IQ or DQ (developmental quotient) is based on combining the two scores. Because the test norms are based on what the majority of children can do at a particular age, the average child will achieve the same scores for mental and motor ability. The child's overall IQ score will be adversely affected by a delay in either area. In one study of children with Down syndrome between 12 and 36 months of age, motor scores lagged behind mental scores by as much as 10 months [19]. As the investigators point out, this mismatch may lead to serious underestimation of mental competence and of the readiness to acquire cognitive skills if the mental and motor scores are used to compute a DQ in the usual way.

THE WIDE RANGE OF DEVELOPMENT

The most important point to emphasize when considering the progress of any child with Down syndrome is that the impact of the condition is variable. This is true of both the physical and mental effects. Some children are much more seriously handicapped than others, so the range of development is very wide. However, there is no reliable way to predict the progress of an individual baby in the first year or two of life. Several investigators have looked for features that might be related to mental progress. Some studies suggest that birth weight and hypotonia correlate with later developmental outcome [20,21] on the basis of sample data. Caution should be exercised in using this kind of group data for prediction in individual cases because the authors know of a number of cases where severely hypotonic babies in the first year of life have been some of the most cognitively and linguistically advanced children at 5 years of age. For parents, any hint that their baby may do less well could lead to them lowering their expectations and could create a self-fulfilling prophecy.

DEVELOPMENT IN THE FIRST FIVE YEARS

In the first years of life, all the usual developmental milestones are likely to be delayed to some degree. The delay will not usually be the same in all areas of development in an individual child, with social and emotional development usually the least affected and either language or motor skills being the most delayed. Each area of development will be considered separately, giving norms for common milestones based on the data from the large Manchester cohort of 181 children born between 1973 and 1980, studied by Cunningham [22] and his colleagues. These families were some of the first in the United Kingdom to receive home-based early intervention.

Motor Development

Motor development is likely to be affected by the hypotonia said to be present to some degree in all the babies [23]. All the gross motor skills are achieved later with the average for sitting being 9 months (range 6–16 months), for pulling up to standing being 15 months (range 8–26 months), and for walking being 19 months (range 13–48 months). The norms for the attainment of these three milestones in ordinary children are sitting at 7 months (range 5–9 months), pulling to standing at 8 months (range 7–12 months), and walking at 12 months (range 9–17 months). These figures illustrate a point that applies to all areas of development in children with Down syndrome: that the variation in development is much greater than in the ordinary population. For example, a baby with Down syndrome may be expected to sit up at any time within a 10-month period, whereas an ordinary baby will be likely to achieve sitting within a 4-month period.

Delays in motor skills will of course have effects on the baby's experiences and development in other areas. Being able to sit extends the baby's view of the world and the range of play activities he or she can explore. Similarly, being able to crawl and walk will greatly extend the baby's scope for exploration of the physical world and the opportunities for social interaction and experience. The late appearance of a milestone in any area of development is likely to distort the normal intermeshing of progress within and between developmental areas, so changing the pathways and processes of future growth.

Social and Emotional Development

Most babies with Down syndrome show the least delay in social and emotional development, smiling when talked to at 2 months (range 1.5–4 months), smiling spontaneously at 3 months (range 2–6 months), and recognizing parents at 3.5 months (range 3–6 months); each of these milestones show only a 1-month delay on average. Although some studies suggest that the intensity of affective responses such as smiling and laughing may be slightly less than that shown by ordinary babies [24,25], parents respond warmly to the onset of smiling and eye contact [26]. The Down syndrome babies begin to enjoy pat-a-cake and peek-a-boo games at about 11 months (range 9–16 months), which is about 3 months later than ordinary babies. Studies in the second year of life show the babies to be skilled in social communication even using social skills to attempt to distract an adult from a task the baby does not want to attempt [17]. The babies are warm, cuddly, and normally responsive to physical contact, unlike babies with some other types of disabilities such as autism.

This normal emotional responsiveness continues into adult life, and as studies of teenagers have shown [15], it develops into appropriate empathy, making the person with Down syndrome a sensitive and socially aware person to live with.

Self-Help Skills

Feeding is an area that can cause quite a lot of anxiety for a variety of reasons. Some babies do not seem interested in feeding, and this can be a great strain in the first year. Digestive problems, both constipation and diarrhea, can also be a worry for a minority of babies, and mothers need support and practical help during this time. The average age for taking solids is 8 months (range 5–18 months), for finger feeding is 10 months (range 6–14 months), and for drinking from an open cup is 20 months (range 12–30 months). For some children, establishing mature chewing and drinking patterns is quite a problem especially if they have been tube fed. Such feeding problems need sensitive and ongoing support because feeding problems often become a battle of wills between mother and baby with consequences for other aspects of their relationship. Equally important is the adverse effect that abnormal chewing, drinking, and swallowing patterns may have on the mobility of tongue, lip, and mouth movements necessary for speech production. On average, the children are able to feed themselves quite independently by 30 months (range 20–48).

Progress in toilet training is delayed by about 1 year with the average age for bladder control during the day being 36 months (range 18–50+) and for bowel control being 36 months also (range 20–60+). There is evidence from at least two studies that firm consistent training routines lead to earlier achievement of continence [26,27]. Most children are using the potty or toilet without help by 4–5 years.

Most children make steady progress with dressing skills, starting by taking off the easy items like socks and shoes, being able to undress themselves by about 36 months (range 24–60+ months) and to dress themselves by 4–5 years, though with help with fastenings.

Cognitive Development

The development of thinking, reasoning, and understanding in children with Down syndrome has mainly been described in terms of early milestones and later IQ scores. The only aspect of cognitive development that has been investigated in detail is that of sensorimotor development in the first 3 years of life [29–31].

Early milestones that reflect the beginning of the baby's exploration of the world are delayed. For example, the average age for Down syndrome babies to reach out to grasp a dangling ring is 6 months (range 4–11 months), which is about 2 months later than ordinary babies, for whom the average is 4 months (range 2–6 months); however, as with all areas of development, the ranges overlap, which means that some babies with Down syndrome will acquire this skill as soon as some ordinary babies. The average age for passing a toy from hand to hand is 8 months (range 6–12 months) for the baby with Down syndrome, pulling a string to obtain a toy is 11.5 months (range 7–17 months), finding an object hidden under a cloth is 13 months (range 9–21 months), putting three or more objects into a cup or box is 19 months (range 12–34 months), building a tower of 2-inch cubes is 20 months (range 14–32 months), and completing a simple three-piece jigsaw is 33 months (range 20–48 months). However, as Wishart pointed out [17], these milestones traditionally taken as evidence of increasing cognitive development are very dependent on motor competence for correct performance.

Dunst [30] in a series of detailed studies of progress through the sensorimotor period showed that babies with Down syndrome show slow but ordinary progress; that is, they progress through the stages in the same order as ordinary babies. Of the tasks that he looked at, vocal imitation showed the most slowing in the second and third years. The acquisition of these sensorimotor tasks has been shown to be sensitive to the quality of the infants' environment for all children, and Dunst presents evidence to show that although babies with Down syndrome are delayed when compared to middle-class American children they are more advanced than ordinary children living in deprived institutional settings in Greece [32].

Play

Another way in which a child's growing understanding of the world may be demonstrated is in the range of play activities he or she engages in. Studies of play in children with Down syndrome suggest that their play follows much the same pathway as in other children. Some differences have been reported; they may be less likely to manipulate and explore objects compared to peers of the same developmental level, although this could be due to poorer fine motor skills needed for manipulation. Most investigators report that play is appropriate for the children's cognitive level [33,34] except perhaps for a tendency for pretend play to show slower development. In one study, for example, the children produced fewer pretend uses for objects [35]. However, McConkey and Martin [36] demonstrated that the infants showed higher levels of pretend actions when their mothers were playing with them rather than merely watching. They attribute this effect to the mothers spontaneously modeling appropriate play for the children. Phemister et al. [37] found no differences in the proportion of time that mentally handicapped children and ordinary children played with toys when observed at home, but those who were studied in day centers, schools, and hospital wards spent significantly less time in attentive play and in interactions with adults. Instead, they had higher levels of self-stimulation and inactivity. This study illustrates the importance of remembering that the infant's environment may be affecting behavior and cautions against always assuming that delays relate to some inherent differences in the child's makeup.

Language Development

Language development is often the area of greatest delay for children with Down syndrome, though not invariably so. The average for first-word production is 18 months, a delay of some 4 months (Fig. 2.2). The baby then builds up a single-word vocabulary more slowly than the ordinary child but acquires the same range of first words [38,39]. At about 30 months (range 18–60 months),

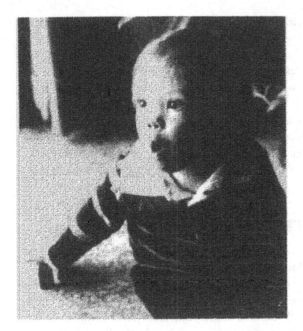

Figure 2.2 Eighteen-month-old practicing "o-o-o."

the children begin to put two words together, and they go on to use the same range of two-word phrases as normal children, using them to communicate the same range of ideas [40–42].

Beyond the two-word stage, the children have increasing difficulty in acquiring the rules of grammar and sentence construction. They can understand many more sentence types than they can produce in their own speech [43–45]. They also have difficulty in producing clear speech [46,47], and this can persist into teenage and adult life when the combination of articulation problems and speaking with immature sentence constructions may make their speech hard for strangers to understand. In a recent study, although 80% of teenagers were understood by parents and teachers, less than 30% of the same group could be understood by people who were not familiar with them. This will be quite a limitation when out and about in the community [15,48].

Despite these difficulties, the children do make good use of the language they have and do understand conversational rules. In fact, their ability to respond appropriately to questions and to keep a conversation going are slightly ahead of ordinary children at the same stage of language development [49,50].

They learn appropriate strategies for repairing conversations when misunderstood, often making use of gesture [51–53].

Some children progress quite fast with their language skills, and by school age, they are talking in sentences and even reading, whereas other children go more slowly, and their first words are spoken at 3 or 4 years. A small number of children (about 5%) acquire only very limited speech and may not progress beyond being able to use a small number of single words and signs [15].

For the children most delayed in learning to communicate, frustration may be a considerable problem and lead to difficult behavior. The link between poor communication and behavior problems has been demonstrated in a number of studies [15,54].

An Overview at 5 Years

By 5 years of age, almost every child will be walking, running, and climbing stairs quite competently. Most will exhibit toilet training during the day—although they may still have occasional accidents and be less reliable at night. Most children will feed themselves quite competently, although they may need their food cut up and may still be a little clumsy and messy. Most will be able to take off many items of clothes and put some on, but they will not be able to manage fastenings, so they will still need some help with dressing. Most children are happy and sociable and present no more behavior problems than other children of their age, although they will not be as self-sufficient and will need more supervision.

Progress in understanding and in language is more difficult to summarize. Some children are talking quite well at 5 years, in short sentences and may be beginning to read. Some are able to go to school in ordinary classes. Most children are talking in short phrases of one to three words and can make themselves understood at home and at school even though their language development is rather behind that of the normal 5 year old.

About 10% of children with Down syndrome will be rather more delayed than the rest. A few children are not talking at all by the age of 5 years. They may be the ones with the more severe hearing or auditory perceptual problems and may be helped to communicate by learning to sign. Similarly, a few children will still be incontinent and very dependent, needing help with feeding, dressing, and all daily activities. Often, the more severely delayed children are those with the most severe and persistent medical problems and sensory defects [15,55].

However, it is important to reiterate the caution that there are no reliable predictors of later development in the first 3 years and to emphasize that the rate of progress in one area of development may bear little relationship to progress in another area in the same child. This is particularly true of the relationship between motor skills and other areas of development. Some of the most cognitively and linguistically able children that the author has worked with have been very delayed in their gross motor progress, perhaps not walking until 3–4 years of age. Similarly, the reverse is not uncommon, that is, children whose motor progress is good and who are walking by 18 months of age but whose cognitive and linguistic progress do not proceed at the same pace.

THE EARLY SCHOOL YEARS

An estimate of the expected range of development during this period can be obtained from examining the results of two studies in the United Kingdom, one looking at a representative group of twenty-two 8–9-year-old children in Oxfordshire [55] and another looking at thirty-seven 6–8-year-old children in South Wales [28]. However, the reader should bear in mind that these children were born between 1964 and 1974, before the advent of family support and preschool services, and most were educated in schools for children with severe learning difficulty. In the author's view, there have been so many changes in the quality of parent support, the education offered, and public acceptance and attitudes, that the findings of any research that was carried out before 1980 or that examined children born before then should be interpreted with caution. The findings may not describe the possible range of developmental progress for this group of children and may turn out to be of historical value only. However, for the moment, they are the only data available.

In the Oxfordshire study, the children were assessed by standardized intelligence tests and the Reynell Language scales. The intelligence test scores varied, ranging from less than 20 to 79, giving a mean IQ of 48 for the group. Two girls (9%) scored in the normal range with scores greater than 75; 7 (32%) were mildly retarded with scores between 50 and 74; and 11 (59%) were more retarded with scores less than 50. There was a significant difference between boys and girls in this study, like most other studies reporting IQ measures [12,27].

In the Oxfordshire study, the teachers and parents completed the American Adaptive Behavior Scale that measures the child's range of everyday skills and achievements. For most children, their ratings on the IQ test and the American Adaptive Behavior Scale were quite closely related, although there were some exceptions. Some children had a greater range of everyday skills than would have been predicted from their IQ scores, presumably because they had been specifically taught these skills. One of these children was being fostered by his teacher. Two children did poorly on everyday skills compared to their IQ scores; both had congenital heart disease and suffered symptoms that would hamper physical activity. The American Adaptive Behavior Scale scores again covered a wide range. The children with the highest scores were very little different from normal children of the same age in self-help skills, social functioning, and the ability to communicate. At the other extreme, those with the lowest scores were very dependent, requiring help with all toilet functions, feeding, and dressing, and they had poor communication and little play repertoire.

In addition to considering the general abilities of the children in her study, Gath looked at their language development and behavior. All the girls had some skills in verbal communication, but some boys were quite severely limited, four having a limited vocabulary or poor articulation. Five boys had no speech, one was beginning to sign, and she found that the children with poor communication skills were more likely to have behavior problems. Seven of the eight boys rated as having behavior problems were those who had no language skills at all or very little.

Shepperdson's [56] data shows the same wide range of development as Gath's. She also points out that Down syndrome children follow the same pattern as normal children in that those from stimulating homes do better than those from the most disadvantaged homes. She found some disadvantaged families who had declined to take advantage of early intervention services and concluded that the lack of support and advice had resulted in some extremely retarded children. This had created self-perpetuating situations in that as the child became increasingly difficult or unrewarding to take out and to play with, less was offered, resulting in even worse attainments [28].

Academic Attainments in the Early School Years

There has been very little progress in recording the range of academic skills that may be achieved in the early school years since the author's own review published in 1985 [57]. In the United Kingdom the majority of children are still being educated in special schools, although this situation is changing fast in many parts of the country. The author is aware of many youngsters now in integrated mainstream school places who are achieving much higher levels of language and literacy skills than was thought possible for children with Down syndrome, but there are few published studies that document these changes in a quantifiable way. In special schools, the teaching of reading, writing, and number skills may not be a priority in the early school years [4,56]. Because so many children are still not having the opportunity to learn to read and write, it is not possible to estimate the potential range of literacy skills of children with Down syndrome at this time.

Two studies that have been able to compare the progress of children in mainstream schools with children in schools for moderate learning difficulty both demonstrate the benefits of full integration for the attainment of academic skills.

Casey et al. [3] followed the progress of 36 children with Down syndrome for 2 years, assessing their progress at 6-month intervals. The children were between 3 years 8 months and 10 years of age at the outset. Half the children were being educated in mainstream schools and half in schools for children with moderate learning difficulties. After 2 years, the mainstream children performed better on all the variables measured, expressive language, comprehension, numeracy, verbal fluency, drawing ability, and reading, making significantly greater progress in numeracy, comprehension, and mental age. The progress made by the mainstream children is not attributable to differences between the groups at or before the baseline because only one difference at this stage was significant; all the girls performed better on expressive language than did the boys. This initial sex difference disappeared 2 years later. However, the investigators suggest that the girls' superior expressive language skills at the outset may explain their superior reading progress. Twice as many girls as boys achieved reading scores at the outset and almost twice as many 2 years later. By the end of the study, only one girl in each group was a nonreader; both were the youngest and least able. By contrast, three boys in the mainstream and six in the moderate learning difficulty setting were still nonreaders. The observation that mainstream schools seem to facilitate the development of numeracy skills to a greater extent than special schools has been shown in other studies with retarded non-Down syndrome children in the United States [58,59].

The most recent study to report on the academic attainments of children with Down syndrome and the factors that may affect their acquisition takes a detailed look at the progress of 117 children aged 6–14 years in the Manchester cohort [4]. Multiple regression analysis was used to investigate the independent effects of a wide range of social, demographic, child, and family variables on the children's attainments in reading, writing, and number skills over and above the effect of mental age. Those that were significant were type of school, gender, father's locus of control score, and the chronological age of the child.

Children in mainstream schools were likely to have the highest academic attainments, followed by those in units in mainstream schools, those in schools for moderate learning difficulties, and those in schools for severe learning difficulties even after allowing for the difference in the mental ages of the children in the different types of schools. The girls tended to be doing better academically as in the study by Casey et al. [3], and scores were increasing with age, suggesting that the children gained in skills over time, presumably through greater quantity of instruction. As the investigators point out, the age-related gain may partly be due to the age at which some schools introduced the children to reading, writing, and number work, with some of the younger children having very little experience in these areas; thus, their apparent delay may result from curriculum issues rather than child or family factors.

The teachers in mainstream schools were likely to place more emphasis on academic skills in the curriculum, whereas those in special schools stressed self-help, socialization, and language skills at the early stages. However, the children in the special schools showed no advantages in these areas, the mainstream children doing just as well.

One intriguing finding in this study was the relationship between the father's scores on a measure of locus of control and the child's academic attainments. Higher academic attainments were associated with higher father's scores on this measure; that is, the father's view that events or outcomes were within his influence rather than external to it. Fathers who scored highly were those who took an active role with the child, instigated activities, took part in decision making about the child, and took responsibility for the child equally with the mother. The importance of the father's involvement for children's well being is a neglected area of research.

Overview at 10 Years

It is clear then that there is the same wide range of progress in the early school years and that the range of skills the child will have acquired becomes increasingly dependent on the learning opportunities available as well as inherent ability. Some children will be making good progress with language and literacy skills, although most find number skills more difficult. The findings of the Manchester cohort [7] study indicated that the children had a range of friends and social activities and were little different from other children of their developmental age in this respect. They also reported no more behavior problems overall than normal, although running away was a problem more likely to occur among the children with Down syndrome. There are the minority of more severely retarded youngsters, and as the Gath and Gumley study [55] indicates, those with the greatest delay in learning to communicate are usually showing more difficult behavior, probably as a result of frustration.

TEENAGERS

Research studies of development in the teenage years are scarce compared to the effort that has been devoted to the early years. The following summary is based on the author's survey of 90 teenagers aged between 11 and 17 years and their families at the time of the study (1986) and born between 1967 and 1974 [15]. This is the largest recent study available, but again, the reader should bear in mind that the young people and their families described in these studies have not had the benefit of early intervention or support services and were mainly born before the legislation was enacted that gave them education as a right. The findings of this study are very similar to those reported by Shepperdson [56] and Carr [60] based on smaller samples of children born between 1963 and 1966 in the United Kingdom [60].

The majority of teenagers were described by parents as warm, happy, cheerful, and much loved members of their families. Most were not difficult to live with, as shown by a low incidence of difficult behaviors and the reluctance of most families to part with their son or daughter. Indeed, 48% of the families listed the positive benefits of bringing up a child with Down syndrome [15].

Most of the teenagers were well on the way to independence in all aspects of personal care and hygiene, but the majority needed more help in learning to cook meals and to cope with emergencies to be completely self-sufficient within the home. The majority did not have the necessary skills to travel far from home without supervision. Although most had some speech ability and could be understood by parents and teachers, communication was clearly a problem for many once they were in the outside world. Poor communication creates difficulties in dealing with feelings, and half the group still played out their worries in fantasy play. Poor communication is also bound to limit the way they can relate to others in social situations and establish friendships.

Very few teenagers had any useful reading, writing, or number skills or money skills. Few could tell the time, and only a minority knew essential personal information well enough to cope if they were lost.

Most of the teenagers were socially isolated, with few real friends or social activities outside school. Parents reported that they had become more lonely as they got older. Although they had the normal range of teenage interests, they were rarely able to actively pursue them by going to discos or playing sports out of school. Most of their leisure time was spent in passive and solitary activity. Most were quite unable to cross roads or go about the neighborhood on their own. About half created fantasy friends to talk to and play games with. Most were very dependent on their families for their social lives.

Health was generally good at this age. Most did not suffer from more infections than normal. Some had permanent sensory problems. About 16% were rated as having persistent health problems, and these had affected their development. There was no evidence of mental illness. Sexual development was proceeding with few problems, although parents were anxious to receive more information on this topic.

Overview of Teenagers

There was the same wide variation in development among teenagers as has been reported for younger children, with some teenagers rather more able than this overview suggests but some were much more dependent. The summary describes the typical range of development for some 80% of the group, about 10% being more able and the remaining 10% much more handicapped. The reader will also realize that the academic attainments being reported in the Casey et al. [3] and Sloper et al. [4] studies for younger children are way ahead of those reported for this older cohort. The limited achievements of these teenagers, the poor communication, lack of independence skills, and social isolation were at least partly due to low expectations, segregated schooling, and lack of positive acceptance or community support when they were born.

EFFECTS OF DOWN SYNDROME ON DEVELOPMENT

It is clear from this overview that having Down syndrome does lead to some degree of delay in all areas of development, although the effect of the condition varies widely from child to child. It is also clear that the quality of the child's social and educational experiences have the same differential effect on their progress as they do for any other child as evidenced by the improvement in outcomes reported for the first born and only children, those born to socially advantaged families [15], and those attending mainstream schools [3,4].

WHY THESE DELAYS?

To say the children are delayed because they have Down syndrome is only the first step in answering this question. Why does having Down syndrome lead to these delays? In what ways is this extra chromosome leading to changes in the pathway of development day by day and week by week? Recent research is beginning to provide some answers to the last question. Space does not permit a comprehensive review but rather the selection of some important examples to illustrate the significance of this work.

Interaction Studies

In the first year of life, studies of smiling, vocalizing, eye contact, and turn taking have all revealed important differences when babies with Down syndrome are compared to normal babies [61]. These differences in the way the Down syndrome baby is establishing and using these behaviors may mean that the baby is distorting his or her world in a way that will lead to delay but could perhaps be compensated for by sensitizing mothers to these differences.

A number of studies [24,25] have identified that the onset of smiling is delayed and that the children may need more intensive stimulation to get them to smile, that the smiles may be shorter and less intense yet mothers seem to respond very warmly to the onset of smiling and adjust to the level of arousal that their baby needs [26].

Recent studies have also shown that in the first 2 months, children with Down syndrome are delayed in establishing eye contact with their mothers by about 2 weeks [62,63]. The amount of eye contact increases more slowly than in ordinary infants over the next 3–4 months, reaching a peak some 7–10 weeks late. Once a peak is attained, the infants maintain much higher levels of eye contact with their mothers than do ordinary babies, who by this time are spending more time visually exploring their environment. The different pattern of behavior of the babies with Down syndrome may be good for attachment and social and emotional development but less good for cognitive development. The babies with Down syndrome also show a delay in moving on to use eye contact for joint reference, that is, to draw the mother's attention to what he or she is doing or looking at. This is an important stage in early language development because mothers usually respond by talking to their children, helping them to learn the words for the actions or objects that they are attending to [64].

In development of ordinary infants, vocal output increases up to 4 months, then shows a decrease as the infant begins to listen to and process adult speech, but in infants with Down syndrome, vocal output is significantly lower for the first 3 months, then increases rapidly from 4–6 months without the decrease seen in ordinary infants [65]. For the mothers of ordinary infants, the amount of time they spent in vocal stimulation of the baby decreased over time, but for the mothers of Down syndrome babies, the time they spent in vocal stimulation increased, leading to an increase in vocal clashes rather than turn taking in the Down syndrome pairs. These vocal clashes may be partly due to longer response times shown by babies with Down syndrome. They need more time to process the information and organize their response in the early months [62]. Another study by the same group showed the babies with Down syndrome becoming less attentive to mother's "baby talk" in the second year of life than did ordinary babies [66]. Studies in the second and third years of life show the turn-taking difficulties still persisting [67,68].

The findings of these studies fit well into the pattern of infant development described earlier. Although a little late to start interpersonal responding, the babies seem to concentrate their efforts on the social aspects of development, smiling, looking, and babbling at the important people in their environment at the expense of spending time exploring their physical and visual world and failing to use the social interactions as opportunities for language learning.

Perhaps this explains why less delay is observed in social and emotional development and more delay in cognitive and linguistic development.

Physical Factors

It is important not to forget the physical issues that are also affecting development in the first year. The delays in gross motor development may be partly due to hypotonia but also to more central mechanisms. Delays in reaching and in exploring objects manually require coordination of motor, visual, and cognitive skills. Analyzing the reasons for the range of motor delays and differences seen across the age range in children with Down syndrome is a complex task. At present, it is easier to pose questions than produce answers. For a comprehensive review of the research and issues to be considered, see Henderson [23]. Many children will also be affected by the visual and auditory impairments that are more common in Down syndrome. Poor vision will lead to less visual exploration, as will poor hearing because a child's attention may first be alerted by sounds. The high incidence of hearing loss reported in infancy must have a significant effect on the language development of affected children.

Learning Strategies

Recent work of Wishart in Scotland using object permanence tasks has produced some important findings about the learning style of children with Down syndrome [17]. In a longitudinal study, she demonstrated that the age at which the children first demonstrate understanding of the tasks may not be much delayed but that they are then poor at practicing and consolidating their learning so that they are more likely to fail a task passed on a previous occasion than ordinary babies. They also failed to use the strategies that they had used to solve an earlier task when faced with a new one. They do not seem to have the same inherent strategies as ordinary children for consolidating recently acquired knowledge and seem less able to build effectively on newly acquired knowledge. In these studies, the children are also abnormally sensitive to failure, showing resistance to training or teaching when the task is just beyond their current level of competence but being happy to resume their efforts if an easier task is offered. The children showed this resistance with "switching-out" behaviors, and these were often attempts at social diversions, trying to draw the experimenter into social games and making use of their social skills.

If the findings of these Edinburgh studies apply to the learning of other sorts of tasks, then they have important implications for all educational programs. Careful consideration will need to be given to the level of difficulty of tasks relative to the child's developmental level, to the use of errorless learning techniques, and to providing many opportunities to practice, consolidate, and build on newly acquired skills.

Language Learning

Many investigators have drawn attention to the delay in language development in children with Down syndrome. A decade ago, the assumption would have been that the language skills of these children simply reflected their level of cognitive development. Current research shows a much more complicated picture. The children's language development lags behind their cognitive development [33]. In addition, their expressive language skills lag behind their comprehension of language [39], and this expressive lag continues into teenage years [45].

These findings suggest specific language learning difficulties that are delaying language development over and above any delay linked to cognitive delay in the first years of life. The language delay itself may then be holding back cognitive development.

At the biological level, a major cause of the language learning difficulty in the first years of life is likely to be hearing loss [69]. Hearing loss will have considerable impact on learning to comprehend speech in this early period, and the knowledge that the children are at risk has led to the use of remedial methods that emphasize attending and listening skills and the use of signing [70].

In attempting to explain the expressive delay, there seem to be at least two separate issues to consider. First, a specific speech-motor delay at the outset that delays the production of first words and is probably biological in origin because some children can express themselves in sign up to a year earlier than in speech [70] (Fig. 2.3). Even when they know what they want to say, they cannot say it but can sign it. Second, once the children do begin to talk, they have difficulty with articulation and in mastering the production of grammatically and syntactically correct sentences. They often continue to express themselves in telegraphic key word utterances that are immature in relation to their own level of comprehension of grammar [45]. The combination of the two problems, speaking in key word sentences that lack conventional grammar and not being able to say the words clearly, results in high levels of unintelligibility when speaking to people out in the community at large [48].

At the psychological level, studies have already been described that draw attention to differences in the way in which babies interact with their mothers in the first year of life that may also be contributing to the language delay. As the children get older and can make themselves understood in two- and three-word utterances, parents and teachers can become too helpful, asking questions that

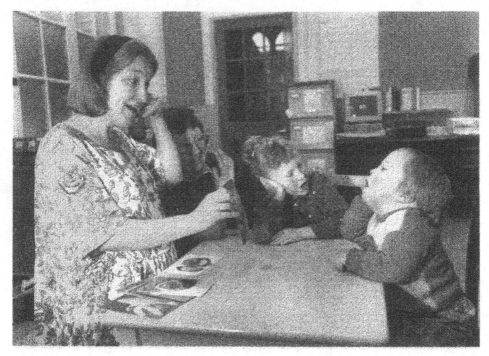

Figure 2.3 Teaching signing while mother and sister observe.

only need a one-word answer, anticipating the child's needs and being too ready to accept and understand these limited utterances. Studies of other language-delayed children show that these adult strategies do hold back the children's progress in mastering syntax and grammar [71]. The delay in auditory memory development discussed in the next section may also have significant implications for language learning.

Cognitive Processes

Much recent research has drawn attention to deficits in auditory short-term memory in children with Down syndrome. In ordinary children, the amount of information that can be held in auditory short-term memory increases steadily during childhood. The work of McKenzie and Hulme [72, 73] in the United Kingdom shows that this increase does not occur in children with Down syndrome. Their slow increase in memory span does not even keep up with their own cognitive development. Using Baddeley's model of working memory

[74], McKenzie and Hulme's results suggest that the children are not using silent rehearsal to retain information in the short-term store referred to as the articulatory loop. This memory impairment will have significant effects on everyday function, not only limiting the retention of spoken information and messages but also affecting the processing and production of language. The processing of sentences will be impaired if the child can only retain a few words at a time, and this may be part of the reason for the difficulty the children show in mastering grammar and syntax. Conversely, the limited production of speech in children with Down syndrome may mean that they are not learning to use and expand the capacity of the articulatory loop in the way that ordinary children do.

A number of studies suggest that visual memory function and the processing of visual information seems to be less impaired than auditory processing and auditory memory function (for a recent review, see Pueschel [75]), and teaching methods should emphasize visual presentation of materials whenever possible. The computer can be a great asset as a teaching aid for this reason. The computer can also be programmed to build in practice and consolidation activities. It has a third advantage in that it is under the child's control, so it does not demand responses too fast and never gets annoyed or impatient!

Functional Organization of the Brain

Another body of knowledge that may have relevance for understanding the development of children with Down syndrome is that concerning the functional organization of the brain. A number of studies have reported that young people with Down syndrome do not show the typical right-ear advantage on dichotic listening tasks assumed to result from left-hemisphere dominance for language. This has been interpreted as possibly indicating atypical localization of language skills in children with Down syndrome. It could be related to delay in acquiring the rules for grammar and syntax. Neville [76] showed that the majority of deaf people do not show the pattern of left-hemisphere specialization found in hearing. She suggests that this is because they usually lack full grammatical competence because four of her congenitally deaf subjects who had perfect English grammar did show the usual pattern of left-hemisphere dominance. Sacks [77] reviewing Neville's work, concludes:

> if language experience is severely delayed, or otherwise aberrant, it may delay the maturation of the brain, preventing proper left hemisphere development, in effect confining the person to a right hemisphere sort of language. Neither language nor the higher forms of cerebral development occur spontaneously; they depend on exposure to language, communica-

tion and proper language use. If children are not exposed early to good language or communication, there may be a delay (even an arrest) of cerebral maturation, with a continuing predominance of right hemisphere processes and a lag in hemispheric "shift."

Visual-spatial skills in children with Down syndrome have recently been reported by Bihrle and colleagues [78] as showing patterns typical of "left-hemisphere" damage. In contrast to children with Williams syndrome, the children with Down syndrome tend to correctly draw the overall shape of figures from memory but lose the detail, whereas the children with Williams syndrome correctly draw the detail but not the overall configuration. Although this finding may be useful in highlighting the children's strengths and weaknesses when drawing and may have implications for teaching, there is no suggestion that it may be another example of delay due to lack of appropriate experience.

Implications for Remediation

The results from each of the areas of research described go some way toward answering the questions set at the beginning of this section, by illustrating some specific ways in which the usual pathways and processes of development are being altered by Down syndrome. Each example has specific implications for remediation with the possibility that such appropriately targeted intervention may be able to reduce delays in development. These implications will be illustrated in the next section.

WHAT CAN WE DO TO IMPROVE
THE CHILDREN'S PROGRESS?

The discussion in this section reflects the author's priorities, taking account of current research and the needs of the family as a whole.

A Normal Family Environment

The first point to emphasize is that the infant with Down syndrome has the same needs as any other baby for a warm, secure, and loving environment to grow and develop with a positive identity and sense of self-worth. He or she needs to be part of a secure, happy family unit, and parents should be encouraged to realize that this normal family life is by far the most important contribution that can be made to the child's development and well being.

Numerous outcome studies have demonstrated that children living at home do better than those in institutions and that in the past some degree of delay could be attributed to unstimulating and emotionally deprived environments. However, the importance of a normal family life has a further implication for service providers because sometimes the demands created by remedial services, especially in the preschool years, may place considerable stresses on young parents and can prevent them from engaging in the activities of other young families in their community. Visits to therapy sessions and home visits can also make the establishment and maintenance of regular sleeping and feeding routines difficult. Such routines not only make life easier for the whole family, they also help to make life predictable and convey security to the infant. Any benefit of the therapy for the child may be more than outweighed by the disadvantages for the family as a whole if parents and therapists do not carefully consider the impact on everyday life for all members of the family.

The Importance of Physical Health

A first priority must be to ensure that the baby and young child are as fit and healthy as possible. This is the message of this book as a whole. Beyond good medical care, the author's next priority would be to promote physical fitness through physiotherapy in infancy and then a range of exercise and sporting activities such as gymnastics, athletics, dancing, and swimming. These activities not only promote good body control and fitness, they also enhance self-esteem and confidence and increase the opportunities for community integration. In the author's teenage study, those young people with a sporting or leisure skill were more likely to have age-appropriate, ordinary friends and an independent social life.

Communication and Play

To promote psychological development, communication and play are the areas that the author encourages parents to focus on. Being able to communicate is fundamental to all aspects of being human; it is equally important for social, emotional, and cognitive aspects of development. In the first months of life, babies learn that it is fun to communicate as they engage in mutually rewarding smiling and babbling games with parents. They move on by the end of the first year, to use single words and gestures for more precise communication. In the second and third years, they usually master the basics of their native language, and this skill enables them to learn rapidly about all aspects of the world and the people around them. For any child, delay in language development will lead to delay in all other areas of development. The research already discussed has identified a number of reasons for the difficulties that children with Down syndrome experience in learning to talk, all of which have specific remedial implications discussed below.

Children's play activities usually reflect their cognitive level, and they learn through play and exploration, as they discover what can be done with toys and play materials such as sand, water, and paint. Pretend play enables the children to play out the activities they experience in their world. Joining in the child's play and encouraging new play activities is an enjoyable way for parents to help their child's cognitive and language development. Many play activities provide natural opportunities to talk about the objects and actions the child is focusing on. Play activities can also encourage fine and gross motor skills. The most important benefit of capitalizing on play as a learning situation is that it should be fun for both parent and child and occur naturally during their times together.

The aim should be to highlight the value of the time parents spend in play with the youngster, not to distort and spoil these times by turning them into forced teaching sessions.

NOT JUST DELAYED

An important point to emphasize is that in designing remedial programs, the recent research discussed in the chapter certainly suggests that the child with Down syndrome cannot simply be regarded as if delayed. Progress in some areas of development may be thought of as delayed in that the child progresses through the same stages in the same order but even so the processes by which the child is acquiring the stages may be different.

The studies of the babies' behavior in the first year of life show that they are often not giving the same cues and inviting the same type or amount of responses from their caretakers. In other words, they are creating different worlds for themselves, worlds that may be less effective learning environments, particularly for cognitive and linguistic development. Parents need to be informed about these differences and encouraged to compensate in responsive and sensitive ways in the course of their ordinary interactions with the baby.

Talking Needs to Be Taught

In the author's view, the evidence concerning the child's language learning difficulties requires intervention that is more specifically tailored to the child's strengths. Communication methods should attempt to compensate for the hearing, auditory perception, processing, and memory difficulties when teaching comprehension and to make use of visual materials and cues to support the speech that the child is being expected to understand (Fig. 2.4). In the light of the evidence for specific speech production problems, children should be

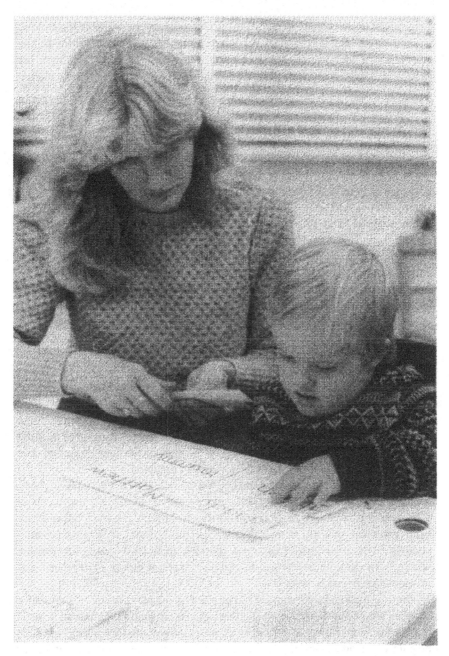

Figure 2.4   Mother present as boy is learning his name, "daddy," and "mummy."

encouraged to use a sign language [70]. In infancy, this may enable the child to maintain communication at the level of his comprehension while waiting for the emergence of adequate spoken production. Later, signing will help him or her to be understood when speech is unintelligible as a result of poor articulation and lack of grammar and syntax.

Teaching Reading to Teach Talking

Reading and symbol systems can be used to teach both comprehension and production of speech from preschool years. Reading has been used to teach language to language-disordered children for many years [79]. Children with severe language delay are taught a sign language as their first language and then taught to read. The author has been successfully using this approach with children with Down syndrome for the past 10 years. Children are taught a sight vocabulary of words selected because they will be used in their everyday communication, and the words are then built into grammatically correct sentences describing the child's own experiences. The child can then practice talking in full sentences by reading them, at a stage when he or she is unable to generate full sentences spontaneously in speech [70]. Other teachers report similar results to our own with preschool children, observing the effect of reading practice on speech production [80,81].

The author has used the same approach with teenagers [82]. In a study designed to improve the grammar and syntax used in their speech, the visual method that used print and pictures in the training sessions was much more effective than the auditory method that used pictures only to support the sentence practice. The two children who showed the greatest benefit of the print were the least able and were nonreaders at the start of the study, and both had extremely limited auditory short-term memory spans.

For all age groups, reading is used as a meaningful everyday activity, teaching the children vocabulary that they can use in talking and writing about their own lives and activities. The majority of children can read and comprehend sentences that are more difficult than those they can produce spontaneously in their speech. Practice at putting their own news into written sentences to share with the class or with their families produces improvements in spontaneous production.

Quite a small sight vocabulary can be used to enhance speech skills, and for children who cannot manage print, symbol systems such as Rebus can be used in the same way. However, many preschool children with Down syndrome can be taught to read as early as 3 years of age. The youngest child the author has worked with learned 30 words in a month at 2.5 years of age. Many children go on to achieve useful levels of literacy and read books for pleasure.

Writing

The children are encouraged to write as they are exposed to reading, tracing over words initially, because it is the author's belief that only practice of the skill required will lead to competent performance. There are many simple word-processor programs available for the computer that allow the child to produce good written work without the need to be able to spell initially, because they can choose whole words on an overlay keyboard. Throughout this approach, the emphasis is on language teaching because the children will need help to master grammar and syntax as they proceed.

Number and Money Skills

It seems to be generally agreed that the children find number skills more difficult than reading [83]. Some guidelines to teaching number skills have emerged from research studies. Gelman and Cohen emphasize the need to use teaching methods that help the child learn counting principles by varying the tasks and not simply teaching by rote [84]. In the author's experience, teaching is more successful when children can relate number work to real tasks such as counting for purchases in shops, and they benefit from having their own pocket money at the same ages as other children to practice in real situations.

Behavior Management

Numerous studies highlight the stress caused by difficult behavior in the lives of children and families, which suggests that this should be a priority area in the minds of all service providers. Many behavior problems could be prevented if parents and professionals were alerted to their significance and learned appropriate management techniques. Parents need to be encouraged to set firm standards for acceptable behavior and to establish clear routines for mealtimes and bedtimes. Prevention is preferable to cure!

Because there is an established link between difficult behavior and poor communication skills, another preventive strategy is to build up the child's communication skills from the first year of life. Parents and professionals should be encouraged to be sensitive to the frustrations that can arise when a child cannot make himself or herself understood and, thus, has little control over his or her life.

Also, difficult behavior can be a sign of insecurity and uncertainty. If a child is not able to understand all that is going on in his or her world because of slow development, then the security of predictable routines may be important. The behavior of adults can be frightening and unpredictable if you cannot understand their speech or intentions. It is important to give the child explanations, choices, and time to anticipate what is about to happen in his or her life.

Integration into the Social World

Ordinary development requires ordinary experience, and this includes mixing with playmates and school friends, going to clubs, and going out and about in the neighborhood. Why should a child be denied access to the ordinary world of his peers simply because of disability?

Segregation will certainly alter the ordinary pathways of development. The study of teenage life reported earlier in this chapter illustrates how easily youngsters with Down syndrome can become socially isolated if they lack the skills to communicate, to travel independently, and if they have few local friends as a consequence of being bused to segregated special schools. The local school is the stepping stone from the family to the wider community for most children.

The results of the recent studies of integrated education clearly have implications for planning education. In addition to the positive benefits reported for the children's academic and language skills, they are more likely to have friends and be integrated into the social world of their neighborhood. Children attending local schools are also more likely to learn to travel independently from home to school, to use money each day for travel and meals, and to be offered the full range of curricular activities including work experience placements. Taking a life perspective, the youngsters with Down syndrome will learn normal social behavior and expectations, and equally important, the ordinary youngsters will learn to value and to relate to those with disabilities. The special needs of the more severely delayed youngsters can still be met on mainstream sites with proper planning and resources. Is it too idealistic to expect that schools should reflect and encourage the values and attitudes toward the disabled that we would wish to see in adult society?

DESIGNING EARLY INTERVENTION AND EDUCATION PROGRAMS

Clearly, the discussion throughout this chapter suggests that much can be done to enhance the development of children with Down syndrome and implies the need for specialist support and teaching from birth to help them overcome their learning difficulties. Early intervention is not a new idea but, unfortunately, it has not met with universal approval [5]. Over the past 20 years, however, a number of countries have developed intensive early education programs to help preschool children with Down syndrome and their families [2]. The focus of most of the early programs was the child, and the main aim was to accelerate their development.

These programs developed in response to the increasing acceptance that the early environment and experience of any child affected their development. Studies of children reared at home were showing better outcomes than for children reared in hospitals [85]. In addition, researchers were providing evidence that people with very low IQs could learn provided that tasks were broken down into small steps and taught in a structured way, thus allowing for practice and overlearning [86]. This led to the acceptance of the view that people with mental handicaps did not learn in the same way as others but could learn if carefully taught the skills that others acquired without explicit teaching.

Many of the first early education projects were model programs set up by researchers and offering an intensive nursery school program [87,88]. According to the previously mentioned principles, the children were taught on behavioral lines. The curriculum was based on the stages of normal preschool development, teaching the children to progress through the stages seen in ordinary development. In other words, treating them as simply delayed [5]. Many of the programs reported significant gains for the children they were working with [87,88].

However, in the 1980s, a series of reviewers urged caution in the light of their findings [89,90]. Many of the published studies could be criticized on methodological grounds. Very few had random samples or control groups, and the numbers of children reported on were often small. The gains were usually reported at the end of the intervention period with no long-term follow up to determine whether the advantages continued during the school years.

Two of the strongest critics of the early interventionists' claims, Gibson and Harris, draw attention to the assumptions behind the curriculum design of most of these programs [5]. Gibson and Harris rightly identify that most programs teach children as if they were simply delayed. They argue that we will only produce long-lasting gains if we actually design programs based on a knowledge of the specific effects of Down syndrome on development. This is certainly the approach being strongly advocated in this chapter. We are only just beginning to try this approach and need to establish careful evaluation of outcomes, although this is extremely difficult to do in any really rigorous way for both ethical and practical reasons.

The Needs of the Family

The other major criticism of early intervention programs is that they have neglected the needs of families in several ways. First, they have tended to focus exclusively on accelerating the development of the child. In doing so, they may have failed to consider the negative effects of the extra demands the teaching or therapy sessions are placing on families and the extent to which parent-child interactions and family life may be distorted.

Second, the actual needs of parents and other family members for support may have been neglected, although professionals should be cautious in making assumptions about these needs. The results of the Manchester family study [7] provide clear evidence that the majority of families with a young child with Down syndrome are leading ordinary lives, doing the same things that other families at their stage in the life cycle do. The lives of most parents, brothers, and sisters are not being noticeably affected by the presence of the special child. The family members have found the coping strategies that they needed to adjust successfully. The families who were showing signs of stress fell into the following categories: families who were coping with unemployment, poor housing, or poverty; families who had difficulty adjusting to the child and where the mother-child relationship continues to be poor; families of children with more severe learning difficulties or serious health or physical problems; and families where the children showed high levels of behavior problems. These findings could be used to identify families likely to be at risk and therefore in need of services.

The work of Crnic in the United States confirms the Manchester findings in that he also reports that the majority of families are leading ordinary lives without any adverse effects on parents or siblings [91]. These two studies draw attention to the importance of looking at representative samples of families in the population. The widely held view that all families suffered as a result of rearing a child with a disability was presumably based on the experience of professionals coming into contact with the vulnerable families who do experience stress. Mink's research suggests that as a group families with children with Down syndrome experience less stress than families of other children with severe learning difficulties [92]. Several possible reasons for this finding have been put forward: the early identification and consequent early support, the available information on future development, and the presence of self-help groups. The responsiveness and emotional warmth of the children may also be a significant factor.

Both Cunningham in the United Kingdom [7,93] and Turnbull in the United States [6] advocate that parents be encouraged to see themselves as consumers of services, choosing those appropriate to their own needs and aspirations for their child and family, recognizing that the family is a system and that all members will be affected by the choices.

Families' Views of Services

Families have clear views about good and bad service provision once they have had some experience. The Manchester families believed that good service providers showed positive and optimistic attitudes to their children, met their family's needs and their children's needs, involved parents, treated them as competent, and liaisoned effectively with other services [7].

When families are asked to reflect on their coping strategies and sources of help that they value, cognitive strategies are top of the list, that is, the ability to interpret stressful situations in a positive way so that stress is minimized. In one study, consultation with professionals ranked equally with alcohol, cigarettes, and television, and only slightly above medication in terms of usefulness [94]. The practical support offered by neighbors and extended family are usually highly valued. The natural development of these social support networks can be disrupted if too much professional help is offered.

The families in the longitudinal study of Shepperdson [16] reported less stress as the children became older, even though as teenagers they were still quite dependent and caring for them placed restrictions on parents' lives. Because they were much-loved members of the family, they were not perceived as a burden and their needs were not resented, emphasizing again that something is only a stress if perceived as such.

Implications for Services

To implement the recommendations for services set out in this chapter, a multidisciplinary team is needed, especially in the early years. The team will need the expert input of a pediatrician, physiotherapist, speech therapist, and special teacher as a core, with the support of others such as a psychologist, dietitian, occupational therapist, and counselor as needed. There will be some overlap of roles because a speech therapist, teacher, or occupational therapist may be competent in the areas of feeding and play, for example. It is therefore essential that the team functions well, free from professional jealousies and rivalries, recognizing and respecting the overlap of skills in some areas.

From the families' point of view, a key worker is essential. This person is their constant point of contact with the team, can coordinate the service to meet their needs, and act as an advocate for them with the services. In the United Kingdom, it is now common practice to provide a home-visiting teacher in the preschool years, sometimes called a teacher counselor in recognition of the inevitable dual role, supporting the family in addition to meeting the child's special educational needs. This service is highly valued by families. The teacher visits weekly, gets to know the family well, and is usually the ideal person to be the key worker and advocate at this stage. Key workers should be chosen by the family and not by the professionals because they must command the confidence and respect of the family.

THE CHALLENGE

Two themes run through this chapter, normality and special needs. First, normality has been emphasized. Most families do pick themselves up after the birth and diagnosis of an infant with Down syndrome, and go on to lead normal lives. The children's development is influenced by the same advantages and disadvantages as that of all children. The services need to ensure that they value and preserve this normality in the lives of the children and families.

Second, special needs have been stressed. The children have a whole range of specific learning difficulties that delay their progress, and they need special help to overcome them. In this respect, it will not do to see them as just delayed normal children. Some families have extra special needs and may experience considerable stress affecting all family members, and they need help focusing on their particular needs. All families have some special needs if only to enable them to learn about their special child and how to access the services available to them.

The challenge for service providers in the next decade is to find ways of meeting the special needs of children and families while preserving and fostering normality.

REFERENCES

1. Cicchetti D, Beeghly M, eds. Children with Down Syndrome: A Developmental Perspective. Cambridge, UK: Cambridge University Press, 1990.
2. Gunn P, Berry P. Education of infants with Down syndrome. Eur J Psychol Educ 1989;4:235–246.
3. Casey W, Jones D, Kugler B, Watkins B. Integration of Down's syndrome children in the primary school: A longitudinal study of cognitive development and academic attainment. Br J Educ Psychol 1988;58:279–286.
4. Sloper P, Cunningham CC, Turner S, Knussen C. Factors related to the academic attainments of children with Down's syndrome. Br J Educ Psychol 1990;60:284–298.
5. Gibson D, Harris A. Aggregated early intervention effects for Down's syndrome persons: Patterning and longevity of benefits. J Ment Defic Res 1988;32:1–17.
6. Turnbull AP, Summers JA. From parent involvement to family support. In: Pueschel S, Tingey C, Rynders J, et al, eds. New Perspectives on Down Syndrome. Baltimore, MD: Paul H. Brookes, 1987.
7. Byrne E, Cunningham CC, Sloper P. Families with children with Downs Syndrome: One Feature in Common. London: Routledge, 1988.
8. Marfo K, Kysela GM. Early intervention with mentally handicapped children: A critical appraisal of applied research. J Pediatr Psychol 1985;10:305–324.
9. Sameroff A. Early influence on development: Fact or fancy? Merrill-Palmer Q 1975;21:267–294.

10. Bellugi U, O'Grady L, Lillo-Martin D, et al. Enhancement of spatial cognition in hearing and deaf children. In: Volterra V, Erting C. From Gesture to Language in Hearing Children. New York: Springer Verlag, 1989.

11. Neville HJ. Neurobiology of cognitive and language processing: Effects of early experience. In: Gibson K, Peterson AC. Brain Maturation and Behavioural Development. Hawthorn, NY: Aldine Gruyter Press, 1989.

12. Carr J. The development of intelligence. In: Lane D, Stratford B, eds. Current Approaches to Down's Syndrome. London: Holt, Rinehart & Winston, 1985.

13. Booth T. Labels and their consequences. In: Lane D, Stratford B, eds. Current Approaches to Down's Syndrome. London: Holt, Rinehart & Winston, 1985.

14. Connolly JA. Intelligence levels of Down's syndrome children. Am J Ment Defic 1978;83:193–196.

15. Buckley SJ, Sacks BI. The Adolescent with Down's syndrome: Life for the Teenager and Family. Portsmouth, UK: Portsmouth Polytechnic, 1987.

16. Shepperdson B. Growing up with Down's Syndrome. London: Cassell, 1988.

17. Wishart JG. Early learning in infants and young children with Down syndrome. In: Nadel L, ed. The Psychobiology of Down Syndrome. Cambridge, Mass: MIT Press, 1988.

18. Fagan JF. The relationship of novelty preferences during infancy to later intelligence and later memory. Intelligence 1984;8:339–346.

19. Laveck B, Laveck GD. Sex differences among young children with Down syndrome. J Paediatr 1977;91:767–769.

20. Cullen SM, Cronk CE, Pueschel SM, et al. Social development and feeding milestones of young Down's syndrome children. Am J Ment Defic 1981;85: 410–415.

21. Reed RB, Pueschel SM, Schnell RR, Cronk CE. Interrelationships between biological, environmental and competency variables in young children with Down syndrome. Appl Res Ment Retard 1980;1:161–174.

22. Cunningham CC. Down's syndrome: An Introduction for Parents. London: Souvenir Press, 1982.

23. Henderson SE. Motor skill development. In: Lane D, Stratford B, eds. Current Approaches to Down Syndrome. London: Holt, Rinehart & Winston, 1985.

24. Emde RN, Brown C. Adaptation to the birth of Down syndrome infants. J Am Acad Child Psychiatry 1978;17:299–323.

25. Buckhalt JA, Rutherford RB, Goldberg KE. Verbal and non-verbal interaction of mothers with their Down syndrome and non-retarded infants. Am J Ment Defic 1978;82:337–343.

26. Berger J, Cunningham CC. Aspects of the development of smiling in young infants with Down's syndrome. Child Care Health Dev 1985;12:13–24.

27. Carr J, Hewett S. Children with Down's syndrome growing up. Assoc Child Psychol Psychiatry News 1982;10:10–13.

28. Shepperdson B. Families with Down syndrome children. Unpublished report. Institute of Health Care Studies, University College of Swansea, Wales, 1984.

29. Morss JR. Early cognitive development: Difference or delay? In: Lane D, Stratford B, eds. Current Approaches to Down's Syndrome. London: Holt, Rinehart & Winston, 1985.

30. Dunst CJ. Sensor-motor development of infants with Down syndrome. In: Cicchetti D, Beeghly M, eds. Children with Down Syndrome: A Developmental Perspective. Cambridge, UK: Cambridge University Press, 1990.

31. Wishart JG. Performance of young non-retarded children and children with Down's syndrome on Piagetian infant search tasks. Am J Ment Defic 1987;92: 169–177.

32. Paraskevopoulos J, Hunt JMcV. Object construction and imitation under differing conditions of rearing. J Genet Psychol 1971;119:301–321.

33. Cunningham CC, Glenn SM, Wilkinson P, Sloper P. Mental ability, symbolic play and receptive expressive language of young children with Down's syndrome. J Child Psychol Psychiatry 1985;26:2:255–265.

34. McConkey R. Play. In: Lane D, Stratford B, eds. Current Approaches to Down's Syndrome. London: Holt, Rinehart & Winston, 1985.

35. Riguet CB, Taylor ND. Symbolic play in autistic, Down's and normal children of equivalent mental age. J Autism Dev Disord 1981;11:439–448.

36. McConkey R, Martin H. The development of object and pretend play in Down's syndrome infants: A longitudinal study involving mothers. Trisomy 21 1985:1:1.

37. Phemister MR, Richardson AM, Thomas CV. Observations of young normal and handicapped children. Child Care Health Dev 1978;4:247–259.

38. Miller J. The developmental asynchrony of language development in children with Down syndrome. In: Nadel L, ed. The Psychobiology of Down Syndrome. Cambridge, Mass: MIT Press, 1988.

39. Cardoso-Martins C, Mervis CB, Mervis CA. Early vocabulary acquisition by children with Down's syndrome. Am J Ment Defic 198;90:2:177–184.

40. Coggins T. Relational meaning encoded in the two-word utterances of Stage I Down's syndrome children. J Speech Hearing Res 1972;22:1:166–178.

41. Layton T, Sharifi H. Meaning and structure of Down's syndrome and non-retarded childrens' spontaneous speech. Am J Ment Defic 1978;83:5:439–443.

42. Owens RE, MacDonald JD. Communicative uses of the early speech of non-delayed and Down's syndrome children. Am J Ment Defic 1982;86:5:503–510.

43. Bridges A, Smith J. Syntactic comprehension in Down's syndrome children. Br J Psychol 1984;75:187–196.

44. Fowler A. Language abilities in children with Down syndrome: Evidence for a specific syntactic delay. In: Cicchetti D, Beeghly M, eds. Children with Down Syndrome: A Developmental Perspective. Cambridge, UK: Cambridge University Press, 1990.

45. Jenkins C, Buckley S. Expressive delay in children with Down's syndrome: A specific cause for concern? Paper presented at the Child Language Seminar, University of Manchester, England, April 1991.

46. Dodd B. A comparison of the phonological systems of MA matched normal, SSN

and Down's syndrome children. Br J Disord Commun 1976;2:27–42.

47. Rondal J. Language delay and language difference. Special Educ Can 1980;54:27–32.

48. Bray M, Woolnough L. The language skills of children with Down's syndrome aged 12 to 16 years. Child Lang Teach Ther 1988;4(3):311–324.

49. Leifer JS, Lewis M. Acquisition of conversational response skills by young Down's syndrome and non-retarded children. Am J Ment Defic 1984;88:610–618.

50. Coggins T, Carpenter RL, Owings NO. Examining early intentional communication in Down's syndrome children. Br J Disord Commun 1983;18:98–106.

51. Coggins T, Stoel-Gammon C. Clarification strategies used by four Down's syndrome children for maintaining normal conversational interaction. Educ Train Ment Retard 1982;17:65–67.

52. Schere NJ, Owings NO. Learning to be contingent: Retarded children's responses to their mothers requests. Lang Speech 1984;27:255–261.

53. Peskett R, Wootton AJ. Turn-taking and overlap in the speech of young Down's syndrome children. J Ment Defic Res 1985;29:263–273.

54. Gath A. Down's syndrome in the first nine years. In: Nichol AR, ed. Longitudinal Studies in Child Psychology and Psychiatry. Chichester, UK: Wiley, 1985.

55. Gath A, Gumley D. Down's syndrome and the family: Follow-up of children first seen in infancy. Dev Med Child Neurol 1984;26:500–508.

56. Buckley S. Attaining basic educational skills: Reading, writing and number. In: Lane D, Stratford B, eds. Current Approaches to Down's Syndrome. London: Holt, Rinehart & Winston, 1985.

57. Shepperdson B. Growing up with Down's syndrome. London: Cassell, 1988.

58. Bradfield HR, Brown J, Kaplan P, Rickert E, Stannard R. The special child in the regular classroom. Except Child 1973;39:384–390.

59. Corman L, Gottlieb J. Mainstreaming mentally retarded children: A review of research. Int Rev Res Ment Retard 1978;9:251–257.

60. Carr J. Six weeks to twenty-one years old: A longitudinal study of children with Down's syndrome and their families. J Child Psychol Psychiatry 1988;29:407–431.

61. Berger J. Interactions between parents and their infants with Down syndrome. In: Cicchetti D, Beeghly M, eds. Children with Down Syndrome: A Developmental Perspective. Cambridge, UK: Cambridge University Press, 1990.

62. Berger J, Cunningham CC. Development of eye-contact between mothers and normal versus Down syndrome infants. Dev Psychol 1981;17:678–689.

63. Gunn P, Berry P, Andrews RJ. Looking behaviour of Down syndrome infants. Am J Ment Defic 1982;87:344–347.

64. Clark EV. Building a vocabulary: Words for objects, actions and relations. In: Fletcher P, Garman M, eds. Language Acquisition: Studies in First Language Development. New York: Cambridge University Press, 1979.

65. Berger J, Cunningham CC. The development of early vocal behaviours and interactions in Down's syndrome and non-handicapped infant-mother pairs. Dev Psychol 1983;19:322–331.

66. Glenn SM, Cunningham CC. What do babies listen to most? Development study of auditory preferences in non-handicapped infants and infants with Down's syndrome. Dev Psychol 1983;19:332–338.

67. Buckhalt JA, Rutherford RB, Goldberg KE. Verbal and non-verbal interaction of mothers with their Down syndrome and non-retarded infants. Am J Ment Defic 1978;82:337–343.

68. Jones OHM. Prelinguistic communication skills in Down syndrome and normal infants. In: Field T, Goldberg D, Stern D, Sostek, eds. High-Risk Infants and Children: Interactions with Adults and Peers. New York: Academic Press, 1980.

69. Cunningham CC, McArthur K. Hearing loss and treatment in young Down's syndrome children. Child Health Care Dev 1981;7:357–362.

70. Buckley SJ, Emslie M, Haslegrave G, LePrevost P. The Development of Language and Reading Skills in Children with Down's Syndrome. 2nd ed. Portsmouth, UK: Portsmouth Polytechnic, 1991.

71. Wood D, Wood H, Griffiths A, Howarth I. Teaching and Talking with Deaf Children. Chichester, UK: Wiley, 1986.

72. McKenzie S, Hulme C. Serial recall in Down's syndrome, retarded and normal children. Unpublished manuscript. York, UK: University of York, 1985.

73. McKenzie S, Hulme C. Memory span development in Down's syndrome, severely subnormal and normal subjects. Cogn Neuropsychol 1987;4:303–319.

74. Baddeley A. Working Memory. Oxford: Oxford University Press, 1986.

75. Pueschel S. Visual and auditory processing in children with Down syndrome. In: Nadel L, ed. The Psychobiology of Down Syndrome. Cambridge, Mass: MIT Press, 1988.

76. Neville HJ. Neurobiology of cognitive and language processing: Effects of early experience. In: Gibson K, Petersen AC. Brain Maturation and Behavioural Development. New York: Aldine Gruyter Press, 1989.

77. Sacks O. Seeing Voices. London: Pan Books, 1989.

78. Bihrle AM, Bellugi U, Delis DC, Marks S. Seeing either the forest or the trees: Dissociation in visuo-spatial processing. Brain Cogn 1989;11:37–49.

79. Hutt E. Teaching Language Disordered Children: A Structured Curriculum. London: Arnold, 1986.

80. Oelwein PL. Pre-school and kindergarten programs: Strategies for meeting objectives. In: Dmitiev V, Oelwein PL, eds. Advances in Down Syndrome. Seattle, Wash: Special Child Publications, 1989.

81. Norris H. Teaching reading to help develop language in very young children with Down's syndrome. Presented at the National Portage Conference. 1989. Cambridge: UK.

82. Buckley SJ. Enhancing the language skills of teenagers with Down's syndrome: A comparison of methods. In preparation.

83. Pieterse M, Center Y. The integration of eight Down's syndrome children into regular schools. Aust N Z J Dev Disab 1984;10:11–20.

84. Gelman R, Cohen M. Qualitative differences in the way Down syndrome and

normal children solve a novel counting problem. In: Nadel L. ed. The Psychobiology of Down Syndrome. Cambridge, Mass: MIT Press, 1988.

85. Cunningham CC. Early stimulation of the severely handicapped child. In: Craft M, ed. Tredgold's Mental Retardation. London: Cassell, 1979.

86. Clarke AM, Clarke ADB, Berg M. Mental Deficiency: The Changing Outlook. 3rd ed. London: Methuen, 1973.

87. Haydn AH, Haring NG. The acceleration and maintenance of development gains in Down's syndrome school-age children. In: Mittler P, ed. From Research to Practice in Mental Retardation. vol 1. Baltimore, MD: University Park Press.

88. Pieterse M. Recent developments and future trends in the early education of the handicapped. Recent Dev Spec Educ Disab 1979;10:11–20.

89. Gibson D, Fields D. Early infant stimulation programmes for children with Down syndrome: A review of effectiveness. Adv Dev Behav Pediatr 1984;5:331–371.

90. Dunst CJ. Overview of the efficacy of early intervention programs. In: Bickman L, Weatherford DL, eds. Evaluating Early Intervention Programs for Severely Handicapped Children and Their Families. Austin, Tex: Pro-ed, 1986.

91. Crnic KA. Families of children with Down syndrome: Ecological contexts and characteristics. In: Cicchetti D, Beeghly M, eds. Children with Down Syndrome. Cambridge, UK: Cambridge University Press, 1990.

92. Mink IT, Nihira K, Meyers CE. Taxonomy of family lifestyles: 1. Homes with TMR children. Am J Ment Defic 1983;87:484–497.

93. Cunningham CC, Davis H. Working with parents. Milton Keynes, UK: Open University Press, 1985.

94. Brotherson MJ. Parents' self-report of future planning and its relationship to family functioning and stress in families with disabled sons and daughters. Lawrence: University of Kansas. Unpublished dissertation, 1985.

II

PREVENTIVE MEDICINE BY AGE GROUPS

3

The Neonate

NEONATAL DIAGNOSIS

When Down syndrome is suspected in the newborn period, the physician completes several important tasks once the suspicion is confirmed.

1. Inform the parents in a supportive way that their child has Down syndrome.
2. Guide parents to educational and resource material.
3. Refer parents to an infant intervention program and to a support group or another family with a child with Down syndrome.

Down syndrome can usually be detected at the bedside (Fig. 3.1), but a chromosome analysis must be done to confirm the diagnosis and to determine recurrence risk. Although more than 300 clinical signs have been described in Down syndrome [1], the clinician only needs to know some of the important distinguishing features. No one infant has all the signs, and there is no one single sign that is pathognomonic of Down syndrome. Table 3.1 will be a helpful guide [2].

The brachycephalic skull, also seen in normal babies, is consistently found in infants with Down syndrome. The fontanels tend to be enlarged. When infants with Down syndrome cry, they can have the purse-string sign, not seen in babies without Down syndrome (Fig. 3.2). Upward slanting palpebral fissures, epicanthic folds, and Brushfield spots (Fig. 3.3) distinguish the eye of the infant with Down syndrome. Maxillary underdevelopment is one sign that

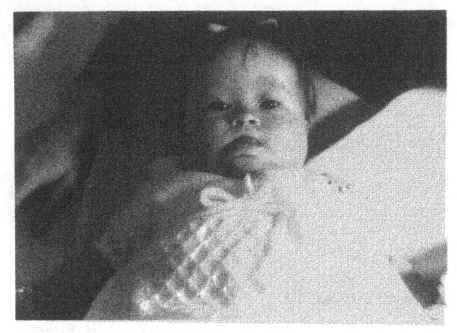

Figure 3.1 An alert neonate with Down syndrome.

probably helps the physician to recognize a Down syndrome face at a glance. The auricle is small and often dysplastic. Tongue protrusion is often prominent. Brachymesophalagia V, sometimes accompanied by clinodactyly, usually is quite striking. The four-finger line is seen more frequently in males (Fig. 3.4). Often hypotonia is marked (Fig. 3.5). There is a gap between the first and second toes (Fig. 3.6).

After making the diagnosis of Down syndrome, the physician has the critical task of informing the parents. This is difficult because parents will experience a great deal of anxiety when they hear that something is wrong with their newborn. The specific words and manner of the physician will have a profound impact on the parents. Even after 20 years, parents recall the exact words used by the physician when they were informed of the diagnosis of Down syndrome [3]. Therefore, before conveying any information to the parents, it is important that the physician carefully plan what he or she will say and the words he or she will use.

In preparation for the process of informing parents, the physician should find it helpful to review current medical information about Down syndrome. Helpful resources include information provided by a regional genetics center, if

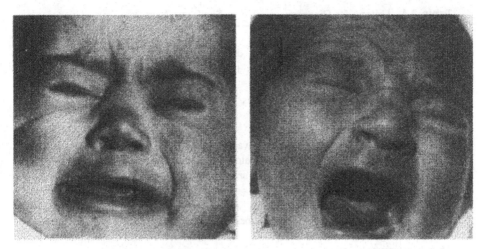

Figure 3.2 The purse-string sign seen on the lids of a crying infant with Down syndrome compared to an infant without Down syndrome. (Reprinted with the permission of Developmental Medicine and Child Neurology)

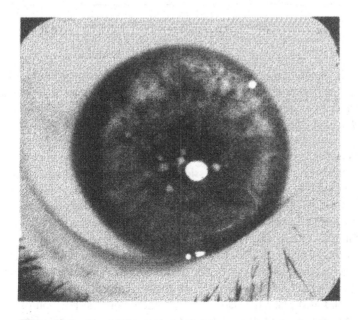

Figure 3.3 Brushfield spots in the iris.

Table 3.1 Criteria for Diagnosis of a Down Syndrome Neonate

 1. Brachycephalic skull
 2. Anterior fontanelle greater than 2.5 × 2.5 cm
 3. Occipital fontanelle greater than 1 × 1 cm and presence of a sagittal fontanelle
 4. Purse-string sign of eyelids
 5. Upward slanting of palpebral fissures
 6. Epicanthic folds
 7. Brushfield spots (speckled iris)
 8. Spokelike appearance of the retinal vasculature
 9. Dysplastic shape of auricle that is below two standard deviations in length
10. Underdevelopment of the maxillary area
11. Lingual hypotonia or dyskinesia
12. Abundant neck skin
13. Brachymesophalangia V or absent mesophalangia V
14. Four-finger line on palm
15. Diastasis recti
16. Small penis (male) or labial index sign (female)
17. Gap between the first and second toes
18. Poor neck traction response
19. Poor muscle tone of extremities
20. Poor or absent Moro's reflex

Source: From Ref. 2.

available, as well as the national parent group. The following are some guidelines for the physician for the process of informing the parents:

1.   Prepare a list of local parent support groups and locate reading material for the parents. For example, in the United States, the National Down Syndrome Congress or the National Down Syndrome Society (see Appendix D, p. 327) are excellent resources for parents or professionals to contact. Both can provide current reading material for parents or professionals (also, see Appendix D). In addition, they can provide lists of infant stimulation programs, local parent support groups, and counselors. Another excellent source of family support can be other parents who have a child with Down syndrome and are experienced in talking to new families. Other parents provide information about the day-to-day experience of raising a child with Down syndrome. Delaying discussion of the diagnosis with the parents until the next day when the geneticist consults or even later when the chromosome report is available heightens the parents' anxiety. Delay could also place the parents in the uncomfortable position of telling their friends and relatives that their new baby is normal and then a few days later calling them back with a new diagnosis.

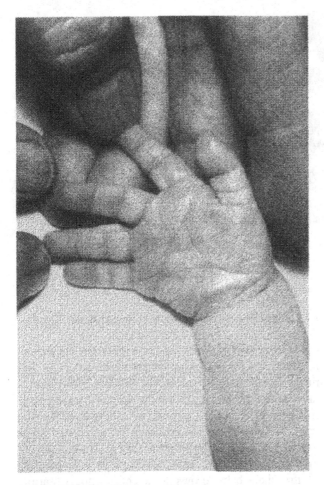

Figure 3.4 The four-finger sign.

2. Talk to both parents in a quiet, private area, and present information in a frank but hopeful manner. A quiet and secluded room is necessary so that the discussions with the family will not be interrupted. Have the baby present to demonstrate normal as well as abnormal features. It is important to show the family that their baby has more "normal" features than features associated with Down syndrome. It is important to be frank and tell parents that some babies have medical problems such as congenital heart defect. However, leave the parents a feeling of hope by reporting that most types of congenital heart

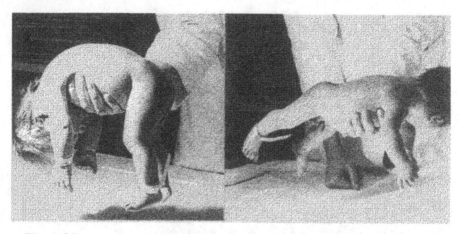

Figure 3.5 A hypotonic infant makes an inverted U when suspended by an adult hand (the Landau posture).

defects can be corrected and usually do not interfere with the quality of the child's life.

3. Allow time for parents to ventilate feelings of depression, anger, or guilt. Mothers may fault themselves for not taking the prenatal vitamins or for having intercourse during pregnancy. Tell parents that families often blame themselves. Ask about their special concerns. Inform the parents that the cause of Down syndrome is unknown, but it is not related to something that they did or did not do during pregnancy. Parents grieve at the loss of the anticipated baby and at the need to adjust to a new baby with special needs [3]. Have a box of facial tissues at hand, and allow a few quiet moments. Share with the parents that most families find that their baby grows to a child who is warm, compassionate, and a source of joy. Or share a parent's description that having a child with Down syndrome is like getting on a plane to go to London, England, but learning on arrival you are in Rome, Italy. Although Rome was not the intended destination, it turns out to be not so bad after all [4]. Some parents express angry feelings in hostile comments about hospital staff or physicians. Acknowledge the parents' feelings, and tell them other families have felt that way also. Allow time for them to talk about how they feel. Arrange for other individuals, such as a social worker or experienced nurse, to talk to the family. Sometimes a person from outside the hospital is helpful, such as a member of the clergy.

4. Discuss briefly reasonable future expectations. Parents' most heartfelt

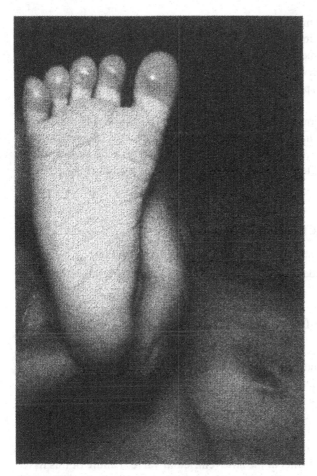

Figure 3.6 A gap between the first and second toes.

question usually is "What will my child be like when he or she is grown?" Although a specific answer is unknown, a general response is imperative. One parent's response may help: "Tell the new parents that by and large, your child will read . . . your child will attend their neighborhood school and take part in many of the activities enjoyed by any child . . . your child will be successfully employed in the community, not necessarily in sheltered situations. Your child will be a delightful individual with his or her own special likes and dislikes and will present his or her own special sets of concerns for caring family members" [5].

5.   Briefly outline management plans. Discuss community resources available, such as infant intervention programs, counseling services, financial assistance programs, and parent support groups. If necessary, provide information about adoption services for the family who feels they will not be able to care for a child with special needs, even after extensive counseling and full information.

6.   Schedule a follow-up conference for additional questions that may arise after the parents have had time to adjust to their child's special needs. Ask if other family members, such as grandparents, would like to attend such a conference. Parents often find a brief letter summarizing your discussion to be helpful.

SPECIFIC MEDICAL CONCERNS

Potentially life-threatening disorders sometimes diagnosed in the newborn with Down syndrome include congenital heart disease, gastrointestinal obstruction, and leukemia.

Congenital Heart Diseases

Congenital heart disease occurs in 40% of persons with Down syndrome and represents the most common cause of death in childhood. In one series, endocardial cushion defect was the most common form of congenital heart disease occurring 52% of the time, ventricular septal defect occurring 28%, tetralogy of Fallot occurring 7%, and patent ductus arteriosis occurring 2% [6]. The endocardial cushions are masses of mesenchymal tissue in the heart of the developing embryo that give rise to part of the atrial and ventricular septa and to the septal leaflet of the atrioventricular valve. Failure of this tissue to develop properly can leave a communication between the left and right sides of the heart at the atrioventricular level as well as incompetence of the mitral and tricuspid valves. Clinically, the infant presents with signs of congestive heart failure, growth failure, recurrent pneumonia, and usually a loud holosystolic murmur. Occasionally, an infant may present with growth failure without heart failure or murmur. The chest roentgenogram shows an enlarged heart and increased pulmonary vascular markings. The electrocardiogram reveals a left-axis deviation and right ventricular hypertrophy. Infants with Down syndrome require early diagnosis and treatment because this heart lesion progresses more rapidly to pulmonary vascular obstructive disease than the same heart lesion in a child with normal chromosomes [7]. Cardiac disease is covered in greater detail in Chapter 9.

Congenital Gastrointestinal Disease

Duodenal obstruction occurs more frequently in infants with Down syndrome than in infants with normal chromosomes. It is usually due to duodenal atresia, duodenal stenosis, or compression from an annular pancreas. The infant with duodenal obstruction presents with vomiting that may be bile stained. Abdominal distension limited to the upper quadrant often occurs with a visible peristaltic wave. The abdominal radiograph is characterized by a "double bubble sign."

Hirschsprung disease, or aganglionic megacolon, also occurs more frequently in infants with Down syndrome. The newborn presents with vomiting, distended abdomen, and failure to pass a meconium stool within the first 48 hours of life. The barium enema is usually diagnostic. When a colostomy is done before enterocolitis develops, mortality is significantly reduced [8]. Imperforate anus also has a relatively high incidence among a neonatal population of Down syndrome [9].

Other malformations that can occur singularly or in combination include: esophageal atresia, pyloric stenosis, diverticulum of the stomach, and malrotation of the bowel [10]. For further details of gastrointestinal problems, see Chapter 10.

Hematological Diseases

Although leukemia occurs rarely in the newborn, the incidence of this life-threatening problem is higher in infants with Down syndrome than in others [11]. Clinical symptoms include skin lesions (petechiae, purpura, and bluish nodules), hepatosplenomegaly, and respiratory distress. A bone marrow biopsy must be done to make the diagnosis. The leukemoid reaction (transient myeloproliferative disease) presents a similar clinical picture but is differentiated by resolution over a few weeks or 3 months at the most. Follow-up hematological monitoring is indicated because a recent report suggests that some cases of transient myeloproliferative disease evolve into acute non-lymphoblastic leukemia [12].

Other disorders described in newborns include polycythemia, thrombocytopenia, and erythroblastosis fetalis (see Chapter 15). To detect hematological disorders, the following laboratory studies are advised: complete blood count, differential, platelet count, and nucleated red blood cell count.

Ophthalmological Problems

Nystagmus and strabismus occur frequently in the newborn period and require consultation to rule out corneal opacities. Other reported anomalies in the newborn affect the iris, fundus, and lens. An abnormality detected on physical examination or poor visual tracking requires further investigation (see Chapter 14).

Urogenital Abnormalities

Urogenital abnormalities described in Down syndrome include micropenis, cryptorchidism, and hypospadias. A renal scan helps rule out associated anomalies of the kidneys and ureters. If indicated, referral to a urologist with pediatric experience is necessary for further evaluation and treatment.

Endocrine Screening

Persistent primary congenital hypothyroidism occurs in 0.7% of newborns with Down syndrome [13]. This is a figure that is 28 times more frequent than in a non-Down syndrome population. T_4 (thyroxine) and TSH (thyroid stimulating hormone) levels are standard screens for congenital hypothyroidism. This screening, so important for all infants, is particularly relevant for infants with Down syndrome (see Chapter 12).

Ear, Nose, and Throat Problems

Because of the increased incidence of congenital sensorineural hearing loss, a hearing screen is recommended before discharge. Middle ear effusions may be present in as many as 15% of newborns with Down syndrome and may be difficult to detect because of a narrow ear canal (see Chapter 8). Consider appropriate referral if the newborn hearing screen indicates questionable or definite hearing impairment.

Oral-Motor Deficits and Feeding

Oral-motor deficits refers to anatomic and neuromotor control problems that may interfere with feeding and speech development. The smaller oral cavity causes spilling of liquids out of the side of the mouth. Hypotonia causes the tongue to flatten out during sucking rather than to form a groove around the nipple [14]. A tongue groove is required to transport liquids to the back of the mouth as well as to form a tight seal during sucking. An infant with these oral-motor problems will present with feeding difficulties such as a weak suck and fatigue before being filled, or will spit, gag, and leak fluid excessively. These problems usually resolve in a few weeks as tongue control improves.

Some simple interventions can assist an infant with mild feeding problems

[14]. First, make sure that the infant is fully awake before feeding. The very young baby with Down syndrome often is placid and sleepy and may not have a loud and lusty hunger cry. In addition, it is important to provide extra support for the infant during feeding. Often two pillows under the baby are required. Last, have the mother support the infant's chin during feeding. This helps steady the jaw until muscle control improves.

Most infants can breast feed successfully and gain two important benefits: added immunity and further stimulation to oral-motor development. The following are some suggestions for mothers with infants who have some initial difficulties with breast feeding [14].

1. Clear the mouth and nose of mucus with a syringe before feeding to help facilitate breathing during feeding.
2. Express some milk from the breast at the beginning of feeding to encourage the infant to grasp the nipple.
3. Feed frequently at 2–3-hour intervals to stimulate the milk supply.
4. Burp the infant frequently at 3–4-minute intervals to expel swallowed air.

The majority of feeding problems resolve within 3–4 weeks as motor control improves. A few infants with severe feeding problems require a consultation from a lactation or feeding specialist.

Extremities

Brachymesophalangia V with clinodactyly occurs frequently but does not interfere with function. Occasionally, infants have polydactyly (extra digits) that is classified as preaxial (radial or thumb side) and postaxial (ulnar or little finger side). The postaxial polydactyly is usually simple to treat in the nursery by ligation with a suture. Preaxial polydactyly is more complicated and requires a referral to a specialist when the infant is about 6 months of age.

GENETIC COUNSELING

Genetic counseling involves informing the parents about the clinical condition of Down syndrome, recurrence risk, and prenatal detection. (The specific data that may be needed in genetic counseling are in Chapter 1.) Occasionally, it may be confusing about who should do the genetic counseling, the child's physician or the consultant who determined the chromosomal karyotype of the infant. Parents benefit from both being involved in the counseling. The geneticist is especially helpful for translocation cases and for the rare family who has one child with Down syndrome and no apparent risk factors and then has a second child with Down syndrome. The primary physician helps by assisting parents in clarifying their initial questions as well as answering questions after their child's discharge.

Although the list of potential medical problems may seem long, most of the problems are remediable. In addition, most physicians are comfortable in diagnosing and managing medical problems. However, physicians may feel less certain about ways to provide support to a family adjusting to a young infant with special needs. The next section discusses some guidelines for providing family support.

PARENT-INFANT ATTACHMENT

Attachment refers to the process that occurs between a family and child before, during, and after the delivery. Attachment is defined as "a unique relationship between two people that is specific and endures through time" [15]. When a child is born with visible abnormalities, the parents' attachment may be more difficult to establish.

The following guidelines help promote the attachment process:

1. Allow both parents to observe the newborn child as soon as possible. The time following the birth of a child is very important in the process of parent–infant attachment. At this time, the parents have the opportunity to hold and touch their baby for the first time. Unless the baby has serious medical problems after delivery, allow the parents extra time to be with their newborn. Immediate removal of the newborn increases the parents' anxiety and does not allow important time for the attachment process.

2. If possible, arrange for an experienced and supportive nurse to be assigned to the family. Parents are often confused by the different nursing and medical staff who are involved in the care of their newborn. Assigning a nurse to the family will give the parents a specific person to contact and discuss concerns. The nurse will be able to further explain to the parents the baby's special diagnostic testing, feeding routine, as well as other concerns that arise.

3. Meet with the nursing staff caring for the child and family so that their own feelings can be ventilated and so that help for the family can be coordinated. Encourage the staff to be sympathetic, supportive, and positive.

4. Arrange visits for the mother if the baby has to be transferred to another hospital. Keeping the mother and father in contact with their infant promotes the attachment process.

When a child is born with Down syndrome, the infant, the mother, and the father are our patients. All three need continuous and intelligent support.

DOWN SYNDROME PREVENTIVE MEDICINE CHECKLIST: NEONATAL

A. Early day 1

1. Establish diagnosis.
2. Laboratory orders: chromosomal karyotype, thyroxine (T_4), thyroid stimulating hormone (TSH), complete blood count, differential, platelet count, nucleated red blood cell count.
3. Admission orders: instruct staff to observe for signs of congestive heart failure and gastrointestinal obstruction, genetic consultation, pediatric cardiology consultation, newborn hearing screening.
4. Discuss diagnosis and management plans with family.

B. Late day 1

1. Meet with staff to coordinate family support.
2. Conduct a follow-up meeting with family and other relatives. Refer family to local support group to aid new parents, if available.
3. Check infant's feeding, weight, and passage of stool.

C. Day of discharge

1. Review laboratory results, consultation evaluations, recommendations, and clinical course of infant.
2. Conduct a follow-up meeting with family to discuss results of tests, answer questions, and make follow-up plans after discharge.
3. Provide letter summarizing discussions about Down syndrome.

REFERENCES

1. Coleman M. Down's syndrome. Pediatr Ann 1976;7:90–103.
2. Coleman M. Chromosomal disorders. In: Coleman M, ed. Neonatal Neurology. Baltimore, MD: University Park Press, 1981:276–292.
3. Carr J. Six weeks to twenty-one years old: A longitudinal study of children with Down's syndrome and their families. J Child Psych 1988;29:407–431.
4. Kingley E. Personal communication, Sept. 1987.
5. Mitnick BM. Answering questions. Down's Syndrome: Papers and Abstracts for Professionals 1989;12:7.
6. Buckley LP. Congenital heart disease in infants with Down syndrome. In: Pueschel SM, ed. The Young Child with Down Syndrome. New York: Human Sciences Press, 1983:353.
7. Clapp SK, Perry BL, Farooki ZO, et al. Down's syndrome, complete atrioventricular canal, and pulmonary obstructive disease. Am J Cardiol 1989;59:454–458.

8. Klein MD, Caran AG, Wesley JM, Drengowski PA. Hirschsprung's disease in the newborn. J Pediatr Surg 1984;19:370–374.

9. Zlotogora J, Abu-Dalu K, Lernau O, Sagi M, Voss R, Cohen T. Anorectal malformations and Down syndrome. Am J Med Genet 1989;34:330–331.

10. Scala PS. Gastroenterology. In: Pueschel SM, Ryngers JE. Down Syndrome: Advances in Biomedicine and the Behavioral Sciences. Cambridge, Mass: Ware Press, 1982:207–210.

11. Miller RW. Neoplasia in Down's syndrome. Ann NY Acad Sci 1970;171:637–644.

12. Wong KY, Jones MM, Srivastava AK, Gruppo RA. Transient myeloproliferative disorder and acute nonlymphoblastic leukemia in Down syndrome. J Pediatr 1988;112:18–22.

13. Fort P, Lifshitz F, Bellisario R, et al. Abnormalities of thyroid function in infants with Down syndrome. J Pediatr 1984;104:545–549.

14. Danner SC, Ceruti ER. Nursing Your Baby with Down's Syndrome. Rochester, NY: Childbirth Graphics, 1984:3.

15. Klaus MH, Kennell JH. Maternal-Infant Bonding. St. Louis, Mo: CV Mosby, 1976:2.

4

The Infant: Two to Twelve Months

The period of early infancy may well be the one where the principles of preventive medicine are most important of all for the very young child. It is in this period where decisions regarding cardiac, infectious, audiological, and the other medical problems help determine the future health of the child. This is also the period in which the infant learning programs have their greatest effect, and how well designed they are and how faithfully they are performed have a significant effect on the level of functioning of the child (see Chapter 2).

Before going into the various medical problem areas, it is good to start with the strengths of this period, particularly regarding the central nervous system. The brain is still very close to normal in some ways in this age group. (This does not imply that some major deficits are not already in place [see Chapter 13] but that this is the age group in which intensive stimulation apparently can make a major difference in later levels of functioning.) Just to consider a couple of examples—in the visual cortex, the dendritic tree is either normal or more advanced in very young children with Down syndrome compared to non-Down syndrome infants of comparable age [1]. Also the cholinergic marker enzymes (choline acetyltransferase [ChAT] and acetylcholinesterase [AChE]) have normal or above normal enzyme activity in infants with Down syndrome between 3 and 12 months [2]. Whether this suggests that children with Down syndrome begin life with a normal complement of cholinergic neurons or whether these normal values are the result of compensation for some cholinergic neuron loss is not established. However, it does indicate that any cognitive deficit detected at this age is unlikely to be a consequence of reduced brain cholinergic

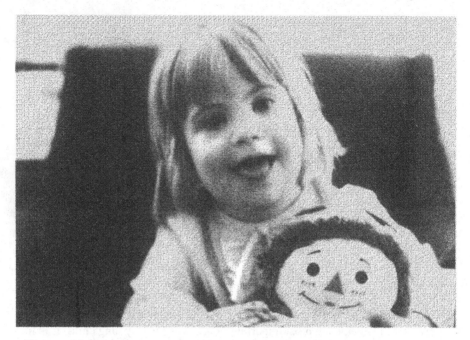

Figure 4.1 Tongue protrusion is most commonly seen in infancy.

function. This is relevant because acetylcholine is such an important neuro-transmitter for so many basic brain functions. The authors raise the question of whether this finding of normal cholinergic enzyme activity opens the possibility of early therapeutic intervention to prevent the development of later brain cholinergic changes. The concept of early therapeutic intervention is explored further in Chapter 21.

MEDICAL PROBLEMS IN THE FIRST YEAR

The age with the highest probability of death for a child with Down syndrome is within the first year of life, and there is no difference in the survival rate between males and females [3]. What chance does an infant with Down syndrome have of surviving that first year? A detailed study from Queensland between 1976 and 1985 showed a survival rate of 87.4% at 1 year of age and no significant difference in such patterns over the period studied [4]. Cardiac anomalies were cited as the cause of death in almost 60% of the infants, and respiratory infection was the other major etiology. There were two deaths from leukemia in this study.

Cardiac Disease

Thus, in this age group, it is important to be on the alert for clinical signs of congenital cardiac disease. It is best if the infant has already had a routine cardiac evaluation in the neonatal period, with any cardiac diagnosis having been established then. Cardiac murmur, which is caused by abnormal blood flow patterns, may not be detectable in the neonatal period but may develop later. This is an important point to stress in the examination of infants less than 1 year of age.

Congenital cardiac disease burdens the body in many ways. The heart beats faster, tachycardia, and more forcefully as can be appreciated by palpation of the infant's chest. There is increased sweating, secondary to the high concentration of catecholamines. The circulatory stress causes water retention, collecting first in the lungs and liver. The water in the lungs causes tachypnea, and the fluid also causes an enlarged liver. The effect in the lung decreases the supply of oxygen, resulting in a pale skin hue. If there is a significant right-to-left cardiac shunt, the skin may have the color of cyanosis also.

If congenital cardiac disease is suspected, referral to a specialist is needed. In the cardiac clinic, precise anatomic diagnosis is the first step followed by medical or surgical therapy as indicated (see Chapter 9).

A special problem with infants with Down syndrome is that they have a tendency to develop pulmonary vascular obstruction relatively early compared to other children with similar congenital cardiac lesions [5]. This lends urgency to early diagnosis in this patient group. If the pulmonary vascular obstruction becomes too developed, it can prevent needed surgery. The principle of preventive cardiac medicine—early diagnosis and prevention of pulmonary complications—is particularly relevant in infants with Down syndrome. Studies indicate that delayed initial referral to a cardiologist was the major impediment to adequate cardiac care [6].

Respiratory Infections

The other major cause of death in the first year of life is respiratory infections. In a study by Oster et al., an increase in respiratory disease in Down syndrome was noted 62 times greater than a matched non-Down population [7]. Infections in general were 12 times greater in Down syndrome. These statistics highlight the immunodeficiency of patients with Down syndrome, especially regarding agents causing respiratory infections (see Chapter 15).

Symptoms of snoring, mouth breathing, nasal drainage, and sleep apnea alert the clinician to upper respiratory problems. Upper airway obstruction may be one factor predisposing the child with Down syndrome to respiratory disease. In one recent study, 6 out of 12 children were found to have severe and previously undetected upper airway obstruction during sleep [8]. In five children, the obstruction occurred in the pharynx, and in the sixth child, a bilateral choanal stenosis was found.

Gastroesophageal reflux is a problem in Down syndrome, which is an additional complication to the often already compromised upper respiratory system. In children with Down syndrome, the esophageal plexus ganglia have fewer neurons, which helps explain this dysfunction [9].

Pneumonia and tracheitis often can be bacterial infections in infants with Down syndrome [10]. In fact, these infections can be life threatening especially during the ages of 2–12 months if they are not promptly and vigorously treated. That treatment of respiratory infections once they start needs to be aggressive in infants with Down syndrome is undisputed. If appropriate, prevention techniques directed to the individualized problem, such as choanal dilatation, can give good results. Tonsillectomy and adenoidectomy are sometimes recommended. However, it needs to be remembered that adenoid tissue is physiologically important to the child with Down syndrome, and its removal can result in hypernasality [11].

The Leukemias

The age of onset for the leukemias is bimodal, peaking first in the newborn period and then again after 3 years of age (see Chapter 15). In the age group of 2–12 months, there are two types of disease patterns usually seen in infants with Down syndrome.

Patients with congenital leukemia surviving past 2 months of age are already diagnosed and under treatment by this time. In addition, there is another group of infants who have the persistence of the transient leukemoid reaction of the newborn (also called transient leukemia). These patients are being observed carefully. By 3 months of age, most transient leukemoid reactions have disappeared. However, in roughly one-fourth of these patients, leukemia may return when they are older, raising the question of whether the termination of the transient reaction may have been a spontaneous regression of a clone of malignant cells [12].

Audiological Problems

The occurrence of ear infections, or otitis media, in children with Down syndrome is among the highest of any populations who are at risk for this disease [13]. There are three types of otitis media: acute, serous, and chronic. Acute otitis media presents with pain in the ear, hearing loss, bulging and redness of the eardrum, and often a fever. Serous otitis media is a noninfected accumulation of fluid in the middle ear with no observable symptoms. Sometimes it is difficult to diagnose without an examining microscope and pneumatic otoscope, particularly in infants with Down syndrome. Chronic otitis media is characterized by a perforated eardrum and drainage from the middle ear.

Serous otitis media, which is so difficult to diagnose, is associated with mild and fluctuating hearing losses in the first 2 years of life. Even normal children may be seriously handicapped from recurrent or constant otitis media that occurs in these first 2 years. Although the conductive hearing losses that accompany the otitis are mild, they occur during critical periods for the development of listening and language skills. Later testing at third grade has shown deficits in sequential auditory memory, sound blending, and selective auditory attention in a population of normal children with middle ear disease in very early childhood [14]. In children less than 2 years of age with Down syndrome, slight hearing losses may be missed by parents or physicians. Serous otitis media is an insidious problem because of its often total lack of observable symptoms [13].

The infant with Down syndrome may not only be affected by ear infections but also may have an additional handicap from the anatomy of the ear itself (see Chapter 8). When these two factors are combined, the result is a very high incidence of hearing loss in this patient group. Balkany et al. reported that 64% of all individuals with Down syndrome have a binaural hearing loss and that another 14% had a monaural loss [15]. Other studies confirm these disturbingly high figures [16,17].

What is the etiology of so much hearing loss? Downs and Balkany state, "It is probable that most of these hearing losses resulted from otitis media which *initially presented itself in the first year of life*" (italics ours). They have coined the term *minimal auditory deficiency syndrome* to describe the syndrome that develops from recurrent bouts of otitis media beginning in the first year of life [13]. In addition, some of the hearing loss may be congenital and related to the anatomy of the ear.

The treatment for this auditory problem involves a sophisticated understanding of the individual infant's needs. It is important to break the cycle of recurrent suppurative otitis media. If four or more episodes occur in a 12-month period, it is possible that a single infection moves in and out of quiescent to exacerbative episodes and back again. Prophylactic low-dose antibiotics may be needed [13]. Failure of such treatment in 2 or 3 months then can lead to placement of tympanostomy tubes. Without this vigorous and prophylactic approach, chronic otitis media and even cholesteatomas can develop as has been noted in so many institutionalized patients with Down syndrome.

Regarding serous otitis media, decongestants and antibiotics have been shown to be of no value [18]. Criteria for the placement of tympanostomy tubes include a hearing loss of greater than 15 dB in both ears for 2 months or more.

When treatment does not prevent recurrence of middle ear effusion or when a constant hearing loss of greater than 15 dB remains in both ears, the use of hearing aids should be considered [13]. Hearing aids also are an excellent alternative to myringotomy and tubes when the external auditory canals of infants with Down syndrome make placement of tubes very difficult. The success already seen in some programs can be gauged by the extraordinary recent assessment by Gordon that early aggressive treatment with grommets or hearing aids is likely to be *more effective than infant enrichment programs* in preventing the declining developmental quotients often charted in individuals with Down syndrome [19].

Monitoring Thyroid Function

In the first year of life, the monitoring of thyroid function is very important and not always understood or easy to interpret. The signs and symptoms of hypothyroidism can, in some cases, be confused with those of Down syndrome itself, making the diagnosis difficult on clinical grounds alone (see Chapter 12). Thus, the importance of laboratory testing to accurately determine thyroid function looms large.

In the neonatal period, reviewed in the previous chapter, persistent primary congenital hypothyroidism was found to be 28 times more frequent in infants with Down syndrome compared to the general population [20]. During the rest of the first year and thereafter, cases of confirmed primary hypothyroidism continue to present one by one [21].

In addition to these infants whose laboratory testing meets classical criteria for hypothyroidism (increased thyroid-stimulating hormone [TSH] and decreased thyroxine [T_4]), there is another group of infants who have normal T_4 values yet have elevations of TSH. In a study of children with Down syndrome less than 3 years of age, Cutler et al. found that 27% had some degree of elevation of TSH [22]. In later age groups, 3–21 years, the phenomenon of elevated TSH with normal T_4 still exists in children with Down syndrome but only 10% of the patients have it according to Pueschel and Pezzullo [23]. Lejeune et al. also reported elevated TSH in a prospective study of 78 patients aged 16 months to 16 years [24]. In this same study, these investigators also reported a significant decrease of $3,3',5'$-T_3(rT_3), a hormone whose biochemical and physiological role in thyroid function is poorly understood.

A retrospective survey by Sharav et al. of 147 patients with Down syndrome confirmed that high TSH levels were predominantly in young patients, mostly less than 4 years of age [25]. In this study, the first year of life had the highest percentage of patients with the high TSH levels. These investigators also found that the mean T_4 value was significantly higher among the patients with the high TSH values. This study is interesting because a comparison was made between TSH levels and growth patterns. The investigators found that shortness of stature was more pronounced in the high TSH group and that this group always remained shorter than the normal TSH group. In fact, all growth parameters (height, weight, and cranial circumference) correlated inversely with TSH concentration. Because this type of thyroid dysfunction was most apparent during the most active phase of growth, that is, during early infancy, Sharav et al. speculated that these values may reflect an unusual prolongation of the normal physiological process. Another theory suggests that there may be resistance to thyroid hormone at the membrane level in the young cells of infants with trisomy 21 [26].

There is no consensus on whether patients with high TSH without low T_4 levels should receive treatment at all or, if they should receive treatment, what kind. The documentation of even more deviant cranial circumference growth in the patients with elevated TSH level is worrisome.

Hidden Gastrointestinal Diseases

Early infancy is a time when any gastrointestinal anomalies in a child need to be identified and dealt with. At least 10% of infants with Down syndrome have congenital malformations of the gastrointestinal tract [27]. Esophageal atresia, duodenal obstruction, and imperforate anus usually present in the newborn period, but many of the other anomalies of the upper and lower gastrointestinal tract are not immediately obvious. In an infant with either unexplained intermittent vomiting or a developing pattern of chronic constipation, other congenital malformations should be considered and testing conducted (see Chapter 10).

Regarding the upper gastrointestinal tract, a late presentation of duodenal stenosis, diverticulum of the duodenum, and jejunal stenosis can become symptomatic after 2 months of age. In the case of the lower gastrointestinal system, there is aganglionic megacolon (Hirschsprung's disease), rectosigmoid aganglionosis, and localized congenital stenosis of the rectum to consider in the early infancy age group with constipation.

Ophthalmological Problems

In the ages 2 to 12 months, the care of an infant with Down syndrome requires addressing ophthalmological problems if they are present. The development of strabismus may have long-term negative implications for the child if it is neglected. More than one out of every three infants with Down syndrome develops strabismus [28]. In children with Down syndrome, strabismus almost always begins at an early age and is usually of the primary, central type. If left untreated, strabismus may result in the loss of binocular fusion and binonocular depth perception as well as eventual loss of vision in the one eye subjected to continuous suppression. Early treatment of strabismus is a classic example of the practice of effective preventive medicine.

Congenital cataracts should have been detected by 2 months of age; they often interfere with vision. Relatively rare in Down syndrome, cataracts can underlie nystagmus, a more common problem. More often in this patient group, nystagmus is probably of central origin or related to refractive error.

Blepharoconjunctivitis often begins in infancy; it can become chronic if not treated.

For a review of ophthalmological diseases, see Chapter 14.

Tongue Visibility

Two to twelve months is often the age where parents become concerned about the appearance of their child with Down syndrome, particularly the protruding tongue. The tongue is vital for speaking and eating. Several factors have been reported to contribute to the characteristic posture of the tongue and mouth in infants with Down syndrome. These include a small oral cavity, an enlarged tongue (macroglossia) particularly in the region of the lingual tonsil, and mouth breathing due to underdevelopment of frontal and paranasal sinuses [29]. There is a case on record of three episodes of acute macroglossia in an adult with Down syndrome due to a congenital malformation of the lingual lymphatics [30]. Another possibility that might be causing the real or apparent tongue enlargement in patients with Down syndrome is hypotonia secondary to a neurogenic etiology. Abnormalities of the neuromuscular junctions of the tongue studied from surgical specimens have been reported by Yarom et al. [31].

Both medical and surgical approaches to reducing tongue visibility currently are being tested. Cheek and tongue tapping, lip brushing, ice stroking, and behavior modification are some of the medical approaches [29]. Partial glossectomy is one surgical approach [32].

An informal observation by the authors of this monograph suggests that an excellent infant learning program with its effect on the central nervous system often is accompanied by many long-term gains for the child, including less and less visibility of the tongue. One point is clear—the 2–12-month age group is at a critical age for establishing the many educational and medical approaches that assist the infant with Down syndrome to move into a higher functioning childhood and future adulthood.

DOWN SYNDROME PREVENTIVE MEDICINE CHECKLIST: TWO TO TWELVE MONTHS

A. History
Check infectious history, especially upper respiratory disease and otitis media. Ask about symptoms of cardiac disease. If constipation is present, use dietary changes or gentle laxative. If no results, consider bowel anomalies, such as Hirschsprung's disease.
B. Examination
Complete a careful cardiac evaluation. Visualize tympanic membrane. Include neurological and musculoskeletal examination, including possibility of dislocated hips.
C. Laboratory
Measure thyroid-stimulating hormone (TSH) and thyroxine (T_4) levels at 12 months.
D. Referral to team specialists or outside consultations
Pediatric ophthalmological examination recommended within the first 6 months. Auditory evaluation, including auditory brain stem-evoked potential, if indicated, is recommended within the first 6 months. If unsuccessful in visualizing the tympanic membrane, refer to an ear, nose, and throat specialist. At the discretion of the pediatric cardiologist, a follow-up examination and echocardiography may be indicated.
E. Educational recommendations
This is the critical age for infant evaluations and enrollment in infant learning programs. Support the family in their educational program, including reviewing its importance to the future of the child.

REFERENCES

1. Becker LE, Armstrong DL, Chan F. Dendritic atrophy in children with Down's syndrome. Ann Neurol 1986;20:520–526.
2. Kish S, Karlinsky H, Becker L, Gilbert J, Rebbetoy M, Chang L-J, DiStefano L, Hornykiewicz O. Down's syndrome individuals begin life with normal levels of brain cholinergic markers. J Neurochem 1989;52:1183–1187.
3. Baird P, Sadovnick A. Life expectancy in Down syndrome. J Pediatr 1987; 110:849–854.

4. Bell JA, Pearn JH, Firman D. Childhood deaths in Down syndrome: Survival curves and causes of death from a total population study in Queensland, Australia, 1976 to 1985. J Med Genet 1989;26:764–768.

5. Chi TPL, Krovetz LJ. The pulmonary vascular bed in children with Down's syndrome. J Pediatr 1975;86:533–538.

6. Sondheimer HM, Byrum CJ, Blackman MS. Unequal care for children with Down's syndrome. Am J Dis Child 1985;139:68–70.

7. Oster J, Mikkelsen M, Nielsen A. Mortality and life-table in Down's syndrome. Acta Paediatr Scand 1975;64:322.

8. Southall DP, Stebbens VA, Mirza R, Lang MH, Croft CB, Shinebourne EA. Upper airway obstruction with hypoxaemia and sleep disruption in Down syndrome. Dev Med Neurol 1987;29:734–742.

9. Nakazato Y, Landing BH. Reduced number of neurons in esophageal plexus ganglia in Down syndrome: Additional evidence for reduced cell number as a basic feature of the disorder. Pediatr Pathol 1986;51:55–63.

10. Cant AJ, Gibson PJ, West RJ. Bacterial tracheitis in Down's syndrome. Arch Dis Child 1987;62:962–963.

11. Kavanagh KT, Kahane JC, Kordan B. Risks and benefits of adenotonsillectomy for children with Down syndrome. Am J Ment Defic 1986;91:22–29.

12. Lazarus KH, Heerema NA, Palmer CG, Baehner RL. The myeloproliferative reaction in a child with Down's syndrome: Cytological and chromosomal evidence for a transient leukemia. Am J Hematol 1981;2:417–423.

13. Downs MP, Balkany TJ. Otologic problems and hearing impairment in Down syndrome. In: Dmitriev V, Oelwein PL, eds. Advances in Down Syndrome. Seattle, Wash: Special Child Publications, 1988;19–34.

14. Kessler ME, Randolph K. The effects of middle ear disease on the auditory abilities of third grade children. J Acad Rehabil Audiol 1979;12:6–20.

15. Balkany TJ, Downs MP, Jafek BW, Krajicek MJ. Hearing loss in Down's syndrome: A treatable handicap more common than generally recognized. Clin Pediatr 1979;18:116–118.

16. Keiser H, Montague J, Wold D, Maune S, Pattison SM. Hearing loss of Down syndrome adults. Am J Ment Defic 1981;86:467–472.

17. Brooks DN, Wooley A, Kanjilal GC. Hearing loss and middle ear disorders in patients with Down's syndrome (mongolism). J Ment Defic Res 1972;16:21.

18. Bluestone CD. Otitis media in children: To treat or not to treat? N Engl J Med 1982;306:1399–1404.

19. Gordon AG. Language deficit and hearing loss in Down's syndrome. Child Care Health Dev 1987;13:137–139.

20. Fort P, Lifshitz F, Bellisario R, Davis J, Lanes R, Pugliese M, Richmond R, Post EM, David R. Abnormalities of thyroid function in infants with Down syndrome. J Pediatr 1984;104:545–549.

21. Coleman M, Abassi V. Down's syndrome and hypothyroidism: Coincidence or consequence? Lancet 1984;i:569.

22. Cutler AT, Benezra-Obeiter R, Brink SJ. Thyroid function in young children with Down syndrome. Am J Dis Child 1986;140:479–483.

23. Pueschel SM, Pezzullo JC. Thyroid dysfunction in Down syndrome. Am J Dis Child 1985;139:636–639.

24. Lejeune J, Peeters de Blois MC, Bergere M, Gillot A, Rethore MO, Vallee G, Izembart M, DeVoux JP. Thyroid function and trisomy 21: TSH increase and rT_3 deficiency (in French). Ann Genet 1988;31:137–143.

25. Sharav T, Collins RM, Baab PJ. Growth studies in infants and children with Down's syndrome and elevated levels of thyrotropin. Am J Dis Child 1988; 142:1302–1306.

26. Ozand PT. Resistance to thyroid hormone in Down's syndrome. Down's Syndrome: Papers and Abstracts for Professionals 1985;8:4–7.

27. Carter CO. A life table for mongols with the causes of death. J Ment Defic Res 1958;2:64.

28. Shapiro MB, France TD. The ocular features of Down syndrome. Am J Ophthalmol 1962;54:398–406.

29. Purdy AH, Deitz JC, Harris SR. Efficacy of two treatment approaches to reduce the tongue protrusion of children with Down syndrome. Dev Med Child Neurol 1987;29:469–476.

30. Padgham ND, Bingham BJG, Purdue BN. Episodic macroglossia in Down's syndrome. J Laryngol Otol 1990;104:494–496.

31. Yarom R, Sagher U, Havivi Y, Peled IJ, Wexler MR. Myofibers in tongues of Down syndrome. J Neurol Sci 1986;73:279–287.

32. Olbrisch RR. Plastic surgical management of children with Down syndrome—indications and results. Br J Plastic Surg 1982;35:195–200.

5

The Child: One Year to Puberty

The child with Down syndrome between one year of age and puberty presents many challenges to the physician and the family. Physicians find that congenital anomalies and respiratory infections continue to be an important cause of mortality, although less compared to the first year of life [1]. Infections are an important cause of morbidity and result in frequent office visits and occasional hospitalization for management [2]. Families continue to adjust to their child's special needs as he or she graduates from infant therapy programs to preschool and eventually to school programs. Each new educational stage presents unique challenges to families. This chapter summarizes important medical problems that confront the physician treating children with Down syndrome. The last part of the chapter presents ways to help families as they strive for the best possible services for their child.

RESPIRATORY INFECTIONS AND MIDDLE EAR EFFUSIONS

Frequent upper respiratory infections with serous otitis media may result in many visits to the physician's office for evaluation and treatment. Chronic middle ear problems result from a combination of two factors: (1) Intrinsic factors include underlying anatomic defects of the veli palatini muscle, deformity of the stapes, and deficits in the immune system [3]. (2) Extrinsic factors include exposure at intervention programs to young children as well as therapists with viral infections.

Management requires a single or combination antibiotic when the single drug is not effective. An audiological evaluation is suggested after a documented episode of otitis media to rule out an accompanying hearing loss.

Consider the following management strategies for the child with particularly severe or frequent middle ear problems:

1. Look for an underlying correctable problem such as chronic sinusitis, nasal polyp, or inhalant allergies.
2. Use prophylactic antibiotics when upper respiratory infections are epidemic in the community.
3. Immunize older children with Pneumovax and the influenza vaccine. This will provide immunity for some of the infections responsible for upper respiratory infections.
4. Switch child to a home-based program to avoid contact with infected infants during the peak incidence of upper respiratory infections.
5. Consider tympanostomy tubes for the child with persistent middle ear effusion and hearing loss after several courses of antibiotics [4].
6. An augmented hearing device can assist the young child with fluctuating hearing loss due to middle ear effusions. (In cases of limited time span, it even can be an inexpensive unit consisting of a small microphone, an amplifier, and head phone purchased at a nearby electronics supply store.) It can be used during class and speech therapy to help amplify the therapist's or teacher's voice. This device helps by compensating for a fluctuating hearing loss. With more consistent and documented hearing loss, a more complex hearing device is needed. All hearing devices should be fitted by a professional (see Chapter 8 regarding auditory problems).

AIRWAY OBSTRUCTION

A school-aged child with innocent sounding symptoms of bed wetting and sleeping in class could have a serious sleep apnea associated with airway obstruction [5]. This condition is more common in Down syndrome and can usually be treated effectively, resulting in a happier and more alert child. Anatomic, as well as neurological factors are related to sleep apnea in children with Down syndrome. Congenital anatomic problems, such as a large posteriorly placed tongue, and acquired anatomic problems, such as tonsillar and adenoid hypertrophy, predispose to obstruction. Generalized hypotonia that results in poor pharyngeal muscle control also is a predisposing factor. An upper respiratory infection or obesity may be the trigger that combines with the predisposing factors to cause partial airway obstruction during inspiration and lowered oxygen content of the blood.

Symptoms in the young child include snoring at night and restless sleep. During the day, the child may have drowsiness and behavior problems. Other features may include failure to thrive, congestive heart failure, and pulmonary hypertension [5]. The diagnosis can be made after a thorough sleep study that documents hypoxemia or reduced oxygen in the blood during sleep. Another diagnostic test that may be necessary is endoscopy to look for anomalies of the upper airway. The diagnostic evaluation and management is best left to special apnea evaluation teams of physicians at the medical center. Management often includes surgical treatment to correct anatomic factors predisposing to apnea and medical treatment to control the triggering factors.

CARDIAC PROBLEMS

Congenital cardiac problems have usually been diagnosed by 1 year of age, but occasional patients still present throughout childhood. It is important to remind parents of children with congenital heart disease to keep follow-up appointments with the cardiologist and to use prophylactic antibiotics when indicated.

ORTHOPEDIC PROBLEMS
Atlantoaxial Subluxation

The topic of atlantoaxial subluxation has stirred great interest among physicians, parents, teachers, and therapists. The death of a person due to atlantoaxial subluxation and subsequent complications while participating in the Special Olympics focused national attention on this medical problem [6].

Asymptomatic atlantoaxial subluxation (atlantoaxial instability) refers to the condition demonstrated by a radiograph of the cervical spine taken in flexion, neutral, and extension positions showing a distance greater than 5.0 mm between the posterior-inferior aspect of the anterior arch of the atlas and the adjacent surface of the odontoid process. There are no neurological signs or symptoms of cord compression present. The cause of the subluxation is believed to be due to congenital laxity of the transverse ligament.

Symptomatic atlantoaxial subluxation refers to the condition demonstrated by an abnormal radiograph of the cervical spine plus symptoms of cord compression (neck pain, torticollis, urinary incontinence, and inability to walk) plus signs of cord compression (hyperreflexia in the lower extremities, ankle clonus, and bilateral extensor plantar responses). About 15% of persons

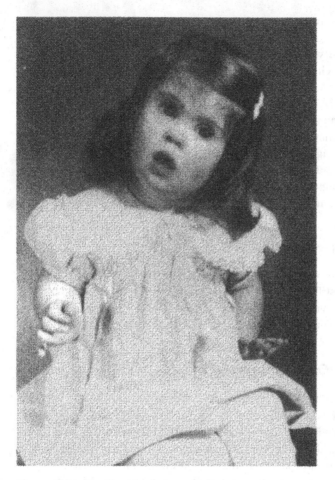

Figure 5.1 Good health care keeps children with Down syndrome attractive and better able to learn.

with asymptomatic atlantoaxial subluxation identified radiographically develop symptomatic atlantoaxial subluxation [7]. Symptomatic atlantoaxial subluxation may be associated with the following:

1. Congenital anomalies of the cervical spine such as a hypoplastic odontoid process
2. Trauma associated with sudden flexion or extension of the neck

3. Surgery when an anesthetic agent is induced by an endotracheal tube when the neck is in an extreme extension position
4. Upper respiratory or deep cervical infection causing possible synovial effusion that results in further instability of the atlantoaxial joint [6].

Management of symptomatic atlantoaxial subluxation includes immediate immobilization to prevent further trauma to the neck. Surgical repair consists of posterior fusion of C1 (cervical spine) and C2 [6]. Postoperative management requires a halo cast or traction until fusion occurs. Like all surgery, there is some risk in this procedure.

Management of individuals with symptomatic atlantoaxial subluxation is known. However, there are some unanswered questions about managing individuals with asymptomatic atlantoaxial subluxation:

1. What is the natural history of asymptomatic atlantoaxial subluxation? If a person has a negative radiograph of the spine at 4 years of age, does the radiograph need to be repeated later?
2. Should fusion surgery be done in a person with asymptomatic atlantoaxial subluxation to prevent the neurological complications of cord compression?

Current research should provide some answers to the previously mentioned management questions. Until final information is available, the following guidelines are suggested:

1. Every person with Down syndrome requires a cervical radiograph at the age of 3 years, and this should be repeated again before and at the end of puberty.
2. The radiograph needs to be read by an experienced radiologist.
3. A person with asymptomatic atlantoaxial subluxation requires special precautions:
   a. The person should avoid contact sports, somersaults, trampoline exercises, and diving [8].
   b. The radiograph needs to be repeated in 2 years to monitor progression of the instability.
   c. Careful yearly neurological examinations are indicated to detect progression.
   d. The patient's family should be instructed in the clinical signs of impending trouble and who to notify if torticollis, neck pain, weakness of a limb, or an abnormal gait develops.

For a review of the current discussion about recommendations in the literature on atlantoaxial subluxation, see Appendix B and Chapter 11.

Dislocation of the Hip

Hip dislocation can be troublesome to adults with Down syndrome. However, in the case of younger patients, compared to children with normal chromosomes, hip dislocation occurs with the same frequency in children with Down syndrome. Ligament laxity and hypotonia predispose to hip dislocation. The person with Down syndrome and dislocation of the hip often presents with gait disturbance, delayed ambulation, or a hip click on physical examination.

Referral to a specialist is advised.

Pes Planus

Pes planus refers to a severe flat foot due to lowering of one or more of the pedal arches. Pes planus occurs more frequently in children with Down syndrome than in ordinary children and can progress to a more severe foot deformity such as hallus valgus (lateral deviation of the great toe) and secondary bunion formation. Pes planus is classified as hypermobile or rigid. The hypermobile flat foot refers to a foot flat only in weight bearing and usually requires no intervention. The rigid flat foot is flat in weight bearing as well as in non-weight bearing situations and requires prescription shoes or other orthoses. Surgery is necessary if there is extensive involvement.

Metatarus Varus

Metatarus varus refers to a forefoot that turns in or is C shaped. This occurs unilaterally or bilaterally and can be detected at birth. Early treatment is indicated and consists of serial casting and special shoes.

Patellar Instability

Patellar instability refers to a patella or knee cap that dislocates frequently. Patellar instability is due to joint laxness and may follow even mild sports activities. Bracing is the first line of management, with surgery reserved for severe or chronic problems.

For a review of other orthopedic problems in this patient group, see Chapter 11.

THYROID DIFFICULTIES

Hypothyroidism continues to be a potential problem throughout childhood. Yearly evaluations of T_4 (thyroxine) and TSH (thyroid-stimulating hormone) levels are recommended because hypothyroidism may present with gradual onset of signs and symptoms such as increased weight, lethargy, decline in academic performance, and slowing of growth. Replacement therapy is indicated for the child with clinical symptoms and a low T_4 and high TSH level.

Occasionally, mild elevations of TSH are seen with normal-to-high T_4 levels [9]. This condition is sometimes referred to as thyroid dysfunction and is associated with significant growth failure in children less than 4 years of age [10]. Although guidelines for managing thyroid dysfunction are still evolving, the following are some suggestions to be used until more definite information is available:

1. Repeat T_4 and TSH screening to determine whether the infant's laboratory values return to normal ranges or progress to hypothyroidism.
2. Consider referral to an endocrinologist for further diagnostic testing to rule out a central nervous system lesion such as a hypopituitary disorder.

In some centers, replacement therapy has been considered for thyroid dysfunction when the TSH is ⩾8MIU/ml. Such centers start with a very small dose of levothyroxine to avoid an adverse reaction such as hyperactivity or sleeplessness. Monthly evaluations of T_4 and TSH levels are indicated to monitor the therapy. In other centers, the concept of treatment of a patient with normal levels of T_4 (no matter what the level of TSH is) is rejected.

Hyperthyroidism is much rarer but also presents in children with Down syndrome. For a review of endocrine disorders, see Chapter 12.

GROWTH AND NUTRITION

Growth charts developed for children with Down syndrome were recently published [11] (see Appendix A). The special charts are useful in detecting unusual growth failure within the Down syndrome group. Growth failure is defined as height and weight below the 5th percentile for age or growth rate that falls to the next lower percentile line when plotted on the appropriate growth chart. Growth failure is frequently secondary to a congenital malformation (most frequently of the heart or gastrointestinal tract), an endocrinopathy, or poor caloric intake.

A pediatric nutritional assessment may help to detect low calorie intake or feeding disorders that cause poor nutritional intake. A nutritional assessment begins with a 3-day food diary provided by the family that documents the amount, time, and type of food the child eats. The daily food intake is analyzed by the physician or nutritional specialist for adequacy of calories, vitamins, and minerals as compared to the Required Daily Allowances (RDA) described for children [12]. One method of determining required daily calories is by centimeter of height, based on the standard of 16.1 calories per centimeter of height for boys and 14.3 calories per centimeter of height for girls.

Oral-motor deficits may delay advancement of the texture of the diet and also inhibit the nutritional intake. An oral-motor deficit such as poor neuromotor control of tongue movements causes the infant to gag and reject food of increased texture such as chopped table food. The physician should ask about the child's feeding abilities and, if indicated, observe the mother feeding the child. An older infant who will only tolerate a reduced textured diet of strained baby food may not be getting a nutritionally appropriate intake. For example, a 12-month-old infant may readily take strained green and yellow vegetables and refuse and gag when offered chopped meat or other food of increased texture. The result is a diet low in protein and high in carotene resulting in carotenemia and a characteristic yellow tinge to the skin. Referral to an experienced nutritionist and feeding specialist may help advance the child's diet and improve the nutritional intake.

Constipation is a common problem that often responds to dietary management. For example, increased fluids such as apple or prune juice may be helpful. Adding fiber, such as bran, to the diet can also be helpful. Constipation that does not respond to dietary management or is unusually severe requires further medical assessment to detect an underlying medical problem such as gastrointestinal anomalies (see Chapter 10) or hypothyroidism (see Chapter 12).

Obesity is another common problem seen in children after 2 years of age. A full dietary investigation is indicated as well as exploring the child's feeding behavior and exercise activities. Occasionally, an underlying medical problem such as hypothyroidism may contribute to obesity. Management requires a thorough investigation for possible etiological factors and then a comprehensive intervention program for the child and family (see Chapter 17).

Malabsorption of nutrients from the gastrointestinal tract may cause symptoms of loose, foul-smelling stools. Occasionally, the signs and symptoms may be subtle, such as poor weight gain. If indicated, screen for malabsorption by carefully monitoring growth and checking yearly a serum vitamin A level or checking a stool for excessive fat content (see Chapter 10).

DENTAL CONSIDERATIONS

The average age for tooth eruption is 13.6 months for a child with Down syndrome and is 6–7 months for children with normal chromosomes. Missing teeth, or partial anodentia, is also frequent. Delayed tooth eruption and fewer teeth do result in one benefit, fewer dental caries in children with Down syndrome than in other children [13]. Periodontal disease is more common probably because of the immunodeficiency of these children (see Chapter 16). The first dental assessment by a pediadontist is recommended at 1 year of age, with at least yearly visits after that.

OCULAR CONSIDERATIONS

Blepharitis is a common inflammation of the eyelid due to an adeno virus or *Staphylococcus aureus*. The condition usually responds readily to antibiotic ophthalmic solutions. Persistent infections require further evaluation to rule out an underlying problem such as a blocked tear duct. Strabismus also is frequent and often due to a lens opacity or severe myopia [14]. An annual ophthalmological evaluation is indicated for early detection of correctable ocular problems, such as refractive error (see Chapter 14).

FAMILY EDUCATION AND SUPPORT

Although medical problems are challenging to the family and physician, the family often seeks the physician's advice on nonmedical problems such as finding a good preschool program and financial benefits available from government agencies. The physician acts as an advocate as well as a resource for the child and family. For example, the physician can guide the family to appropriate community resources to apply for financial aid. The following section discusses some of the specific concerns of families and some recommended community resources in the United States.

Infant Programs: Birth to Two Years

The young child presents many concerns to the family. Often the encounter with school and special education programs is an unhappy experience because it reminds the family that their child has special needs. In addition, families must learn a new vocabulary with terms such as *least restrictive* and *mainstreaming*. These new educational terms probably are also new to many physicians. This section provides the physician some background information about special education programs from a medical perspective. This section also discusses the special support needs of families as they experience these challenging years.

Special education begins early in a child's life with infant learning programs (see Chapter 2). Infant programs are "organized programs of enrichment designed to provide developmentally appropriate activities to babies and toddlers who have or who are at risk for a variety of conditions that may interfere with their ability ultimately to have a full and productive life" [15]. In the United States, these programs have a legal mandate under the 1989 Education of Handicapped Children Act, Public Law 99-457. Although this law spells out specific guidelines for development of infant intervention programs, the role of the physician is not as clearly defined. The following will provide a general overview of infant intervention programs to guide the physician.

Although goals often vary at different programs, most attempt the following:

1. Provide activities to stimulate developmental skills such as fine motor, gross motor, visual perceptual, and language skills.
2. Include the family in the program so that they can do the infant interventions at home.
3. Provide education to families to help them cope with feeding problems, transporting, and so on as the issues arise.

Intervention programs may be home based, where a therapist makes regular home visits, or center based where the family is required to bring their child to a center for the intervention. Services may be provided by an infant intervention specialist, one trained to do several types of therapy, or a professional trained in a specific type of therapy, such as a physical therapist (gross or large motor movement), occupational therapist (fine motor or hand movement), or speech pathologist. The cost for such programs may be borne entirely by the family and any insurance that may provide coverage or may be partially or entirely supported by local or federal grants or tax support.

The physician can help by directing the family to appropriate intervention programs. Lists of local programs are available from local groups organized to help retarded children or from the National Down Syndrome Society (see Appendices C and D). The following factors affect the family's selection of an intervention program: the family's finances, the child's additional health problems, family availability of time, and transportation needs.

The following are some general guidelines for helping a family select an intervention program:

1. For families with no insurance coverage, that is, no third party coverage either through welfare or Blue Cross or Blue Shield, consider referral to a tax-supported or grant-supported program.
2. For children with serious medical problems such as severe, frequent respiratory infections or severe congenital heart disease, consider a home-based interventionist so that the child will have decreased exposure to other children who may have viral infections.
3. For families who have difficulty with transportation, consider a home-based program, which also may be beneficial.

4. For infants with global delays, recommend an infant interventions specialist. As the child matures, a physical therapist, occupational therapist, and speech specialist should all evaluate the child to determine whether more intensive therapy is indicated.
5. For parents who refuse all intervention programs, consider scheduling an office visit to evaluate their coping and denial. For the family with mild coping problems, having them talk with another family often helps them to accept an intervention program. For the family with serious problems, consider referral to an experienced counselor.

For the family who enrolls their child in 3 or 4 extensive programs a week, consider an office visit to review their needs and expectations. Most children require two therapy sessions a week.

The Preschool-Aged Child

Families with a child with Down syndrome share many problems experienced by all families who have a preschool child: arranging child care if mother works, balancing an individual child's needs against those of the other children, and making the paycheck stretch to meet day-to-day needs of the children. Although a preschool-aged child with Down syndrome brings added responsibilities and stresses, most families report that the benefits outweigh the problems [16].

A survey revealed some of the special situations families encounter raising a child with Down syndrome [16]. Parents reported that one dilemma is that their child requires more time, leaving less time for the siblings. Time is quickly used up for trips to the infant interventions programs, physician's visits, parent group meetings, and so on. Another common family predicament is the decreased likelihood that the mother will return to work. If she does return to work, she often changes to a job that demands less time and energy. A few mothers report ongoing personal stress, anxiety, and poor health. Some parents found that the child stresses the marriage. The stressed mothers reported that they get insufficient support from their spouses and that their sex life often stops because of anxieties about possible pregnancies.

Overall, most families believed that the other children benefited from having a sibling with Down syndrome. A few parents noted that siblings expressed jealousy over the extra time spent with the child with Down syndrome and complained that the sibling got into their things. Most parents believed that their children benefitted because they gained compassion and tolerance for others. The siblings also do academically and socially as well as their peers [17].

Families also find that the severity of difficulties encountered are less than expected. As their child becomes older and more independent, the parents found that they made more friends through the child. Parents also expressed pride for their child's achievements as well as the child's kindness, affection, and humor [16].

The physician can provide support to families by suggesting community resources that can assist the family with these occasional dilemmas. Often, families can benefit from respite care services. Respite care programs exist in most communities and provide trained people to provide in home or out of home child care. The trained respite care worker can be especially helpful for a child with significant medical problems such as congenital heart disease or seizures. In addition, respite programs often provide up to 2 weeks care in emergency situations such as hospitalization of a parent. Information about a community's respite care programs is available from the local Association for Retarded Citizens or Down syndrome parent group. The National Down Syndrome Congress in the United States can also provide information about local respite programs.

Another community resource that can assist families is case management service, which is a social service that helps persons with developmental disabilities find appropriate services in or outside of their community. The most important help provided by a case manager is coordination of services. A family may often be overwhelmed by the number of different service programs available in the community or by how to deal with the professionals that deliver intervention services. The case manager can assist the family in finding the appropriate program as well as deal with communication blocks and other problems that arise in dealing with the intervention specialists. Information about case management services is available through local development disability program directors or the National Down Syndrome Congress in the United States.

In addition to community services that aid families, parents also want to know what they can do at home to improve their child's development. Microcomputers can help children gain developmental skills. A home computer may benefit a child in several ways [18]:

1. Improve communication skills. Newer programs provide a synthesized voice in response to a child's selections of objects on the screen.
2. Increase motivation. Children's interaction with a computer can be entertaining and engaging.
3. Enhance self-esteem. As a child learns how to control a computer, it can provide a sense of accomplishment.

The first question to ask when exploring the potential for a computer is whether a child is ready developmentally for a computer. A child needs to have visual motor skills at about a 2–2.5-year level to be able to begin to profit from having a home computer. A rule of thumb for parents in determining whether their child is ready to operate a computer is when he can use a remote control for television. The next step is selecting specific developmental skills that can be enhanced by the computer, such as improving articulation or specific prereading skills. By talking to the child's therapists or teachers, parents can learn what is needed.

Parents appreciate any suggestions about what they can do to help stimulate their child's development. Another equally important concern of parents is their child's behavior. It is important to inquire because some parents do not voluntarily ask questions about their child's behavior because they believe the physician deals only with medical concerns.

Occasional behavior problems seen in the preschool-aged child include head banging, temper tantrums, sleep disturbances, and oppositional behavior. It is helpful to set up an office visit to meet with both parents when they are having difficulty dealing with a specific behavior disorder with their child. When approaching behavior problems, it is important to rule out any underlying medical problems that trigger or promote a problem behavior. For example, head banging may be the chief complaint for a young child with acute serous otitis media or sinusitis. Excessive drowsiness and lethargy may accompany hypothyroidism. Sleep disturbances such as loud snoring and frequent night waking may be due to sleep apnea caused by an upper airway obstruction.

Once medical problems are ruled out, it is helpful for the parents to chart for 1–2 weeks the time, frequency, and circumstances of two or three more severe problems. Review these data to see what specific events precede the behavior as well as the consequences. Evaluate the possibility that the problem behavior is actually due to a skill deficit. Often some very simple interventions can help parents gain control of their child's problem behaviors. For example, ignoring temper tantrums while improving communications skills will usually decrease the problem in a short time. Time out, that is, placing a child on a chair in a corner for a 2- or 3-minute period, is helpful in managing antisocial behaviors such as hitting and pushing other children. Problems that do not resolve after one or at the most two office sessions should be referred to an experienced child psychologist in the community. Behavior control by medications is contraindicated in the preschool-aged child.

The School-Aged Child

The school years are often very difficult for parents because they must decide about educational placement options in the community's schools. The family often turns to the physician for guidance in dealing with the school and special education programs. The physician plays an important role in the special education of children, particularly in being an advocate for the child and assisting the family. The following section will help guide the physician in collaborating with the school and special education programs.

The Education for All Handicapped Children Act, Public Law 94-142, passed in 1975, requires states of the United States to provide an education for all handicapped children and guarantees parents the opportunity to participate in their child's programming. A handicapped child is defined as a person less than 22 years of age with one or more of the following handicaps: hearing or visual impairment, learning disabled, orthopedic handicap, speech disorder, severe behavior handicap, or other chronic health problems that affect a child's academic performance. Special education refers to specifically designed instruction to meet the learning needs of a child with a handicap. The school provides a continuum of special education services in the least restrictive

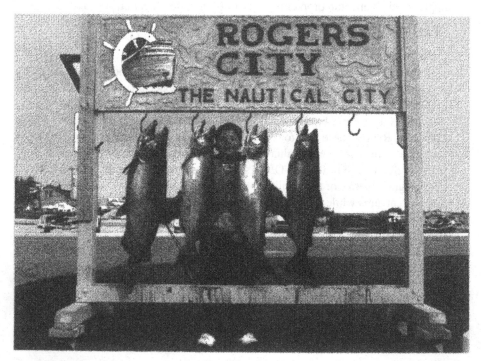

Figure 5.2 Children with Down syndrome can participate in all recreational and family activities.

environment. Least restrictive environment refers to services for children that are as close as possible to education provided to children without handicaps. For example, the least restrictive environment would be supplemental services that involve consultation with a teacher about a student in his or her class. A more restrictive environment would be special class placement where a student is placed in a self-contained classroom for special instruction. The most restrictive special education option refers to an instructor who provides education in the child's home.

The special education process consists of several distinct steps:

1. Identification. A student is identified by teacher, parents, or physician as having possible special education needs.
2. Assessment. An evaluation is completed by the school psychologist, physical therapist, or other professional to determine the student's learning strengths and weaknesses.
3. Individual Education Plan (IEP) development. A conference with the parents and school personnel is held to review the evaluation results and make specific remediation plans as indicated.
4. Instruction. The education program is actually implemented.
5. Periodic review and reevaluation. Meetings are held formally and informally to review progress and to make adaptations as indicated.

When parents approach the physician about a placement decision for their child, the physician can do several things to help the child and the school. It is important that all medical problems are identified and, when possible, remediated. For example, chronic middle ear effusions can cause fluctuating hearing loss and interfere with classroom learning. Hypothyroidism also has devastating effects on classroom learning. It is important that these problems are all identified and corrected. If a permanent medical problem is present, such as a seizure disorder, it is critical to explain to school staff the extent of the problem so that they can make appropriate adjustment in the classroom to maximize a student's learning ability. The physician needs to inform the school staff about such specifics as functional limits, safety precautions, and medications required by the child [19].

In placement, as well as other school service decisions, the physician can serve as an advocate for the child, ensuring that he or she gets an appropriate evaluation as well as the appropriate special education service. Some schools are constrained by budgetary limitations and cannot provide all the services needed by a child. It is important to assist the family in the due process to obtain services required or help find services elsewhere.

The physician can also play an important role in helping families involved in formulating the IEP, a process that often is intimidating to parents. The physician can help parents prepare for the IEP meeting by making sure that they have all critical evaluation and testing results to review before the meeting. Review with them important questions to ask at the IEP meeting. Support them in asserting their special concerns and requests for their child's program. Although most parents may not be education professionals, they offer keen insight into the likelihood that a plan for their child will fail because of factors often overlooked by school staff. For full information about parents' rights, contact the school for a list of their rights as outlined by P.L. 94-142.

During the school age years, major behavior problems are rare, but many parents have concerns about their child's social skills deficits. With the majority of children attending community schools, interaction with peers and teachers becomes very important. Because cognitive deficits may often be associated with social skills deficits, parents and professionals have become very interested in ways to improve or train a child's social skills.

Social skills training refers to methods to improve a person's interpersonal interaction. Techniques for training social skills include modeling, role playing, and positive reinforcement techniques for specific prosocial behaviors such as eye contact or initiation of social conversation.

A social skill deficit may present in several ways. Often a child will be withdrawn and will not interact with other children in the classroom or on the playground. Occasionally, a child may use inappropriate attention-getting methods such as hitting or inappropriate language. The behavior problem is due to a social skill deficit.

A social skill such as social conversation can be enhanced [20], although there may be difficulty in use of the new social skill in different settings [21].

This section has outlined some general suggestions for guiding the physician when helping a family with a child with Down syndrome. Sometimes it is difficult to provide extensive assistance to families during a busy office visit. Often a physician can be most helpful by merely listening to the family's concerns and directing them to an appropriate community resource.

ANNUAL DOWN SYNDROME PREVENTIVE MEDICINE CHECKLIST: AGE ONE YEAR TO PUBERTY*

A. Clinical history

    1.   Review parents' concerns.

---

*Lentz G. Down Syndrome Preventive Medicine Checklist. Down Syndrome Papers and Abstracts for Professionals 1989;12:1–9.

2. Inquire about school progress and future educational plans.
3. Inquire about behavior problems.
4. Review Individual Education Plan (IEP) to make sure it is complete and appropriate.
5. Review history of infections, ear problems, constipation, ophthalmological problems, and snoring.
6. Assess need for subacute bacterial endocarditis (SBE) prophylaxis.
7. Monitor total caloric intake, eating behaviors, and exercise.

B. Medical examination

1. General pediatric examination with growth parameters plotted on a growth chart for children with Down syndrome
2. Neurological examination with special attention to long track signs suggesting atlantoaxial subluxation
3. Audiological examination annually or more frequent if there has been numerous ear infections or middle ear fluid
4. Pediatric ophthalmological examination annually unless there are abnormalities indicating more frequent visits
5. Dental evaluations beginning at 2 years of age and yearly after that; check on home tooth brushing program to prevent gingivitis
6. Annual thyroxine (T_4) and thyroid-stimulating hormone (TSH) evaluation to screen for thyroid disorders
7. Cervical spine radiograph in flexion, neutral, and extension views at 3 years of age and repeated at 12 years of age

C. Family support and child education

1. Continue speech and physical therapy evaluations and treatment as indicated.
2. Conduct a complete psychoeducational assessment including social adaptive skills every 3 years.
3. Monitor family's needs for respite care, supportive counseling, and training in behavior management.

REFERENCES

1. Baird PA, Sadovnick AD. Causes of death to age 30 in Down syndrome. Am J Hum Genet 1988;43:239–248.
2. Murdoch JC. Comparison of the care of children with Down's syndrome with the care of matched controls. J R Coll Gen Pract 1984;34:205–209.
3. Schwartz DM, Schwartz RH. Acoustic impedance and otoscopic findings in young children with Down's syndrome. Arch Otolaryngol 1978;104:652–656.

4. Gates AJ, Avery CA, Prihoda TJ, et al. Effectiveness of adenoidectomy and tympanostomy tubes in the treatment of chronic otitis media with effusion. N Engl J Med 1987;317:1444–1451.

5. Silverman M. Airway obstruction and sleep disruption in Down's syndrome. Br Med J 1988;296:1618–1619.

6. Chaudhry V, Sturgeon C, Gates AJ, Myers G. Symptomatic atlantoaxial dislocation in Down's syndrome. Ann Neurol 1987;21:606–609.

7. Pueschel SM, Scola FH. Atlantoaxial instability in individuals with Down syndrome. Epidemiologic, radiographic, and clinical studies. Pediatrics 1987; 80:555–560.

8. Pueschel SM. Atlantoaxial instability and Down syndrome. Pediatrics 1987; 81:879–880.

9. Cutler AT, Benezra-Obeiter R, Brink SJ. Thyroid function in young children with Down syndrome. Am J Dis Child 1986;140:497–483.

10. Sharav T, Collins RR, Baab PT. Growth studies in infants and children with Down's syndrome and elevated levels of thyrotropin. Am J Dis Child 1988; 142:1302–1306.

11. Cronk C, Crocker AC, Pueschel SM, et al. Growth charts for children with Down syndrome: 1 month to 18 years of age. Pediatrics 1988;81:102–110.

12. Palmer S. Down's syndrome. In: Palmer S, Ekvall S, eds. Pediatric Nutrition Problems in Developmental Disorders. Springfield, Ill: Charles C. Thomas, 1978: 25–35.

13. Stark AM. Dentistry. In: Pueschel SM, Rynders JE, eds. Down Syndrome Advances in Biomedicine and the Behavioral Sciences. Cambridge, Mass: Academic Guild Publishers, 1982:199–203.

14. Pueschel SM. Ophthalmology. In: Pueschel SM, Rynders JE, eds. Down Syndrome Advances in Biomedicine and the Behavioral Sciences. Cambridge, Mass: Academic Guild Publishers, 1982:190–196.

15. Denhoff E. Current status of infant stimulation or enrichment programs for children with developmental disabilities. Pediatrics 1981;67:32–37.

16. Carr J. Six weeks to twenty-one years old: A longitudinal study of children with Down's syndrome and their families. J Child Psychiatry 1988;29:407–431.

17. Gath A, Gumley D. Retarded children and their siblings. J Child Psychol Psychiatry 1987;26:715–730.

18. Willner J. Using Computers to Help Children with Down Syndrome. New York: National Down Syndrome Society, 1989.

19. Walker DK, Palfrey JS, Handley-Derry M, Singer JD. Mainstreaming children with handicaps: Implications for pediatricians. Dev Beh Pediatr 1989;10:151–156.

20. Wildman BG, Wildman HE, Kelly WJ. Group conversational skill training and social validation with mentally retarded adults. Appl Res Ment Retard 1986; 7:443–458.

21. Berler ES, Gross AM, Drabman RS. Social skills training with children. J Appl Beh Anal 1982;15:41–53.

6

The Adolescent

What a special time adolescence is. The transition from childhood to adulthood is marked by a longing for and a fear of independence. Physical appearance becomes much more important as puberty brings changes to the body. It is a time of evaluation of the skills developed throughout childhood and a time of new directions more focused toward specific vocational aims.

The first cohort of children with Down syndrome to benefit from home rearing with educational and medical support are now in their teenage years and early adulthood. They are continually challenging our outdated perceptions of the inherent capabilities of adolescents with Down syndrome. The child with Down syndrome, as well as the child's family, often finds his or her adolescence a time of appraisal. The child, sensitive to peer approval, may have to come to terms with short stature and weight problems. The parents may find this time another chance to come to terms with the vocational and social challenges of the level of developmental delay in their son or daughter.

This is the age when the prejudice of society against individuals with Down syndrome, sometimes spilling over to the other teenage siblings of the child, can begin to affect the child directly. It is a time of sensitivity and new opportunity.

PUBERTY

Puberty is announced by the development of secondary sex characteristics. Institutionalized children with Down syndrome have been reported in the past to have significantly delayed puberty [1]. In contrast, the contemporary studies of home-reared youngsters with Down syndrome report that the age of onset of puberty is similar to that of children without Down syndrome [2,3].

The biological effect of the same extra chromosome on children varies depending on the environment in which the child is raised. This could be considered as one more demonstration that institutions are an environment that may have a negative impact on the child's life, in this case on the hypothalamic-pituitary-gonadal axis [2].

Home-reared children go through the normal sequential development of the primary and the secondary sex characteristics, suggesting that their pituitary-gonadal function is intact. Pubic hair develops normally. However, a delay and sparseness in axillary hair development and, in males, facial hair development have been reported [3]. The mustache development may lag behind in some home-reared young men.

Both precocious puberty and delayed puberty have been reported in association with medical diseases in patients with Down syndrome. A Down syndrome child with early puberty could be checked for the possibility of hypothyroidism [4, 5] and one with delayed puberty for celiac disease [6].

In home-reared male children with Down syndrome, the plasma level of testosterone is normal [2,3]. Regarding follicle-stimulating hormone (FSH) and luteinizing hormone (LH) in both sexes, there tends to be elevated levels, and this tendency increases with age. Forty-three percent of home-reared females had primary gonadal dysfunction in one series [2].

Cryptorchidism is found more frequently in some series than in others. The ovaries can have diminished follicles, and a minority of females have little evidence of ovulation. Menstrual cycles tend to be regular. Pregnancies have occurred in a number of women; one man has demonstrated the ability to reproduce (for details of these studies, see Chapter 12).

In a study that recorded parental perceptions, more than half of a home-reared group of adolescents showed an interest in the opposite sex and were attending social gatherings. Masturbation was observed in 40% of the young men and 52% of the young women with Down syndrome. Only a limited number of adolescents were given sex education in this study [7].

Puberty is accompanied by a normal pubescent fat spurt in this patient group, but if the magnitude of the height spurt is diminished, this may add to a tendency to obesity [8]. Obesity does not help their self-esteem at a time when social and vocational issues come into focus (see Chapter 17).

Regarding their social and vocational opportunities, "gentle incompetence" refers to how adolescents with Down syndrome often are gently protected in a social cocoon; their extra chromosome becomes a sign that not much is expected. Mitnick says:

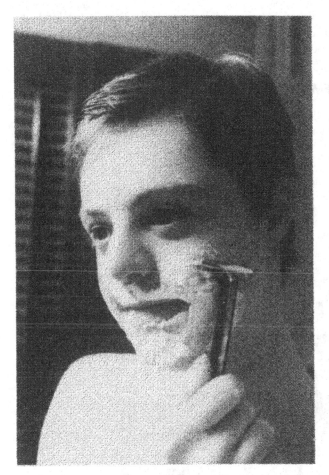

Figure 6.1 Adolescence—a time of transition.

The families love them and "learn" from them (how much more they would learn if they expected butterflies inside the cocoon!)

Professional social agents use the chromosome as a guide for superficial labeling, and thus for a placement in a setting that guards but does not challenge [9].

This is not to suggest that this patient group does not need special care in choosing vocational opportunities. To take one example, there is evidence that there is a slight impairment of the ability to use sensory information for precise motor control. Their ability to adapt grip forces to changes in the properties of lifted objects is diminished in some adolescents [10]. This is the kind of problem that individualized vocational training can identify, and then a program can be developed for modification of responses.

MEDICAL PROBLEMS IN ADOLESCENCE

If Down syndrome children have had good preventive medical attention while growing up, the medical problems special to adolescence should be limited. At

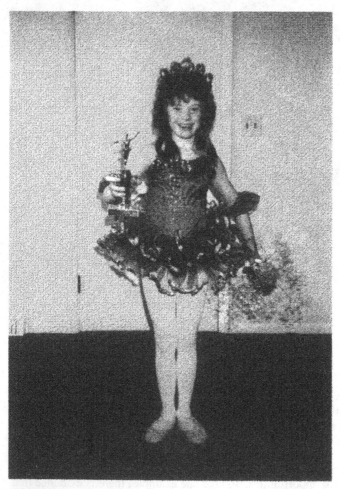

Figure 6.2 There is no limit to the talents seen in children with Down syndrome.

least some of the problems are the problems that they share with other teenagers.

These are the years of intense sports activities. The possibility of atlantoaxial instability needs to be reevaluated at this age (see Chapter 11 and Appendix B). Seizures beginning after 13 years of age in an adolescent with Down syndrome are most often a result of head injury or the delayed sequelae of cardiac disease [11].

The problem of acne does not spare the youngster with Down syndrome. Other skin lesions, such as crusted (Norwegian) scabies or staphylococcal blisters, may occur in up to 50–60% of this age group [12] (see Chapter 18). The skin infections often occur in the perigenital area, buttocks, and thighs and may progress to abscesses if not rapidly treated. This is the age in which the immunological deficiency (discussed in Chapter 15) is less likely to present as a respiratory infection and is more likely to show up in other ways, such as skin or bladder infections. Pueschel reports that with proper skin hygiene, with application of antibiotic ointment if follicular skin eruptions are noted, and sometimes with administration of systemic antibiotic treatment if recurrent multiple abscesses are noted, these infections usually can be controlled [12].

This is the age in which regular dental care becomes even more important (see Chapter 16). Although the major ophthalmological problems should have been well under control by the time of adolescence, the possibility of keratoconus now looms larger as the person grows older [13].

Like any other adolescent, a young person with Down syndrome may become antisocial, moody, or depressed. In addition, psychiatric or behavioral disorders of the adult patterns may begin during adolescence.

ANNUAL DOWN SYNDROME PREVENTIVE MEDICINE CHECKLIST: ADOLESCENT

A. History
Inquire about occurrence of infections, vision loss, seizures, symptoms of hypothyroidism, behavioral disturbances, and problems in handling menstruation.
B. Examination
Monitor for obesity by plotting weight for height. Conduct physical, neurological, and pelvic examinations.
C. Laboratory
Perform annual thyroid-stimulating hormone (TSH) and thyroxine (T_4) level evaluations, serum vitamin A level evaluation (usually at 13 years of age), and echocardiography (usually 19 years of age).

D.   Referral to specialists as indicated
Perform ophthalmological examination and cardiological reevaluation. Dental care twice yearly.
E.   Recommendations
Daily exercise program, healthful diet. Continue speech therapy if necessary. School program: continue academics with additional vocational programming; should encourage independence in daily living activities, sexual education as appropriate. Social life: leisure time activities need to be developed.

REFERENCES

1.   Benda CE. The Child With Mongolism. New York: Grune & Stratton, 1960.
2.   Hsiang YH, Berkovitz GD, Bland GL, Migeon CJ, Warren AC. Gonadal function in patients with Down syndrome. Am J Med Genet 1987;27:449–458.
3.   Pueschel SM, Orson JM, Boylan JM, Pezzullo JC. Adolescent development in males with Down syndrome. Am J Dis Child 1985;139:236–238.
4.   Pabst HF, Pueschel SM, Hillman DA. Etiologic interrelationship in Down's syndrome, hypothyroidism and precocious sexual development. Pediatrics 1967; 40:590.
5.   Floret D. Trisomy 21, myxedema due to thyroiditis with precocious puberty involvement: Study of gonodatrophins and prolactin secretions. Pediatrie 1978; 33:189–200.
6.   Simila S, Kokkonen J. Coexistence of celiac disease and Down syndrome. Am J Ment Retard 1990;95:120–122.
7.   Pueschel SM. Maturation during adolescence. Down's Syndrome: Papers and Abstracts for Professionals 1986;9:1.
8.   Cronk CE, Chumlea WC. Is obesity a problem in trisomy 21? Trisomy 21 1985; 1:19–26.
9.   Mitnick BM. Growing up in the social cocoon: The case for maturational intervention. Down's Syndrome: Papers and Abstracts for Professionals 1988;11: 1–3.
10. Cole KJ, Abbs JH, Turner GS. Deficits in the production of grip forces in Down syndrome. Dev Med Child Neurol 1988;30:752–758.
11. Stafstrom CE, Patxot OF, Gilmore HE, Wisniewski KE. Seizures in children with Down syndrome: Etiology, characteristics and outcome. Dev Med Child Neurol 1991;33:191–200.
12. Pueschel SM. Clinical aspects of Down syndrome from infancy to adulthood. Am J Med Genet 1990;(suppl 7):52–56.
13. Cullen JF, Butler HG. Mongolism (Down's syndrome) and keratoconus. Br J Ophthalmol 1963;47:321.

7

The Adult

The 75-year-old woman with Down syndrome had been cared for throughout her life by her immediate family. She was presently living with her 83-year-old sister [1]. Laboratory tests showed serum autoantibodies against thyroglobulin and thyroid microsomes, but the levels of thyroid-stimulating hormone (TSH) and thyroxine (T_4) were within normal ranges. The electrocardiogram showed complete heart block with a ventricular rate of 40 beats per minute. Other laboratory test results were within the normal range. Her presenting sign was gradual deterioration in her mobility and activity over several months.

The life expectancy of infants born with Down syndrome has improved from 40% of the children still alive at 5 years in 1955 [2] to 90% alive at 5 years today [3]. As a direct consequence of the lengthening life span of individuals with Down syndrome, there is an anticipated increase in the number of adults with Down syndrome [4].

The 75-year-old woman with Down syndrome is one of the oldest patients recorded in the medical literature. She has a mosaic form of the chromosomal syndrome and also is atypical because she was not institutionalized as were many of her peers. Today, the population of adults with Down syndrome mostly consists of two groups. The young adults are the first representatives of a cohort of home-reared well-cared-for generation; the older adults usually were institutionalized and have since been deinstitutionalized in many cases to live in community-based group homes. Although all these persons share the direct genetic effect of extra chromosomal material from the twenty-first chromosome, they are dissimilar in many ways—almost like two separate populations.

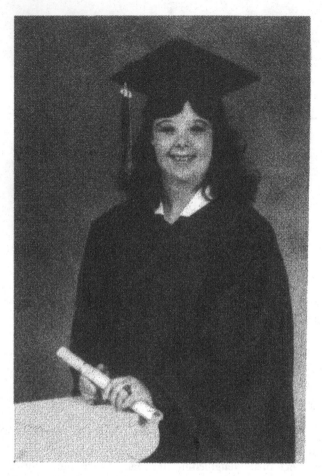

Figure 7.1 Good education is the structure underpinning a successful adult life.

These two contrasting groups of adults are visible evidence that the effect of institutionalization compounds and worsens the effect of the trisomy 21 on the individual.

Adults with Down syndrome, particularly those who live in community-based group homes, need a primary care physician to care for them and to be part of their network of support services, which includes case management, workshops, day programs, and family support services.

Adults with Down syndrome can have complicated medical problems and may require more visits to the physician than non–Down syndrome individuals

[5]. The limited ability of these adults to convey their symptoms and history makes the availability of good medical records a priority in their medical care. On the first visit, extra time may be needed to review records before actually seeing the patient. It is also good to spend a little extra time interacting with the person, reducing his or her anxiety about the visit. Sometimes there are so many problems, it is necessary to focus one's attention on the more serious ones.

MEDICAL CONCERNS IN ADULTS

Cardiac Disease

Heart disease is a major concern throughout the lifetime of a person with Down syndrome. Forty percent of children with Down syndrome have congenital heart disease, with ventral septal defect and atrioventricular canal the most frequent problems. Because many children with Down syndrome and congenital heart disease are receiving treatment and living to the adult years, many may require ongoing special monitoring.

The following are some general guidelines for the physician managing adults:

1. For the adult with no history or symptoms of heart disease, assess cardiac status annually with an electrocardiogram to check for signs of heart failure, and auscultate for changes in heart sounds.
2. For the adult with previously identified heart disease and who has not seen a cardiologist for a long time, a chest radiograph may be indicated to monitor heart size. Because of the complexity of congenital heart disease, a cardiologist should be involved in management.

Persons without congenital cardiac disease may acquire cardiac problems in adulthood. Mitral valve prolapse is seen in about half of the adults with Down syndrome [6] and can be associated with serious complications, such as infective endocarditis and cerebral emboli. Typical ausculatory findings are a midsystolic click and a late systolic murmur that shifts with changes in body position. The diagnosis can be confirmed by a two-dimensional echocardiogram in the parasternal long-axis view [7] (Fig. 7.2). Antibiotic prophylaxis for invasive procedures is indicated for persons with mitral valve prolapse and mitral regurgitation.

In addition to the congenital aspect of cardiac disease in individuals with Down syndrome, there also is laboratory evidence of an increased risk for arteriosclerotic changes that can affect the heart. In studies encompassing both home-reared and institutionalized persons with Down syndrome, total choles-

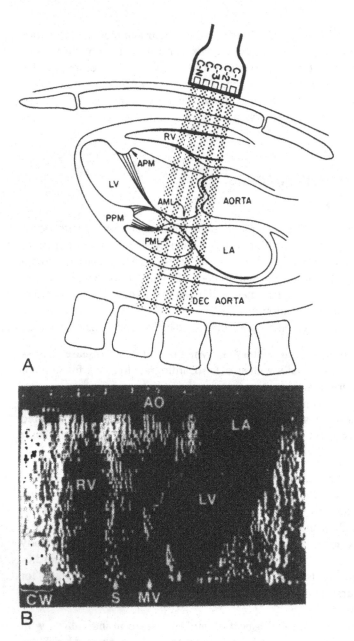

Figure 7.2 Two-dimensional ultrasonography. A. Diagrammatic representation of examination of the heart. B. Ultrasonogram.

terol levels, cholesterol fractions, and lipoprotein levels were evaluated. Compared to non–Down syndrome individuals, the low-density to high-density lipoprotein ratio was found to be higher in children and adolescents with Down syndrome [8].

Dementia

Dementia, that is, regression in intellect and self-care skills, presents a particular challenge in diagnosis to the physician. In a study of adults with Down syndrome between 35 and 49 years of age, intellectual deterioration was reported to occur in less than one-third [9], so dementia is not inevitable after the age of 35 as was once thought. See Chapter 13 for a review of the literature on this subject.

Early signs of dementia may be subtle and include social withdrawal, apathy, decreased self-care skills, and sleep disturbances. Occasionally, dementia can present dramatically with aggressive or self-injurious behavior. Although Alzheimer's disease is more common in the adult, it is important to diagnose any reversible cause of dementia (see Chapter 13). Obtain older psychometric test scores to compare with recent test scores to document changes in skills. A detailed history and a physical examination are critical to diagnose simple medical problems that can present as a dementia: for example, ear cerumen [10], an abscessed tooth, infection, or a toxic reaction to a drug such as phenobarbital or phenytoin. Appropriate laboratory studies include an audiology evaluation to rule out a hearing loss, thyroid screening to detect hypothyroidism, complete blood count to detect anemia, and electroencephalography to detect a seizure disorder.

After a medical evaluation has shown no definite cause, consider referral for further neurological and psychiatric evaluation. If no other cause can be found, and Alzheimer's disease is diagnosed, it is important for the caretakers to know and understand this diagnosis because it has important implications for future care and community management.

Hypothyroidism

Hypothyroidism can present in adults with weight gain, constipation, sleepiness, or occasional behavior disturbances such as apathy, withdrawal, or refusal to participate in social activities. In the adult age group, thyroid testing includes TSH, T_4, triiodothyronine, and thyroid antibodies due to the increased incidence of autoimmune thyroiditis seen in this patient group. In one study of thyroid status in adults with Down syndrome greater than 40 years of age, the investigators noted that, except for obesity, none of the patients showed any of the clinical signs usually seen in individuals with hypothyroidism [11]. This emphasizes again the importance of routine thyroid laboratory screening in individuals with Down syndrome as discussed in Chapter 12.

Presbyacusis

Up to 78% of patients with Down syndrome leave childhood with some hearing loss [12], and the adult with Down syndrome has an additional aging problem with the auditory system. Virtually every person sooner or later develops a complication of aging that results in hearing loss called presbyacusis. However, in the case of adults with Down syndrome, there can be an early onset of this problem [13]. This needs to be kept in mind when an adult Down syndrome patient presents with apparent inattention or withdrawal.

Routine Health Care Needs

Persons with Down syndrome should have the routine health care similar to that recommended for the general population [14]. Women should have a Pap test done at 20 years of age for 2 consecutive years, then every 3 years if negative. A pelvic examination is indicated every 3 years in women until 40 years of age, then yearly. A baseline mammogram should be obtained in women between 35 and 40 years of age, then yearly after 50 years of age. Men and women greater than 40 years of age require a digital rectal exam, and after 50 years of age, they require a stool guaiac test yearly and a sigmoidoscopy every 3–5 years after two consecutive negative annual examinations. Additional yearly examinations for the adult include: blood pressure, hearing screening, visual acuity, and tonometry.

Persons with Down syndrome present several problems that require special attention. Obesity is a common problem that requires yearly checks on weight (see Chapter 17). Nutrition monitoring is indicated to determine whether that person is avoiding excess calorie intake and is getting appropriate exercise. Persons who have been institutionalized or have close contact with persons who have been in institutions are at high risk for contacting hepatitis B [15,16], tuberculosis, and *Shigella* gastroenteritis.

Immunizations

Adults with Down syndrome still have a relative immunodeficiency that has been present all their life (see Chapter 15). Therefore, they should continue to have immunizations during adult life [17]:

1. Tetanus and diphtheria toxoid every 10 years after primary immunization in childhood

2. Rubella live virus vaccine
3. Measles live virus vaccine
4. Poliovirus

Because of the high rates of respiratory infections in persons with Down syndrome, also consider influenza and pneumococcal vaccines. Hepatitis B vaccine is indicated for individuals with negative screening results.

Occasionally, the immunization history is unknown, especially for those persons who have been institutionalized since early childhood. When no immunization information is available, consider rubella or polio antibody screening to detect immune status.

Musculoskeletal Disorders

The musculoskeletal problems of people with Down syndrome are present in all age groups. Primarily, they are troubled by atlantoaxial instability, instability of the hip joint, patellar instability, pes planus, and metatarsus primus varus. These disorders are discussed in Chapter 11.

Based on serum uric acid levels, a great deal of gouty arthritis would be expected in adults with Down syndrome. Instead, it is rare in this patient group. When gout does occur, the metabolic turnover of purines in adults with Down syndrome was reported to be consistent with the findings in normoexcretory gouty patients [18].

Dental Care

Periodontal disease, common in many people, is a particular problem for adults with Down syndrome. The disease may exist even in early childhood and worsens with age. In one study of patients with an average age in the late 20s, bone loss was found in 60% of the dental sites in adults with Down syndrome compared to 9.3% in adults without Down syndrome [19]. Caries is less of a problem (see Chapter 16).

Reproductive Health Care

Questions about the reproductive health of their offspring with Down syndrome are probably most worrisome to parents but are infrequently asked. In regard to questions about normal physiology, women with Down syndrome demonstrate no difference compared to women of the general population in respect to age of menarche, duration of menses, length of cycle, or presence of premenstrual symptoms [20]. Males are generally considered to be sterile, whereas a number of females have become pregnant [21] (see Chapter 12).

The following summarizes management of the reproductive health problems most frequently asked by parents [22]:

1. Menstrual hygiene management. Menstrual hygiene training can be successful with supportive parents and Down syndrome offspring with developmental skills high enough to complete toilet training. An experienced developmental specialist can provide help if needed by the family.

2. Sexual abuse and unwanted pregnancy prevention. First, sexual counseling of the parents, as well as the person with Down syndrome, is indicated. With the parents, counseling focuses on understanding their child's sexuality and setting reasonable goals for its expression. Counseling for persons with Down syndrome focuses on understanding appropriate social behavior and avoiding situations that could lead to sexual abuse. Second, depro-medroxprogesterone acetate given at 3-month intervals is one possible choice for contraception; even longer term products may soon be available.

3. Indications for hysterectomy. Hysterectomy was traditionally performed for menstrual hygiene and contraception, but now it is difficult to arrange because of laws that require informed consent. It is recommended that the parents are counseled about contraception and menstrual hygiene. The final decision for hysterectomy requires a committee review.

A book that may help physicians, as well as parents, on concerns about reproductive health is *Just Between Us* [23].

The gynecological examination often is indicated for routine Pap testing as well as to investigate menstrual discomfort or heavy menstrual flow. This examination may be difficult to do in some women. The following are some suggested guidelines for the gynecological examination [23]:

1. Females with Down syndrome may have extremely anxious feelings about the gynecological examination because of a general fear of medical procedures often done by persons in white coats using excessive physical force. Clinical staff can prepare the female by using photographs and anatomically correct dolls to demonstrate the procedures of a pelvic exam.

2. It is also very important for the physician to take some time to establish an initial relationship with the woman. Taking time to talk and answer questions helps her to relax before the examination.

3. A shortcut for females who are not sexually active is to do a Pap test with only the fingertip in the pelvis. Another shortcut is to do an abdominal ultrasound to identify pelvic organs without the use of the physician's hand or gynecological speculum.

Many females will be successfully examined after following these guidelines. However, a few may require referral to a special interdisciplinary team for sex counseling as well as gynecological examination.

MANAGEMENT OF PSYCHIATRIC AND BEHAVIOR DISORDERS

Overview

Many adults with Down syndrome are gentle and loving people. However, a minority do have behavior problems. Psychiatric and behavior disorders present quite a challenge to physicians, parents, and other professionals caring for the adult. These disorders are more complex than the medical disorders because less is known about their diagnosis, natural history, and management. Treatment is controversial to many nonmedical people who object to the use of medications to control maladaptive behavior [24]. The following section provides an introduction to management of psychiatric disorders as well as some specific suggestions for psychotropic drug use. The next section will deal with the management of severe behavior problems such as destructive and assaultive behavior.

Definition and Epidemiology

A psychiatric disorder refers to a severe, observable disorder of adaptation and meets the criteria as outlined in the *Diagnostic and Statistical Manual of Mental Disorders*, third edition, revised (*DSM III-R*) [25]. The *DSM III-R* is a publication of the American Psychiatric Association and represents a consensus of diagnostic criteria for psychiatric disorders. About 25% of persons with Down syndrome have a psychiatric disorder, which is generally a lower rate than the prevalence of psychiatric disorders in other persons with mental retardation but normal chromosomes [26]. Common psychiatric diagnoses include: adjustment reaction, hyperactivity, autism, depression/affective disorders, personality disorders, and anxiety disorders. A behavior disorder refers to a maladaptive behavior pattern that does not fit a specific psychiatric disorder. Evaluation and management of behavior disorders will be discussed further in the following section.

Diagnostic Approach

The diagnostic approach to the psychiatric disorders begins with the modification of the *DSM III-R* criteria because they are based on persons with normal intelligence. The reason for this modification is that persons with Down syndrome have characteristics that alter the clinical features of a psychiatric disorder. Four of the most important characteristics that can alter the presentation of a disorder include the following [27]:

1. Concrete thinking and decreased communication skills that limit the ability of the person to report clinical symptoms. For example, the person may not be able to describe hallucinations.
2. Lack of social skills and decreased life experiences that minimize symptoms. For example, the person with mania will not be able to express the grandiosity usually associated with that disorder.
3. A person with Down syndrome may become disorganized under stress. Because of concrete coping skills, stress may result in transient psychotic symptoms. For example, a stressed person may begin to talk frequently about an imaginary friend. Initially, it may appear that this imaginary friend represents a hallucination, whereas it is actually a reaction to a stressful situation.
4. Stress often significantly increases occasional behavior problems. For example, stress may increase temper tantrums in a person, from a usual baseline number of one per month to one per day.

The diagnostic approach to a psychiatric disorder also includes a modification of the way clinical information is collected. Because the person being evaluated may have poor communication skills, it is important to interview all significant people connected with that person. The mental status examination must rely on behavior observations such as the ability to carry out simple tasks and to follow directions and the degree of socialization, gestures, and courtesies [28]. Generally, referral to a psychiatrist experienced in working with persons with Down syndrome is indicated when there is a severe problem or confusion over diagnosis.

The last step in the diagnostic approach is the determination of a specific diagnosis. A specific psychiatric diagnosis is required to select an appropriate therapeutic intervention. Psychotropic drugs are usually part of an intervention program for control of a psychiatric disorder and are often necessary for initial treatment. Newer drugs have been found that are more helpful and will be discussed in the following section.

Psychotropic Medication

Psychotropic drugs such as thioridazine, haloperidol, and chlorpromazine have been traditionally the drugs of choice in treating persons with psychiatric disorders. However, this is changing because of their side effects of sedation, depressed cognitive function, akathisia, extrapyramidal signs, and tardive dyskinesia. The following drugs may be more useful in the person with Down syndrome with a psychiatric disorder [24]:

1. Benzodiazepines, such as diazepam, may be very effective in anxiety disorders. Diazepam is most useful for severe, acute anxiety conditions in which an initial reduction in anxiety helps nonmedical interventions such as counseling and relaxation training.
2. Lithium carbonate or carbamazepine is often helpful for severe, life-long hyperactivity. It is important, however, that behavior management be included in treatment of hyperactivity as well as in using medications.
3. Inderal in high doses occasionally helps in managing persons with assaultive behavior.

Once a drug is selected, it is important to collect some baseline data on the target symptom before starting the drug regimen. Once therapy has begun, it is important to check the frequency of the target behavior to guide drug dosage. Staff can assist in data collection. It is also important to educate the family and staff about the common and significant side effects of the drug used. Once the target symptom has been controlled with the drug for at least 30 days, it is important to begin a medication reduction or removal trial. The reason for the trial is to judge whether any side effects are present as well as to see if the person can be controlled without the medication.

Excessive medication usage is a common problem seen in persons recently discharged from institutions. Often these persons may be on either high doses of an individual psychotropic or multiple medications. It is important to decrease or discontinue these medications because they will not be required once a person is in a supportive environment of the community. However, some persons experience serious withdrawal symptoms after long-term or high-dose use.

When any medication has been used to control a psychiatric disorder, it is important to discontinue it or try a medication-free holiday for the following reasons [29]:

1. There may have been complete remission of the psychiatric disorder. Some psychiatric disorders are episodic or nonrecurring, and the person may be symptom free for months or years.
2. Psychotropic drugs may no longer be required to maintain control of the behavior. Behavior management techniques alone may be enough to control the disorder without medication.
3. Medication withdrawal may be needed to reveal certain side effects of the drug therapy. For example, akathisia refers to excessive involuntary motor restlessness that may be caused by antipsychotic medications. However, it may be mistaken for a symptom of worsening of the psychiatric disorder, and the physician may mistakenly elect to increase

the medication's dosage. When the medication is discontinued, the akathisia decreases.
4. Tardive dyskinesia is another medication-related disorder that can be
    diagnosed after medication reduction. Tardive dyskinesia is a distinct
    involuntary movement disorder caused by permanent brain dysfunc-
    tion. It is characterized by excessive chewing movements, tremors of
    the upper extremities, and slowing of gait. Tardive dyskinesia may
    improve with medication withdrawal but sometimes persists.

Withdrawal reaction refers to a physically and biologically mediated behavior response to discontinuing drug therapy. Such reactions generally develop
after a person receives high doses of a psychotropic medication over a long
period of time. It is best to discontinue medication very slowly, that is, by 10%
decrements of the dosage every 2–4 weeks [29].

Discontinuing antipsychotic drugs, such as chlorpromazine or thioridazine,
may produce an anticholinergic withdrawal reaction characterized by nausea,
vomiting, insomnia, sweating, and diarrhea. Although symptoms are usually
mild, a person will sometimes experience acute distress and may need to be
placed on a low-dose regimen of the medication again. Persons may also
develop behavior disturbances during withdrawal and should be treated with
nondrug methods rather than restarting the medication regimen.

Discontinuing all tricyclic antidepressants may also be associated with an
anticholinergic withdrawal reaction. In addition, a hypomanic reaction to
withdrawal has been described [29].

Withdrawal of antianxiety drugs may be associated with a reaction. Abrupt
withdrawal of such medications as diazepam or librium can result in a life-
threatening reaction if the person has been receiving the medication for a long
time [29]. Early symptoms include agitation, nausea, and vomiting. The reaction can progress to rapid heart rate, hypotension, severe nightmares, seizures,
and cardiovascular collapse. Hospitalization is indicated for treatment.

OFFICE MANAGEMENT OF SPECIFIC PSYCHIATRIC DISORDERS

This section discusses management of some specific psychiatric problems that
are commonly seen by the physician. The focus is on common, mild disorders.

Depression

Depression is a common psychiatric disorder especially in older teenagers and
young adults. A depressed person with Down syndrome may have clinical
features that are different from the normal population with depressive or

affective disorder. The physician must rely on clinical features modified from the criteria for depression listed in the *DSM III-R* for persons with Down syndrome [26]:

1. A disturbance of mood characterized by sadness, withdrawal, or agitation.
2. Any four of the following:
    a. Change in sleep pattern
    b. Change in appetite or weight
    c. Onset or increase in severity of self-injurious behavior
    d. Apathy
    e. Psychomotor retardation
    f. Loss of activity of daily living skills
    g. Spontaneous crying
    h. Fearfulness
    i. Family history for an affective disorder
    j. Any unexplained increase in hostility
    k. Increase in irritability

Interviews with the caretakers are often necessary to obtain information about clinical features needed to make the diagnosis. Inquire about recent losses such as death of a close sibling or parent. Other losses may be a move from home to a community-living facility, a change in workshop location, or loss of a significant friend of the opposite sex. Sometimes a loss may be unapparent. For example, a teenager may feel a great loss as the last younger sibling leaves home for college or when other siblings marry or obtain a driver's license. These events help underscore the restrictions often experienced by a person with mental retardation.

During the interview with a depressed person, look for irritability, withdrawn behavior, or emotional lability. It is also helpful to observe how the person interacts with significant others and to determine whether there has been a change as well. It is important to rule out medical problems that may mimic depressive illness such as hypothyroidism, hearing loss, occult infection, or physical or sexual abuse. A sexually abused female may present clinical signs of depression during a physical examination; bruises on the legs and thighs or a vaginal discharge suggest the primary problem of abuse.

Once the diagnosis is established, treatment with low doses of an antidepressant such as amitriptyline may be indicated plus brief supportive counseling.

Hyperactivity

Hyperactive behavior has been discussed elsewhere in children, but this can also be a common problem in adults. Hyperactivity is actually a symptom characterized by a short attention span, distractibility, impulsivity, and excessive motor activity. Sudden onset of hyperactivity or short attention span may accompany a medical problem such as hyperthyroidism or hearing loss. During the interview with caretakers, it is important to determine whether the hyperactivity is situational, that is, related to specific situations or places. Hyperactivity in all situations and activities suggests a medical problem.

After medical problems and psychiatric disorders are ruled out, treatment might first involve a behavior management program. Medications such as methylphenidate and pemoline generally are not helpful. Carbamazepine or lithium carbonate may sometimes help in combination with a behavior management program to control excessive hyperactivity.

Adjustment Disorders

Adjustment disorders are also commonly seen in adolescents and young adults. The most important clinical feature of an adjustment disorder is a severe reaction to a stress that interferes with interaction with other people or with work productivity. Common symptoms include increased temper tantrums and withdrawn or tearful behavior after a major change in a person's daily routine, such as a move to a new living facility. Management is usually successful with supportive counseling. Occasionally, short-term antianxiety medications may be a helpful adjunct to the counseling.

MANAGEMENT OF BEHAVIOR DISORDERS

Although psychiatric disorders are frequently treated with medications, often the physician will evaluate persons with behavior disorders for the possible use of medications to control behavior. A behavior disorder is defined as a pattern of functioning that is maladaptive or disruptive [30]. Although psychiatric disorders represent an underlying biological abnormality, the behavior disorder can be a response to a situational or environmental change. Behavior disorders can be classified as mild, for example, temper tantrums or obstinate behavior, or moderate to severe, for example, violent or self-injurious behavior. The prevalence rate for behavior disorders in persons with Down syndrome is estimated to be 38.6% and is lower than the rate found in other adults with mental retardation [26]. Behavior management techniques are indicated for treatment, whereas psychotropic medication is reserved for the patient who does not respond to behavior modification and for whom the behavior is dangerous to that person or others. The next section discusses interventions for some general behavior disorders and then for some specific behavior disorders.

Behavior Management Principles

Behavior management is based on the principle that all behavior is a response to a stimulus coming from the environment. A reinforcer is an event or object that promotes the frequency of response of that behavior [30]. A reinforcer may be positive, for example, a reward such as food or attention, or negative or aversive, for example, a verbal reprimand. Usually, only positive reinforcement programs are used with persons with behavior problems. Often a behavior problem is due to a communication or social deficit. For example, a temper tantrum may be a way of expressing dislike of a food or a way of avoiding an unpleasant task or situation. A behavior management program uses positive reinforcers to control the temper tantrum while devising ways for the person to increase communication skills and express dislike for certain foods in an acceptable way.

The first step in implementing a behavior management program is to identify a target behavior problem. It must be an important problem for all people involved, and it must interfere with the person's work or social interactions. Eccentric behavior, for example, wearing a certain hat, should be respected and not made a target behavior for an intensive, behavior management program. The problem behavior must be defined in objective, behavioral terms, and it should be defined in terms so that all caretakers can recognize the problem and count its occurrence.

The second step in a behavior management program is to make sure that the person is in a safe and supportive environment [31]. Questions to ask include: Is the home and workshop safe? Are social and recreational opportunities available? Are environmental demands appropriate for the person's developmental level?

The third step is the collection of appropriate data about the occurrence of that behavior. It is important to collect data about the behavior for 2–3 weeks and to record the following: (1) situations where the problem arises, (2) situations where the problem does not arise, (3) antecedents and consequences of that behavior, and (4) the person's overall developmental abilities: intellectual, social, and communicative.

The fourth step is a functional analysis of the data. The objective is to identify a behavior determinant that promotes the problem behavior. A hypothesis is made about what are the main or key determinants of the problem behavior. The behavior determinants are important to identify so that they can be controlled in a behavior management program.

The fifth step involves setting up an intervention strategy to decrease the frequency of the problem behavior. A positive reinforcer is identified that will appeal to the person with the behavior problem. In addition, a program is initiated to deal with any underlying problems that may help promote the problem behavior, for example, a communication deficit that causes a temper tantrum problem. For the person who uses a temper tantrum to express a dislike for a certain food, a behavior management program includes communication and social skills training. The goal of this training is to improve social interaction skills so that the person will not require maladaptive behaviors to express his or her needs. In addition, a positive reinforcer is introduced every time the appropriate behavior is used, for example, a reward with the person's favorite food.

The last step is maintenance of the acceptable behavior. Occasionally, the procedure may need to be used for a long time before the newly acquired skill is sufficient to meet the person's needs.

Failure of a behavior management program may be due to several reasons: (1) an overlooked medical problem that causes the problem behavior, (2) a reinforcer that is not reinforcing to the person with the behavior problem, (3) a reinforcer that is not applied frequently enough, and (4) an incorrect functional analysis or hypothesis about the cause of the problem behavior.

For long-term behavior disorders, another step may be added to the behavior management program: a consequence or punishment for the problem behavior. This may be a verbal reprimand at the occurrence of the behavior, a loss of some object or privilege, or time out, that is, placement away from the area to a nonstimulating area. Punishment must not be the only way to deal with problem behaviors but may be part of a comprehensive behavior management plan. Punishment alone only suppresses, and does not eliminate, a behavior problem. Negative reinforcement must never consist of physically hitting the patient or administering any kind of extreme discomfort or humiliation to the person with Down syndrome.

Management of Some Mild Behavior Disorders

The following are some suggestions for dealing with mild behavior disorders [24]:

1. Stereotypic mannerisms, such as body rocking or repetitive finger movements, often respond to increasing social and recreational activities. Often training is needed to teach leisure or recreational skills to a person with deficits in these areas.

2. For pica behavior (that is, eating inedible objects, such as toys or clothing), improve supervision and limit access to items likely to be ingested. Provide appropriate, accepted items or activities for oral stimulation such as gum, popcorn, and tooth brushing.

3. Temper tantrums can be controlled by modifying activities that are

associated with tantrums. For example, a person may respond with a temper tantrum when asked to do a task that is too complex or not understood. Management consists of modifying the task so that it is understood and appropriate for the person's developmental level. When temper tantrums are used to avoid tasks or situations, use ignoring or time out.

4. Occasional mild hyperactivity, that is, excessive running and jumping, can be controlled by increasing opportunities for physical activities. Other suggestions include time out, ignoring, or relaxation training.

5. Inappropriate verbal behavior refers to loud speech, loud noises, whining, and cursing that can be controlled with ignoring, time out, or reinforcing appropriate verbal responses. Teach appropriate situations for loud verbal responses. For example, loud verbal responses may be acceptable at a football game but not at the workshop. Check auditory acuity.

Management of Severe Behavior Disorders

The physician may occasionally care for a person with severe behaviors such as property destruction, violence, or self-injury. Severe behavior disorders require management by an experienced interdisciplinary team consisting of a behavior psychologist, social worker, psychiatrist, and other intervention specialist. The physician will be working with this team of professionals on a behavior management program that will be developed across all the person living areas: home, workshop, transport bus, and so on.

As part of a team, the physician has several important duties when managing a person with a severe problem:

1. Rule out or treat any underlying medical problems such as hearing loss, occult infection, or hyperthyroidism.
2. Evaluate for underlying neurological problems such as partial complex seizure disorder.
3. Evaluate for a possible medication-induced aggression. Antipsychotic drugs can cause akathisia and can result in hitting out. Anticonvulsants such as phenobarbital are often associated with behavior problems and can often be replaced with newer anticonvulsants such as carbamazepine or valproic acid. Occasionally, diazepam can cause a state of disinhibition leading to assaultive behavior.
4. Consider medications only as part of an overall intervention strategy. Medications should not be the sole method of control. As an alternative to the antipsychotics, consider a trial of a short-acting benzodiazepine such as Ativan. Other drugs that have been shown to help control severe behavior problems in a few published case reports include propranolol, lithium, and carbamazepine.

Mild psychiatric and behavior problems may be challenging, but most can be managed by the physician in one or two office visits. For problems that do not improve after two office visits, refer the person to a behavior management specialist for further assessment and treatment. All severe behavior and psychiatric disorders need an experienced interdisciplinary team for management. To locate specialists in your area, contact a behavior psychologist for suggestions on referrals. Other resources for names of specialists include the local Association for Retarded Citizens or the National Down Syndrome Congress. Both keep lists of local resource people.

SUPPORT FOR THE FAMILY

Although families and persons with Down syndrome come to the family physician for medical evaluation and treatment, they often have greater concerns about appropriate workshop or employee experience, a lack of appropriate support services, need for respite care assistance, and so on. Although the physician may not have answers for these nonmedical questions, it is helpful to know about appropriate resources to refer the family. This section briefly discusses some of the resources available to enhance community living, work, and family support.

Vocational Opportunities

In most communities, adults with Down syndrome have the opportunity to work. This may be with a regular employer who makes some adaptations on the job such as decreased work hours or increased supervision. This type of employment experience is called supported or semi-independent work placement, and salary is usually at the minimum wage. Sometimes a special coach is used while the person learns the required job skills. Another employment experience is the sheltered workshop where a person may do simple tasks such as assembling small piece work. The sheltered workshop offers closer supervision and can also provide further educational and prevocational training. Earnings depend on the type of placement and productivity, but a worker with Down syndrome can average close to $360 per year (in 1986 U.S. dollars) according to one survey of persons with Down syndrome in a county-run sheltered workshop [32]. The wide range of yearly earnings, from $76.55 to $910.98, reflects the variation in productivity as well as skills attained by an adult.

Early vocational planning is very important to provide appropriate preparation for adult employment. Vocational planning begins in midadolescence and should include educational personnel, the parents, the person with Down syndrome, as well as the physician. The physician's role includes the following [33]:

1. Diagnosis and management of medical problems
2. Education and counseling of parents
3. Advocacy for the person with Down syndrome

Important medical problems that can affect vocational plans include the following: vision impairment, hearing loss, seizures, communication disorders, and motor disabilities. All problems that can be corrected should be before formal vocational and prevocational evaluations. The physician also plays an important role in communicating to the family and vocational evaluator any medical problem that can affect vocational goals.

The family has the most important role in their teenager's eventual success in employment. The family provides the key support and advocacy that make the vocational plan successful. The physician can assist by discussing with the family their goals and by ensuring that the goals are appropriate for their teenager's developmental level. The physician can also direct the family to prevocational and vocational services in the community.

Finally, the physician can advocate for persons with Down syndrome in the community. This will include advocating for appropriate vocational opportunities and will encourage an educational program that helps each person reach his or her full potential.

Community Living Facilities

The physician also can be very helpful to the family when they consider a community-living facility for their child who now is a young adult. More community-living options have resulted from the deinstitutionalization movement. The physician can help the family by discussing this option and deciding whether it is appropriate for the family's adolescent or young adult. Many communities offer several types of living facilities:

1. A group home is a regular residence that may house 2–10 persons with developmental disabilities. The house structure usually needs to be modified to meet local regulations and license requirements, such as the addition of emergency exit signs, smoke detectors, and so on. Supervision and care provided may range greatly. In some group living facilities, care may be limited to minimal help with self-care activities such as dressing, toileting, and feeding. Other group care facilities may offer extensive care for persons with severe deficits in self-care skills.

2. Semi-independent living programs provide a person his or her own

living facility with staff nearby for assistance. Often help is required for shopping, budgeting, transportation, and use of banking facilities. This arrangement is best for a person with independent self-care skills.

3.   Nursing homes provide full-time nursing services and are needed by persons with severe, chronic medical problems.

4.   Foster homes provide care in a regular family and home.

5.   Specialized foster and treatment group homes provide specialized care for persons with severe behavior or medical problems.

Public or tax supported community-living facilities often have a long waiting list for entrance. It is important to have the family start planning for group placement several years in advance of the time it will be needed. Guide the family to appropriate local resources so that they can decide if a community-living facility is appropriate for them and their adult child. In the United States, the Association for Retarded Citizens or the National Down Syndrome Congress can supply a list of local agencies involved with the management of a community-living facility in your community.

Some families may find it difficult to place their grown child out of the home. Although community living may not be an acceptable alternative for all families, it is important that all families explore this option. For some families, community placement may suddenly become a necessity because of severe health problems or death of the parents or caretakers. Suggest that the family visit some of the group homes or other facilities available in the community. The family may also benefit from talking to another family who has placed their child in a community facility and has learned first hand some of the pros and cons of group homes.

Help educate the family by having them obtain reading material locally through community agencies such as the Association for Retarded Citizens or nationally through the National Down Syndrome Congress. Guide families in what to look for when they visit group homes or other facilities. Help them prepare a list of questions to ask the group home or facility manager:

1.   How are staff trained? What do they do to update their skills?
2.   How is medical care provided? What arrangements are made for emergency care? Are nursing and nutritional services available?
3.   What specialized services are available such as physical therapy, speech therapy, or other habilitation services?
4.   What leisure time and recreational opportunities are made available?
5.   What kind of medical problems and behavior disorders are present in the other persons living in the group facility? At what developmental level are they?

6. How close to a true home environment is provided? Are the residents all responsible for chores and activities in the group facility?

Deciding about community placement is difficult for families. The physician's important role is to aid the family by listening to their plans and guiding them to appropriate resources when the family is perplexed. Because he or she has often known the family and the grown child for a long time, the physician may be the first person to whom the family will turn to for assistance. It is known that the quality of life in adults is determined by their early educational opportunities and living conditions. Home-raised individuals with Down syndrome do better in adult life—whether they continue to stay at home or go into an institution as an adult [34]. In comparison with adults with many other kinds of mental retardation, those with Down syndrome are reported to be more socially interested and active [34].

DOWN SYNDROME PREVENTIVE MEDICINE CHECKLIST: ADULT*

A. Recommendations for routine medical care

1. Pap test at 20 years of age and then annually for 2 years. If negative, then every 3 years.
2. Baseline mammogram between 35 and 40 years of age, and then annually
3. Digital rectal examination for men and women more than 40 years of age
4. After 50 years of age, a stool guaiac examination for men and women annually. A sigmoidoscopy every 3–5 years after two consecutive negative examinations
5. Annual physical examination to include blood pressure, vision, hearing, and tonometry screening

B. Special medical concerns

1. Monitor exercise and caloric intake to prevent obesity.
2. Obtain a cervical spine radiograph in flexion, neutral, and extension views at 18 and 30 years of age.
3. Evaluate thyroid-stimulating hormone (TSH) and thyroxine T_4 levels annually.

---

*Lentz G. Down syndrome preventive medicine checklist. Down Syndrome Papers and Abstracts for Professionals 1989;12:1–9.

4. When clinically indicated, screen for hepatitis, tuberculosis, and infectious gastroenteritis.
5. Review immunization history to ensure completeness.
6. Obtain an echocardiogram, when clinically indicated, to rule out mitral valve prolapse.

C. Support for the family

1. Review family's vocational plans.
2. Review family's plans for possible community living when their child is an adult.
3. Review family's estate and insurance planning.

REFERENCES

1. Demisse A, Ayres RC, Briggs R. Old age in Down's syndrome. J R Soc Med 1988;81:740.
2. Record RG, Smith A. Incidence, mortality and sex distribution of mongoloid defectives. Br J Prev Soc Med 1955;9:10–15.
3. Bell JA, Pearn JH, Firman D. Childhood deaths in Down's syndrome: Survival curves and causes of death from a total population study in Queensland, Australia, 1976 to 1985. J Med Genet 1989;26:764–768.
4. Editorial. Declining mortality from Down syndrome—no cause for complacency. Lancet 1990;i:888–889.
5. Goldstein H. Utilization of health services over a one year period by an adult population with Down syndrome. Dan Med Bull 1988;35:100–104.
6. Goldhar S, Brown WD, St John M. High frequency of mitral valve prolapse and aortic regurgitation among asymptomatic adults with Down syndrome. JAMA 1987;258:1793–1795.
7. Devereux R. Diagnosis and prognosis of mitral valve prolapse. N Engl J Med 1989;320:1077–1079.
8. Tolksdorf M. Clinical aspects of Down's syndrome from infancy to adult life. In: Trisomy 21: An International Symposium. Berlin: Springer-Verlag, 1981.
9. Fenner ME, Hewitt KE, Torpy DM. Down's syndrome: Intellectual and behavioral functioning during adulthood. J Ment Defic Res 1987;31:241–249.
10. Myers B, Pueschel SM. Pseudodementia in the mentally retarded. Clin Pediatr 1987;26:275–277.
11. Dinani S, Carpenter S. Down's syndrome and thyroid disorder. J Ment Defic Res 1990;34:187–193.
12. Balkany TJ, Downs MP, Jafek BW, Krajicek MJ. Hearing loss in Down's syndrome: A treatable handicap more common than generally recognized. Clin Pediatr 1979;18:116–118.

13. Buchanan LH. Early onset of presbyacusis in Down syndrome. Scand Audiol 1990;19:103–110.
14. Caldroney RD. The periodic health examination. Hosp Pract 1987;22:189–236.
15. Breuer B. Transmission of hepatitis B virus to classroom contacts of mentally retarded carriers. JAMA 1985;254:3190–3194.
16. Troisi CL, Heiberg DA, Hollinge FB. Normal immune responses to hepatitis B vaccine in patients with Down's syndrome. JAMA 1985;254:3194–3199.
17. Fedson DS. Adult immunization: Protocols and problems. Hosp Pract 1987; 22:143–158.
18. Ciompi ML, Bazzichi LM, Bertolucci D, Mazzoni MR, Mencacci S, Macchia D, Mariani G. Uric acid metabolism in two patients with coexistent Down's syndrome and gout. Clin Rheumatol 1984;3:229–233.
19. Barnett ML, Press KP, Friedman D, Sonnenberg EM. The prevalence of peridontitis and dental caries in a Down's syndrome population. J Peridontol 1986; 57:288–293.
20. Goldstein H. Menarche, menstruation, and sexual relations and contraception of adolescent females with Down syndrome. Eur J Obstet Gynecol Reprod Biol 1988; 27:343–349.
21. Scola PS. Genitourinary system. In: Pueschel SM, Rynders JE, eds. Down Syndrome: Advances in Biomedicine and the Behavioral Sciences. Cambridge, Mass: Academic Guild Publishers, 1982:210–212.
22. Elkins TE, Gafford LS, Wilks CS, Muram D, Golden G. A model clinic approach to the reproductive health concerns of the mentally handicapped. Obstet Gynecol 1986;68:185–188.
23. Edwards JP, Elkins TE. Just Between Us: A Social Sexual Training Guide for Parents and Professionals Who Have Concerns for Persons with Retardation. Portland, Ore: Ednick Communications, 1988.
24. Sovner R. Psychotropic drug therapy: An overview. Psychiatr Aspects Ment Retard Newsletter, 1983;2:17–20.
25. American Psychiatric Association. Diagnostic and Statistical Manual of Mental Disorders, 3rd ed, rev. Washington, DC: American Psychiatric Association, 1987.
26. Lund J. Psychiatric aspects of Down syndrome. Acta Psychiatr Scand 1988; 78:369–374.
27. Sovner R. Limiting factors in the use of DSM-III criteria with mentally ill/mentally retarded persons. Psychopharmacol Bull 1986;22:1055–1059.
28. Kuehn J. Mental health consultation of the dual diagnosed individual. Personal communication, 1987.
29. Sovner R. Discontinuing psychotropic drug therapy: Rationale, guidelines, and side-effects. Psychiatr Aspects Ment Retard Rev 1984;3:41–44.
30. Sovner R. Behavior modification IV: Positive reinforcement. Psychiatr Aspects Ment Retard 5:57–62.
31. Flavell JE. Severe behavior disorders: An overview. Presented at a National Seminar on Down Syndrome. November 1987, Akron, Ohio.

32. Rogers PT. Special communication, 1986.
33. Committee on Children with Disabilities. Role of the pediatrician in prevocational education of children and adolescents with developmental disabilities. Pediatrics 1986;78:529–530.
34. Schroeder-Kurth TM, Schaffert G, Koeckritz W, Kernich M. Quality of life of adults with trisomy 21 living in mental retardation homes compared with those staying under parental care. Am J Med Genet 1990;(suppl 7):317–321.

III

WHAT WE KNOW ABOUT PREVENTIVE MEDICAL CARE

8

The Ears

Perhaps there is no more important job for the physician of a child with Down syndrome than protecting the child's auditory apparatus. Optimal care of the ear not only is related to a decrease of medical problems but also can be a factor in the development of the eventual speech patterns of the child [1]. Of even greater import is the suggestion of a few studies indicating that there may be a relationship between disease of the auditory system and later intelligence quotient (IQ) testing of the child [2].

To preserve the individual's cognitive function at the highest possible level is particularly important in the care of children with any form of mental retardation. In the case of the child with Down syndrome, the physician possibly may have the opportunity to actively contribute to the process of cognitive development by assiduously protecting the language input system of this child. It has been shown that the prevalence of auditory abnormalities—as judged by hearing examinations, otoscopic studies, and impedance testing—are higher in children with Down syndrome than in a comparable group of mentally retarded children matched for chronological age (CA) and IQ [3]. Realistically, it is difficult for all auditory abnormalities in children with Down syndrome to be overcome by modern medicine, but major protections of this vital system are possible and efficacious.

In an important and comprehensive recent study of the common medical problems found in children with Down syndrome, hearing losses were documented in a significant number, even though the investigators noted that 25% of the children had no previous history of a known ear infection or prior audiological examination [4]. They recommended that audiological evaluations should be routine even in the absence of clinically apparent ear infections.

Thus, regular auditory evaluation may be the ideal preventive medical approach for a child with Down syndrome instead of waiting for a clinical presentation, such as an episode of otitis media. The decisions about the frequency and type of such evaluations depend on the circumstance of the individual child and the judgment of the physician. Some general guidelines are found in the age recommendations of the preventive medicine checklists (found at the end of Chapters 3–7).

THE EAR AT RISK

Eleven otological problem areas in the anatomy of the ear in patients with Down syndrome have been identified (see Fig. 8.1).

The External Ear

Problem Area One

The longitudinal dimension of the pinna is usually more than two standard deviations below that of other children with normal chromosomes. Maldevelopment of the external ear is one of the diagnostic signs that has been used in early diagnosis of the syndrome. In his 1964 study, Hall published several pages of photographs of the ears of newborns with Down syndrome to help the clinician [5]. In particular, the longitudinal dimension, measured at the greatest vertical axis, has been reported as the most deviant of any anthropomorphic measurement in this patient group [6] and so diagnostic that any newborn with ears less than 3.4 cm should be investigated for the possibility of the syndrome [7]. Although this last study may overstate the issue, the mean longitudinal dimension in newborns with Down syndrome is, in fact, 3.0 cm compared to a mean of 3.6 cm in the normal newborn in a study from the United States [7]. With regard to the child, the actual appearance of the external ear is a minor inconvenience, but what this measurement may presage about the size and malformation of the middle and inner ears has greater clinical relevance.

Problem Area Two

The diameter of the external auditory meatus may be more than two standard deviations below that of age-matched controls and can be narrow to the point of actually being stenotic. Particularly in the newborn period, the finding of an external auditory canal so very tiny and sometimes stenotic prevents adequate

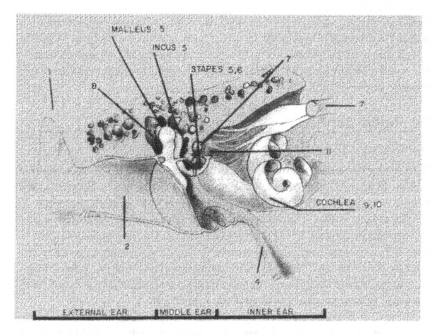

Figure 8.1 The three parts of the ear—external, middle, and inner.

inspection of the tympanic membrane. In one study, up to 80% of Down syndrome individuals had small external auditory canals, whereas 39% had some degree of stenosis [8]. Other studies have confirmed these findings [9]. Excessive accumulation of cerumen sometimes resulting in impaction has also been associated with documented hearing losses [3].

In some medical centers, a special very small otoscopic tool is on hand for the use with neonates with Down syndrome before their discharge from the hospital. This is an important part of the preventive medical care of these infants because middle ear disease can start in the first week of life in some of these neonates [10]. Such a child might later speak incorrectly and pronounce words imperfectly if language is heard from the very beginning through the distortions mediated by middle ear effusions and infections. There is a great deal of focus in the literature (well summarized by Borghi) [11] on speech difficulties being primarily related to structural problems, that is, short palate and large and hypotonic tongue. Relevant as these structural problems are to the speech therapist struggling with poor pronunciation in children who already are speaking, in any individual child they may be only one component of a multifaceted language disability. In some cases, part of the problem might be preventable by sophisticated auditory care before the child says an understandable word. The tiny auditory meatus in a Down syndrome infant is no surprise; it should not stand in the way of adequate otological care.

The Middle Ear

Problem Area Three

There is an increased incidence of upper respiratory infections often associated with an increased incidence of acute or chronic otitis media both with and without middle ear effusions. Abnormal immune mechanisms (discussed in Chapter 15) play a part in the tendency toward upper respiratory infections well documented in children with Down syndrome [8]. Sinusitis and rhinorrhea—sometimes purulent—are not uncommon. Often they are nothing more than a nuisance to the patient. However, developing simultaneously with these clinically more visible infections in many children are the less visible but more damaging infections and effusions of the middle ear.

Middle ear diseases including effusions and otitis media unfortunately are quite common in children with Down syndrome. A study in 1978 of children with Down syndrome in institutions found that 59% had at least a unilateral middle ear effusion at the time of the study [9]. In the patients with stenosis of the external auditory canals—that is, those in whom it was most difficult to visualize the tympanic membrane and make a diagnosis of middle ear disease—the incidence was 80%. An outpatient study revealed that one out of every four of the children studied had a middle ear effusion at the time of the study [12]. Sixty percent of these children living at home and with active disease were being treated surgically with myringotomies and tympanostomy tubes, whereas 40% were treated medically. Myringotomies and tubes often are successful in cases of serous otitis media, but it is estimated that one out of every seven patients with this approach still has reoccurrences [13]. If these reoccurrences are associated with proven hearing loss, the use of a hearing aid should be considered [14].

The importance of accurate diagnostic testing followed by rapid and adequate attempts at therapy cannot be overestimated when the long-term consequences of neglect or inadequate trials of therapy are considered [15]. Good care of the auditory system is one of the areas in which the physician can make a significant contribution to the level of language functioning of an individual with Down syndrome.

Problem Area Four

Brachycephaly and hypotonia in children with Down syndrome are associated with an abnormal vector pull of the tensor veli palatini muscle, which contributes to Eustachean tube dysfunction and leads to an increased prevalence of middle ear effusions. An interesting hypothesis discussed by Schwartz and Schwartz postulates that partial occlusion of the Eustachean tube due to the location and muscle tone of the tensor veli palatini muscle may contribute to inadequate drainage of the middle ear, helping set the stage for effusion and infection [9].

Problem Area Five

The bones of the middle ear—the incus, malleus, or stapes—transmit the sound and may be malformed, either congenitally or because of multiple episodes of otitis media [16]. Deformed or malformed bones of the middle ear have been documented in patients with Down syndrome [14]. As a general rule, the stapes deformities often appear to be congenital, whereas those of the malleus and incus appear to result primarily from inflammation. Malformed or eroded mallei were found in 12 cases of recurrent otitis media and were fused to the incus in one case. In the same study, the incus, mainly the long process, was eroded or malformed in 8 of 12 cases of chronic otitis media [14].

Problem Area Six

There may be permanent fixation of the stapes [16,17]. Malformation of the stapes was found in 7 of 12 cases of chronic otitis media and in all four ears examined for unexplained hearing loss [14]. In three of the four cases, the stapes was affixed by bone to the oval window.

Problem Area Seven

Hypoplasia of the facial nerve that transverses the ear or dehiscence of the facial canal has been described [16,18]. The bony fallopian canal and the facial nerve canal can be dehiscent. The risk of facial nerve injury seems to be increased in middle ear surgery in these patients [14].

Problem Area Eight

The epithelium of the middle ear may be roughened or abnormal because of functional vitamin A deficiency, increasing the chances of chronic effusion. The question of whether there is any absolute or relative vitamin A deficiency in children with Down syndrome is reviewed elsewhere (see Chapter 10). However, if these studies are correct in suggesting that vitamin A deficiency can be a problem in some members of this patient group [19], the effect on the epithelium of the middle ear in the children who actually had such a deficiency would be undesirable.

The Inner Ear

Problem Area Nine

The cochlear spirals are shorter than in controls. Several investigators have described the length of the cochlear spirals as shorter than normal [16,20]. This in itself may have a distorting effect on auditory input. The widths of the coils and other supporting structures appear to be normal.

Problem Area Ten

Vestibular systems and the utriculoendolymphatic valve may be malformed with associated endolymphatic hydrops present. Structural abnormalities of the vestibular system are seen in some patients [20,21]. Smallness of the structures and actual malformations have been described. Endolymphatic hydrops may be present.

Problem Area Eleven

There may be increased pressure in the inner ear because of obliteration of the round window membrane by fibrous tissue [21].

HEARING LOSSES

When an individual is classified as mentally retarded, problems with speech development and pronunciation often are attributed solely to developmental problems in the cognitive area. This was the fate of many children with Down syndrome in past generations.

It is now clear that a compromised auditory system is one factor in the speech and language difficulties of many of these children. In 1972, an article was published describing an abnormality of hearing in 73% [22]. In 1979, Downs and Balkany reported that 64% of all individuals with Down syndrome had a binaural hearing loss and that another 14% had a monaural loss; this makes a total of 78% [14]. Similar figures were found in a study limited to adults in which 50–74% were described with some degree of hearing impairment [23].

Thus, it is clear that the majority of individuals with Down syndrome have impaired hearing. Part of this hearing loss may be due to the effects of chronic effusions and infections of the middle ear—an area where modern preventive medical techniques may salvage additional decibels of hearing. As early as 1969, the relationship of chronic otitis media on language and speech development was under investigation for all pediatric patients [24]. Surely, there is no child who needs the benefit of extra care given to the auditory system more than the youngster with Down syndrome who is already struggling with other handicapping conditions affecting speech and language.

EVALUATION AND TREATMENT

Evaluation may include auditory procedures such as impedance tests and electrophysiological studies. The auditory brain stem evoked response (ABER) is a hearing test checking the auditory system as sound is processed from outside the ear, through the three parts of the ear, through the auditory nerve, and into the brain stem. It evaluates the first 7 milliseconds of sound processing. In patients with Down syndrome, the interpeak intervals I–II and III–IV are reported to be relatively reduced, and the interpeak interval IV–V is prolonged [25]. If the patient with Down syndrome has a high-frequency hearing loss, the latency–intensity function of wave V may be steeper, and its amplitude may be reduced [26].

Treatment programs are based on careful monitoring of the child's auditory function. The hearing should be monitored, beginning before 6 months of age and continuing every 3 months until 3 years of age; every 6 months after that until 8 years of age; and yearly thereafter [27]. Physicians should work closely with speech pathologists and audiologists in carrying out habilitative programs and medical treatment. Appropriate antibiotics, myringotomies, and tympanostomy tubes are mainstays of treatment. However, Downs and Balkany say "one must recognize the peculiar nature of ear disease in these children which seldom results in a permanent cure following medical or surgical treatment" [14].

Special auditory amplification techniques may be needed in addition to ensure the success of language stimulation programs. Hearing aids should not necessarily be limited to the severely and profoundly deaf children with Down syndrome but should include other children with proven amounts of hearing loss. Ideally, the team of a child with Down syndrome should include an otolaryngologist, an audiologist, and a speech pathologist.

If there is any chance that decreasing effusions in the middle ear by medical and surgical means plus amplification if indicated can enhance the transmission of the sounds of human language, the application of such methods is preventive medicine in the very best meaning of that term.

REFERENCES

1. Northern JL, ed. Seminars in Speech, Language, Hearing. New York: Thieme-Stratton, 1980.

2. Libb JW, Dahle A, Smith K, McCollister FP, McLain C. Hearing disorder and cognitive function of individuals with Down syndrome. Am J Ment Defic 1985; 90:353–356.
3. Dahle AJ, McCollister FP. Hearing and otologic disorders in children with Down syndrome. Am J Ment Defic 1986;90:636–642.
4. Van Dyke DC, Lang DL, Miller JD, et al. Common medical problems. In: Van Dyke DC, Lang DJ, Heide F, van Duyne S, Soucek MJ, eds. Clinical Perspectives in the Management of Down Syndrome. New York: Springer-Verlag, 1990:3–14.
5. Hall B. Mongolism in newborns. Acta Paediatr Suppl 1964;154:30–31.
6. Thelander HE, Pryor HB. Abnormal patterns of growth and development in mongolism: An anthropometric study. Clin Pediatr 1966;5:493.
7. Aase JM, Wilson AC, Smith DW. Small ears in Down's syndrome: A helpful diagnostic aid. J Pediatr 1973;82:845–847.
8. Strome M. Down's syndrome: A modern otorhinolaryngological perspective. Laryngoscope 1981;91:1581–1594.
9. Schwartz DM, Schwartz RH. Acoustic impedance and otoscopic findings in young children with Down's syndrome. Arch Otolaryngol 1978;104:652–656.
10. Balkany TJ, Berman SA, Simons MA, et al. Middle ear effusions in neonates. Laryngoscope 1978;88:398–405.
11. Borghi RW. Consonant phoneme and distinctive feature error patterns in speech. In: Van Dyke DC, Lang DL, Heide F, van Duyne S, Soucek MJ, eds. Clinical Perspectives in the Management of Down Syndrome. New York: Springer-Verlag, 1990:147–152.
12. Samuelson ME, Nguyen VT. Middle ear effusion in Down's syndrome patients. Nebraska Med J 1980;65:83–84.
13. Downs MP, Jafek BW, Wood II RP. Comprehensive treatment of children with recurrent serous otitis media. Otolaryngol Head Neck Surg 1981;89:658–665.
14. Downs MP, Balkany TJ. Otologic problems and hearing impairment in Down syndrome. In: Dmitriev V, Oelwein PL, eds. Advances in Down Syndrome. Seattle, Wash: Special Child Publications, 1988:19–34.
15. Balkany TJ, Downs MP, Jafek BW, Krajicek MJ. Hearing loss in Down's syndrome: A treatable handicap more common than generally recognized. Clin Pediatr 1979;18:116–118.
16. Balkany TJ, Mischke RE, Downs MP, Jafek BW. Ossicular abnormalities in Down's syndrome. Otolaryngol Head Neck Surg 1979;87:372–384.
17. Maurizi M, Ottaviani F, Paludetti G, Luungarotti S. Audiological findings in Down's children. Int J Pediatr Otorhinolaryngol 1985;9:227–232.
18. Igarashi M, Takahashi M, Alford BF, Johnson PE. Inner ear morphology in Down's syndrome. Acta Otolaryngol 1977;83:175–181.
19. Palmer S. Influence of vitamin A nutriture on the immune response: Findings in children with Down syndrome. Int J Vit Nutr Res 1978;48:188–216.
20. Walby AP, Schuknecht HF. Concomitant occurrence of cochleoccular dysplasia in Down syndrome. Arch Otolaryngol 1984;110:447–449.

21. Harada T, Sando I. Temporal bone histopathologic findings in Down's syndrome. Arch Otolaryngol 1981;107:96–103.
22. Brooks DN, Wooley A, Kanjilal GC. Hearing loss and middle ear disorders in patients with Down's syndrome (Mongolism). J Ment Defic Res 1972;16:21.
23. Keiser H, Montague J, Wold D, Maune S, Pattison SM. Hearing loss of Down syndrome adults. Am J Ment Defic 1981;86:467–472.
24. Holm V, Kunze L. Effect of chronic otitis media on language and speech development. Pediatrics 1969;43:883.
25. Squires N, Ollo C, Jordon R. Auditory brainstem responses in the mentally retarded: Audiometric correlates. Ear Hear 1986;7:83–92.
26. Widen JE, Folsom RC, Thompson G, Wilson WR. Auditory brainstem responses in young adults with Down syndrome. Am J Ment Defic 1987;91:472–479.
27. Downs MP (guest ed). Communication disorders in Down's syndrome. In: Northern JL, ed. Seminars in Speech, Language and Hearing, vol 1, no 1. New York: Decker, 1980.

9

The Heart

Perhaps the most dramatic complication of Down syndrome where early diagnosis followed by appropriate treatment makes a clear-cut difference is cardiac disease. One of the most frequent type of cardiac anomalies found in children with Down syndrome is complete endocardial cushion defect [1]. Before modern therapy, nearly 100% of these children died by school age [2]. Today, with early and aggressive surgical intervention, up to 70% of these severely affected children survive [3]. This kind of result is indeed a triumph for modern preventive medicine.

Down himself first mentioned the possibility of cardiac disease when he reported "The circulation is feeble" [4]. In 1894, Garrod wrote an article establishing the relationship between congenital cardiovascular anomalies and Down syndrome [5]. Indeed, by 1900, the presence of congenital cardiac disease was used as a differential diagnostic feature in separating Down syndrome from cretinism [6].

Just how frequent is cardiac disease in patients with Down syndrome? This is a difficult question to answer because incidence figures range from 7% to 70% [7]. This great variation reflects selective factors regarding early childhood mortality and other ascertainment methods in various studies. Among unselected fetuses with Down syndrome aborted after prenatal diagnosis, congenital cardiac disease was found in 45%, not including patent ductus arteriosus and some cases of atrial septal defect because of postnatal closure of these structures [8]. In this fetal study, the investigator noted that minor anomalies of the heart were present almost regularly in the 100 cases studied. It is of interest that these minor anomalies occur at the same location and involve the same tissues as gross cardiac malformations. A consecutive study of 184 children with Down syndrome from the Hospital for Sick Children in Toronto disclosed an incidence of 40% [9]. Autopsy studies tend to report a somewhat higher figure, such as 44% [10], 56% [11], and 66% [12]—perhaps reflecting some cardiac disease that is not clinically apparent. In trying to settle on some kind of figure, probably the estimate of Gordon that 40–50% of patients with this syndrome will have some kind of cardiac disease seems reasonable [13].

Many series report that among Down syndrome patients, females have a higher percentage of cardiac disease [14,15]. This is surprising because in the general population there is a slight preponderance of males with congenital cardiac disease. Pinto et al. speculate that because there is very little of the type of congenital cardiac disease usually seen in males (aortic coarctation, stenosis, or complete transposition) the molecular determinants of Down syndrome may increase the incidence of atrioventricular septal defect in females [14].

Diagnosis of cardiac disease in infants with Down syndrome is not always obvious; in fact, clinical cardiovascular examinations in the newborn period may be entirely normal. Poor feeding, easy fatigability, dyspnea, diaphoresis, cyanosis, and a cardiac murmur are alerting signs, but some infants are asymptomatic particularly if they are not experiencing congestive cardiac failure. Because during the first 6 months of life the most rigorous exercise done by an infant occurs during feeding, it is not surprising that effort intolerance often shows up as a feeding problem [16].

Cardiac ultrasound may be performed safely even in fetuses. Presently, it is recommended that all patients with proven trisomy 21 by amniocentesis undergo fetal echocardiography. Certainly, any infant with Down syndrome needs careful evaluation by one or more of the current techniques such as electrocardiography, two-dimensional echocardiography, Doppler flow analysis, and so on (see recommendations, Chapter 3).

What type of cardiac defects occur in children with the various chromosomal types of Down syndrome? As can be seen in Table 9.1, endocardial cushion defects lead most lists with ventricular septal defect a close second. These are the two most common cardiac defects found in Down syndrome. However, in reviewing these figures, it is important to remember that up to one-third of children with Down syndrome with congenital cardiac disease have multiple defects [3].

The data on cardiac status in adults with Down syndrome are sparse compared to the literature on children. Recently, cardiac auscultation and Doppler echocardiography were performed on 35 adults, and the results showed that 71% of these *asymptomatic* adults had positive findings [17]. The most

Table 9.1 Frequency of Anatomic Defects in Children with Down Syndrome Diagnosed with Congenital Heart Disease

	Rowe & Uchida (1961) [9]	Gordon 1990 [13]
Total patients	70	63
Percent of patients with		
Atrioventricular canal	36	33
Ventral septal defect	33	32
Patent ductus arteriosus	10	13
Atrial septal defect	9	10
Tetralogy of Fallot	1	1
Other defects	11	11

frequent finding was holosystolic mitral valve prolapse in 20 individuals, of whom five had associated tricuspid valve prolapse. Also, mild aortic regurgitation was noted in four adults.

ENDOCARDIAL CUSHION DEFECT

Endocardial cushion defect is the single most common form of cardiac malformation found in individuals with Down syndrome (see Fig. 9.1). Alterations in the embryological development of the endocardial cushions results in abnormalities of the atrial septum, the atrioventricular valves (mitral and tricuspid), and the ventricular system [18]. Categorization of endocardial cushion defect into a complete, transitional, or partial form is determined by the degree of ventricular septal deficiency. In the complete form of endocardial defect, there is deficiency of the atrial septum, both atrioventricular valves and the ventricular septum.

Although examination by the physician of a patient with Down syndrome in early infancy may be normal, often there are some clinical clues [18]. Prominence of the left precordium can be noted, and the cardiac impulse may be hyperactive both at the xiphoid and apical regions. The first cardiac sound usually is normal; the second heart sound may split on inspiration. The presence of a low frequency, middiastolic murmur over the xiphoid or cardiac apex suggests a large left-to-right shunt. Regarding systolic murmurs, one at the left sternal border is commonly ejection in nature if a large left-to-right

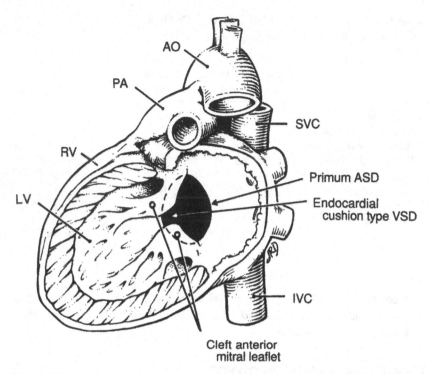

Figure 9.1 Atrioventricular canal defect of the heart. (Drawn by the Department of Medical Illustration, Johns Hopkins School of Medicine, Baltimore, MD)

shunt is present; an apical holosystolic murmur may be present in patients with mitral insufficiency.

Chest radiography may reveal cardiomegaly with enlargement of the left and right atria and left ventricle. Sometimes dilatation of the main pulmonary artery segment and increased vascular markings occur with large left-to-right shunts. The electrocardiogram can be characteristic, demonstrating an abnormal axis of ventricular depolarization as well as chamber hypertrophy.

The two other forms of endocardial cushion defect—the transitional and partial—are seen less frequently in this patient group [3]. The children can have symptoms similar to those of children with complete endocardial deformity. These defects often result in significant morbidity but have less predisposition to the development of pulmonary hypertension and pulmonary vascular disease. Careful physical examination and ultrasound studies are most useful for distinguishing the various types of endocardial cushion defects.

VENTRICULAR SEPTAL DEFECT

This cardiac malformation is the second most common defect seen in children with Down syndrome (see Fig. 9.2); it is almost as common as endocardial cushion defect (see Table 9.1). The membranous portion of the ventricular septum is located in the superior portion of the septum. When viewed from the left ventricle, the membranous defect is immediately inferior to the aortic valve ring.

The clinical manifestations of the defect are related directly to the size of the deformity itself [18]. The majority of ventricular septal defects in infants and children with Down syndrome are large [19]. Usually accompanying a large ventricular septal defect are a large left-to-right shunt and pulmonary hypertension. Infants may present with congestive cardiac failure or pulmonary hyper-

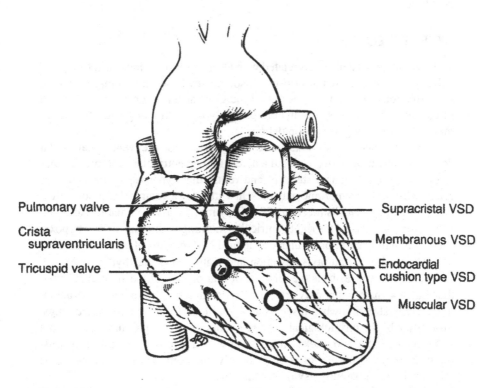

Figure 9.2   Ventral septal defect of the heart. (Drawn by the Department of Medical Illustration, Johns Hopkins School of Medicine, Baltimore, MD)

tension if the child has a large defect. As a result of the large left-to-right shunt, similar symptoms to those seen with the complete form of the endocardial cushion defect may be noted, such as dyspnea, diaphoresis, poor feeding, and failure to thrive. Infants with small defects generally are asymptomatic.

The physical examination of an infant or child with ventricular septal defect often is similar to the examination of a child with endocardial cushion defect, making it difficult to specifically diagnose the exact cardiac anomaly by history and physical examination alone. The electrocardiogram is helpful in distinguishing between the two because patients with isolated ventricular septal defect—of the nonendocardial cushion type—usually have a normal QRS axis [18]. Two-dimensional echocardiography can accurately distinguish the types of septal defects.

Another septal defect—the atrial septal defect of the secundum type—is considerably rarer than the ventricular types but is occasionally seen in this patient group.

OTHER DEFECTS

The other forms of defects associated with Down syndrome include tetralogy of Fallot and patent ductus arteriosus. Also, most of the rare forms of cardiac malformation, such as transposition of the great arteries, have been described in patients with Down syndrome but probably not with any greater frequency than is seen in the general population.

The four classic hallmarks of tetralogy of Fallot are ventricular septal defect, an aortic valve overriding the defect in the ventricular septum, valvular or infundibular pulmonary stenosis, and ventricular hypertrophy. Early in life, infants with Down syndrome may present with only a ventricular septal defect or a pulmonary stenosis murmur [20]. They may be asymptomatic. However, progressive severity of the right ventricular shunting with cyanosis and hypoxic spells gradually begin, particularly at about 12–18 months of age. The electrocardiogram shows right-axis deviation and right ventricular hypertrophy.

The ductus arteriosus is the remnant of that portion of the sixth aortic arch that joins the main pulmonary artery to the dorsal aorta. It is a normal structure in the prenatal period when it serves to shunt blood from the nonaerated lungs. Soon after birth, physiological closure occurs even though anatomic closure is not achieved for 1–6 weeks. In an infant with a persistent ductus arteriosus, the heart remains normal or is only slightly enlarged. There is a continuous murmur in an apparently asymptomatic child.

Other vascular anomalies of the aortic arch and vessels are usually asymptomatic and diagnosed only at autopsy. They have been reported in 15% of fetuses with Down syndrome [8].

PULMONARY ARTERY HYPERTENSION AND PULMONARY VASCULAR DISEASE

A very clinically significant problem in patients with Down syndrome is the presence of pulmonary artery hypertension and thus the future development of pulmonary vascular obstructive disease. Not only does this complication tend to occur earlier in infants with Down syndrome than in normal infants with similar cardiac defects, there are a number of reports of the development of pulmonary vascular obstructive disease in children with Down syndrome who have little or no detectable cardiac malformations [21–23].

There have been a number of different explanations advanced to explain the pulmonary vascular obstructive disease in this patient group. One group of explanations raises the question whether the lung parenchyma itself may be abnormal. Chi and Krovetz suggested that there is a failure of regression of the fetal pulmonary vascular pattern [24], whereas others raised the question of immunologically mediated damage [8]. Differences in the pulmonary capillary bed with abnormalities of capillary loops have been demonstrated [25]. In some cases, the media of small pulmonary arteries has been reported to be thinner [26]. A smaller number of alveoli and a smaller alveolar surface than in controls has been reported [27].

Another set of explanations focus on chronic upper airway obstruction. This obstruction has been postulated to be secondary to excessive secretions, macroglossia or glossoptosis, maxillary underdevelopment [28], tonsilar and adenoidal hypertrophy [29], laryngomalacia [20], or obstructive sleep apnea [22].

In addition, there are other complications of Down syndrome that can aggravate pulmonary artery hypertension. One is gastroesophageal reflux, a phenomenon associated with congenital cardiac disease in Down syndrome patients [31]. Reflux results in further pulmonary complications including bronchospasm and infection. As reviewed in Chapter 15, children with Down syndrome already have a compromised immune system that can make them more susceptible to infections, including pulmonary infections. Such infections can aggravate upper airway obstruction and pulmonary congestion and sometimes cause additional pulmonary parenchymal damage [18].

Clinical evidence to suggest the presence of pulmonary artery hypertension consists of a prominent right ventricular impulse, increased intensity of the pulmonic closure sound, decreased intensity of systolic murmurs, and disappearance of the diastolic rumble. In some patients, there can be improvement in the signs and symptoms of congestive cardiac failure. The chest radiograph in children with severe pulmonary hypertension and pulmonary vascular disease may demonstrate a dilated main pulmonary artery segment and a disorganized "pruning" pattering of the pulmonary blood flow [18].

There is one possible positive finding in the arteriovascular system in patients with Down syndrome. The complete absence of atherosclerosis in adults with Down syndrome has been observed [32] in spite of unfavorable lipoprotein ratios reported in other studies (see Chapter 7).

MANAGEMENT

As in all other organ systems of the body, the key to good treatment starts out with adequate and detailed diagnosis. Supplements to the clinical diagnostic examination such as modern chest radiography, electrocardiography, echocardiography, and cardiac catheterization for angiography can help tease out the exact configuration of the cardiac lesion in each child.

Once the diagnosis is established, medical management of the clinical symptoms can be tried. In addition to the impressive array of cardiac drugs available today, management of anemia, respiratory insufficiency, chronic infections, gastroesophageal reflux, and sleep apnea may be needed [13]. If the child develops congestive cardiac failure, extra monitoring is required.

A decision to intervene with surgery depends on age and weight as well as diagnostic and other health conditions of the young patient. Surgical techniques have improved to the point that, if necessary, cardiopulmonary bypass with deep hypothermia and cardioplegia will allow complete intracardiac repair at essentially any age [13]. The mortality rate of the patients undergoing these operations is not yet adequately studied and depends on many factors, including the type of lesion, age of the child, and other health problems in that particular individual. Early estimates in general are at a 15% mortality rate for the patients undergoing these major surgeries. In at least one institution, children with Down syndrome and congenital cardiac disease did not have a higher mortality rate for surgical treatment when compared lesion by lesion to children without Down syndrome [15]. In contrast to the surgical statistics, one study of unoperated endocardial defect based on actuarial analysis stated that only 54% of the patients survived until 6 months of age, only 35% of the patients survived until 12 months of age, only 15% to 2 years, and only 4% to 5 years [2]. In another study, the figure was similar—50%—at 6 months of age [33].

ACCESS TO CARDIAC CARE

Several studies recently appeared addressing the issue of equal access to medical care for cardiac patients with Down syndrome. The natural history of complete endocardial defect in infants with Down syndrome often is a relentless progression to pulmonary vascular obstructive disease, rendering the patient a poor candidate for surgery because of this complication. Sondheimer et al. compared patients with and without Down syndrome who had this complete defect in one hospital and found that referral to surgery and surgical intervention differed between the two groups [34]. All eight patients (100%) without Down syndrome were referred before 1 year of age, and surgical intervention was possible. In the case of the patients with Down syndrome, 22 out of 28 (79%) were referred in time for the possibility of surgical intervention, leaving six patients too far advanced for surgery because of late referral.

From another point of view, Barrera et al. studied developmental and caretaking patterns related to several variables in the group of infants enrolled in an intervention program [35]. One of the variables assessed was the presence or absence of cardiac disease in this patient group. This study reported that, regarding the home environment, infants without cardiac defects were provided a "better home environment" than infants with cardiac disease. They were not referring to the medical care of these infants but to the family's attitude toward the infant as measured in their study. Reed et al. also noted that parents of children with severe cardiac conditions were much less likely to follow through with furnished guidance, noting that the long rest periods needed by these patients often precluded activities of early stimulation [36].

In contrast to the reports of late referral for medical care, Schneider et al. compared 160 infants with Down syndrome to 540 infants matched for the same cardiac diagnoses but without chromosomal or other extracardiac anomalies [37]. Their conclusion was that for defects of comparable severity, the pattern of cardiac care in the Baltimore–Washington, D.C., area for infants with Down syndrome is timely and comparable to the care given other infants.

As Gordon clearly states:

> It should be clear that neglect of the patient with Down syndrome and cardiac disease is not prudent. Patients who survive with complete atrioventricular canal and pulmonary vascular obstructive disease are significantly worse off than their peers who have received treatment . . . in their early 20s, these children often must use a wheelchair, are persistently short of breath, cyanotic, and polycythemic. They may develop right cardiac failure. Clinical manifestations of their chronic hypoxemia include visual disturbances, severe headaches, dyspnea on any exertion, chest pain, syncope, cardiac dysrhythmias, and, in some cases, associated bleeding tendency. There is no doubt that the quality of life in the unoperated patient who develops pulmonary vascular obstructive disease is poor [13].

The principle of preventive medical care clearly is seen in the handling of the cardiac patient, particularly those with the more severe cardiac defects. Each defect has its optimal age for surgical referral—for example, tetralogy of Fallot in some cases is repaired after 3 or more years of age or after achieving a 15–20 kg weight because the later age may reduce the incidence of residual pulmonary stenosis. In contrast, the complete endocardial defect discussed previously usually needs much earlier repair to attempt to prevent the progression to pulmonary vascular obstructive disease.

The key is early individual diagnosis and thoughtful therapy.

REFERENCES

1. Tandon R, Edwards J. Cardiac malformations associated with Down syndrome. Circulation 1973;47:1349–1355.
2. Berger TJ, Blackstone EH, Kirklin JW, Bargeron LM, Hazelring JB, Turner ME. Survival and probability of cure without and with operation in complete atrioventricular canal. Ann Thorac Surg 1978;27:104–111.
3. Spicer R. Down's syndrome and congenital heart disease. Down's Syndrome: Papers and Abstracts for Professionals 1986;9:2–3.
4. Down JL. Observations on an ethnic classification of idiots. Lond Hosp Clin Lect Rep 1866;3:259–262.
5. Garrod AE. On the association of cardiac malformations with other congenital defects. St Barth Hosp Rep 1894;30:53.
6. Smith GE, Berg JM. Down's Anomaly. Edinburgh: Churchill Livingston, 1976.
7. Pueschel SM. Cardiology. In: Pueschel SM, Rynder JE, eds. Down Syndrome: Advances in Biomedicine and the Behavior Sciences. Cambridge, Mass: Ware Press, 1982, pp. 203–207.
8. Rehder H. Pathology of trisomy 21. In: Burgio GR, Fraccaro M, Tiepolo L, Wolf U, eds. Trisomy 21. Berlin: Springer-Verlag, 1981:57–80.
9. Rowe RD, Uchida IA. Cardiac malformations in mongolism: A prospective study of 184 mongoloid children. Am J Med 1961;31:726.
10. Evans PR. Cardiac anomalies in mongolism. Br Heart J 1950;12:258–262.
11. Berg JM, Crome L, France NE. Congenital cardiac malformations in mongolism. Br Heart J 1960;22:331–346.
12. Warkany J, Passarge E, Smith LB. Congenital malformations in autosomal trisomy syndromes. Am J Dis Child 1966;112:502–517.
13. Gordon LS. Cardiac conditions. In: Van Dyke DC, Lang DJ, Heide F, van Duyne S, Soucek MJ, eds. Clinical Perspectives in the Management of Down Syndrome. New York: Springer-Verlag, 1990:55–71.
14. Pinto FF, Nunes L, Ferraz F, Sampayo F. Down's syndrome: Different distribution of congenital heart diseases between the sexes. Int J Cardiol 1990;27:175–178.
15. Baciewicz FA, Melvin WS, Basilius D, Davis JT. Congenital heart disease in Down's syndrome patients: A decade of surgical experience. Thorac Cardiovasc Surg 1989;37:369–371.

16. Feit TS. Aspects of cardiac disease in Down syndrome. In: Dmitriev V, Oelwein PL, eds. Advances in Down Syndrome. Seattle, Wash: Special Child Publications, 1988:35–44.

17. Goldhaber SZ, Brown WD, Sutton MG. High frequency of mitral valve prolapse and aortic regurgitation among asymptomatic adults with Down's syndrome. JAMA 1987;258:1793–1795.

18. Spicer RL. Cardiovascular disease in Down syndrome. Pediatr Clin North Am 1984;31:1331–1343.

19. Laursen HB. Congenital heart disease in Down syndrome. Br Heart J 1976;38:32–38.

20. Perry LW, Midgely FM, Galioto FM, Shapiro S, Scott L. Down's syndrome and cardiovascular disease. Down's Syndrome: Papers and Abstracts for Professionals 1980;3:1–5.

21. Wilson SK, Hutchins GN, Neill CA. Hypertensive pulmonary vascular disease in Down syndrome. J Pediatr 1979;95:722–726.

22. Loughlin GN, Wynne JW, Victorica BE. Sleep apnea as a possible cause of pulmonary hypertension in Down syndrome. J Pediatr 1981;98:435–437.

23. Levine OR, Simpser M. Alveolar hypoventilation and cor pulmonale associated with chronic airway obstruction in infants with Down syndrome. Clin Pediatr 1982;21:25–29.

24. Chi TPL, Krovetz LJ. The pulmonary vascular bed in children with Down's syndrome. J Pediatr 1975;86:533–538.

25. Krontas SB, Bodenbender JG. Abnormal capillary morphology in congenital heart disease. Pediatrics 1966;37:316–322.

26. Yamki S, Horiuschi T, Sekino Y. Quantitative analysis of pulmonary vascular disease in simple cardiac anomalies with Down syndrome. Am J Cardiol 1983; 51:1502–1506.

27. Conney TP, Thurlbeck WM. Pulmonary hypoplasia in Down's syndrome. N Engl J Med 1982;307:1170–1182.

28. Strome M. Down syndrome: A modern otorhinolaryngological perspective. Laryngoscope 1981;91:1581–1594.

29. Rowland TW, Nordstrom LG, Bean MS, et al. Chronic upper airway obstruction and pulmonary hypertension in Down syndrome. Am J Dis Child 1981;135:1050–1052.

30. Aggarwal KC, Rasogi A, Singhi S. Cor pulmonale due to laryngomalacia in Down syndrome. Indian Pediatr 1981;18:914–916.

31. Weesner KM, Rosenthal A. Gastroesophageal reflux in association with congenital heart disease. Clin Pediatr 1983;22:424–426.

32. Murdoch JC, Rodger JC, Rao SS, Fletcher CD, Dunnigan MG. Down's syndrome: An atheroma-free model? Br Med J 1977;23:226–228.

33. Kirklin JW, Baratt-Boyes BG. Cardiac Surgery. New York: Wiley, 1986.

34. Sondheimer HM, Byrum CJ, Blackman MS. Unequal cardiac care for children with Down's syndrome. Am J Dis Child 1985;139:68–70.

35. Barrera ME, Watson LJ, Adelstein A. Development of Down's syndrome infants with and without heart defects and changes in their caretaking environment. Child Care Health Dev 1987;13:87–100.
36. Reed RB, Pueschel SM, Schnell RR, Cronk CE. Interrelationships of biological, environmental and competency variables. In: Pueschel SM, ed. The Young Child with Down Syndrome. New York: Human Sciences Press, 1984:285–302.
37. Schneider DS, Zahka KG, Clark EB, Neill CA. Patterns of cardiac care in infants with Down syndrome. Am J Dis Child 1989;143:363–365.

10

The Gastrointestinal System

A child who has a mentally handicapping condition combined with other symptoms sometimes does not receive a standard medical evaluation for those additional symptoms. From the newborn period to the end of life, gastrointestinal malformations and disease entities can underlie symptoms hitherto written off as "just part of Down syndrome." Yet, in fact, intermittent chronic vomiting can be caused by undiagnosed underlying congenital duodenal or jejunal stenosis—there is one person in the medical literature with Down syndrome and this congenital problem who did not have a diagnosis until 19 years of age [1]. Although this is an extreme case, undiagnosed chronic vomiting in young children, particularly in 1 and 2 year olds, is seen from time to time in a Down syndrome clinic.

Another example of a symptom that tends to be overlooked is the problem with chronic constipation, which is found in at least 30% of this patient group [2]. Underlying this condition in Down syndrome may be a variety of malformations such as aganglionic segment of the colon, Meckel's or other diverticuli, rectal stenosis, partial anal atresia, or (in infants) imperforate anus. Persistent constipation should not be ignored in anyone, particularly in an individual with Down syndrome.

The actual incidence of congenital malformations of the gastrointestinal tract in this patient group is 10%, based on a review by Carter of 725 autopsy cases [3]. According to Knox and Bensel, gastrointestinal malformations are one of the most significant causes of death in Down syndrome after cardiac malformations and infections. In their clinical study of 110 Down syndrome individuals, Knox and Bensel reported 12% of people with the syndrome have some type of gastrointestinal malformation [4]. To make diagnostic studies even more complicated, it is important to remember when evaluating gastrointestinal symptoms in individuals with Down syndrome that the possibility of multiple gastrointestinal anomalies should not be forgotten [5].

DUODENAL OBSTRUCTION AND OTHER UPPER GASTROINTESTINAL ANOMALIES

Among the congenital malformations, obstructions of the duodenum are the most frequent; they range from 5% to 8% [6–8] (see Fig. 10.1). Vomiting and dehydration are alerting signs. The increased frequency of this obstruction in Down syndrome patients was not noted until as late as 1950 [9–11]. Because some of the patients, particularly infants, must have been dying of it all along, this may be another example of failure of diagnosis. It is distressing that the medical literature sometimes reports that even after diagnosis, there was a refusal to permit surgical intervention to relieve the obstruction, and this may have been the cause of death [12].

The obstruction may be caused by congenital atresia, intrinsic stenosis, or extrinsic stenosis secondary to annular pancreas or malrotation of the bowel with bands [13]. Using polyhydramnios as an alerting sign, sonography has been used to detect duodenal obstruction even before birth [14–16]. In the neonatal period, these lesions may constitute surgical emergencies because they can be life threatening in that period.

Without surgical intervention, infants may die of starvation. However, surgical intervention does not guarantee survival; in a series reported by Puri and O'Donnell in 1981, 59% of the infants died in the first year, most postoperatively or because of associated cardiac disease or infection [17]; in the series by Buchin et al., 56% died [6]. Stauffer and Irving did a study of duodenal obstruction and surgical intervention in all infants with the diagnosis where the patients were classified by their risk factors. Thirty-eight percent of these infants had Down syndrome. A comparison of the Down syndrome and the non–Down syndrome groups showed no difference in early mortality rates, although a greater percentage of infants with Down syndrome had later deaths. In this study, one or more repeated laparotomies were required in six children with Down syndrome and in only two without Down syndrome [18].

Other anomalies of the upper gastrointestinal tract are much rarer. Esophageal atresia has been described in the medical literature [19,20]. In the notorious "Baby Doe" case, an infant with esophageal atresia was allowed to

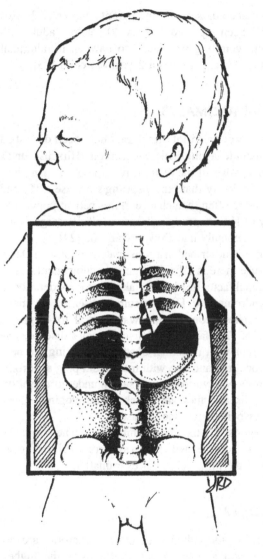

Figure 10.1 The "double bubble sign" of duodenal stenosis of the gastrointestinal tract. (Drawn by the Department of Medical Illustration, Johns Hopkins School of Medicine, Baltimore, MD)

die by attending physicians in accordance with the parents wishes [21]. Two cases of pyloric stenosis have been reported [19]. A 40-year-old adult with Down syndrome and recurrent vomiting was found to have an intraluminal diverticulum of the duodenum [22] and so was a 2-year-old child [23].

LOWER GASTROINTESTINAL ANOMALIES

A number of anomalies of the lower gastrointestinal tract have been described in Down syndrome; these include aganglionic megacolon (Hirschsprung's disease), localized congenital stenosis of the rectum, rectosigmoid aganglionosis, and imperforate anus. It is likely that Hirschsprung's disease (2%) and imperforate anus (3%) occur more often than chance in this patient population [6]. Conversely, in one study of Hirschsprung's disease itself, Passarge found 2% of the individual with this anomaly had Down syndrome [24].

Hirschsprung's disease was first described in a constipated infant with Down syndrome in 1956 [25]. Because there is a familial genetic component to this disease entity [26], this additional factor needs to be taken into consideration in a child with both Down syndrome and Hirschsprung's disease. As many investigators emphasize, persistent constipation was central to diagnosis [4,27–29]. In a recent series of 13 infants with Hirschsprung's disease, five presented with constipation, four with intestinal obstruction during the neonatal period, three with enterocolitis, and one with meconium plug syndrome [30]. Although children with Down syndrome can safely undergo definitive operations for Hirschsprung's disease, they are at risk for developing enterocolitis and complications of associated cardiac disease.

Imperforate anus can be diagnosed in the first examination of a newborn [7]. Because it is found in up to 3% of neonates with Down syndrome [6], ruling out this anomaly should be part of the initial physical examination.

INFLAMMATORY BOWEL DISEASE

Bowel problems occurring in an individual with Down syndrome are not automatically based on congenital anomalies, although this is the highest statistical probability in children and even some adults. Both chronic ulcerative colitis with bloody diarrhea [31] and regional enteritis [32] have been described in adults with Down syndrome. As in any other individual with these symptoms, both genetic and autoimmune factors need evaluation. (The role of autoimmunity in Down syndrome is reviewed in Chapter 15.)

IS THERE EVIDENCE FOR MALABSORPTION
IN DOWN SYNDROME?

From time to time, intense controversies arise regarding Down syndrome therapies, and recently leading the list are the controversial therapies that are based on the concept of malabsorption. As described in Chapter 19, glowing reports of the use of supplementary multivitamins and nutrients to overcome malabsorption in a group of Down syndrome children are published every so often, and such reports require many hours of investigators' time to sort out the evidence and determine whether there is any underlying validity to these claims. What has happened is that after an enormous research effort on the part of many physicians and families, the indiscriminant use of a standard cocktail of vitamins and minerals for all children with Down syndrome is discredited by double-blind studies, and the Down syndrome community sits back waiting for the next dramatic claim of miraculous vitamin therapy to pop up.

The concept of malabsorption is not a hazy, mystical idea but a factual matter that can be investigated by scientific methods. The effect of the extra chromosome on each individual is different. Just as individuals with Down syndrome differ in the amount of cardiac disease that they express clinically, so it is possible that Down patients, each evaluated as individuals, may or may not have malabsorption of one or more nutrients. For example, a study of a patient with Down syndrome and a specific malabsorption of vitamin B_{12} has been published [33]. This, of course, does not mean that other individuals with Down syndrome are deficient in vitamin B_{12}; the importance of individual evaluation of each patient cannot be overstressed.

Exactly what is known about the ability of children with Down syndrome to absorb the nutrients that they eat? Tichy et al. examined the mucosa of the small intestine of three children with Down syndrome, aged 10–14 years [34]. Electron microscopy showed abnormal structure of the apical portions of the enterocytes, manifested by the sparsity of cytoplasmic structures and gross changes in the configuration of the microvillous layers of enterocytes. These investigators also studied the gastric mucosa of this patient group, and their conclusions were that changes as evidenced by electron microscopy suggested degeneration probably related to Down syndrome.

One usual method of checking whether a patient group tends to have malabsorption is by performing a D-xylose absorption and excretion test. Studies of mentally retarded children in general have shown impaired xylose absorption with a significant portion of those being investigated below the normal range [35]. In this study by Chapman et al., children with Down syndrome did not differ from children with other forms of mental retardation. However, in a study by Williams et al., adults with Down syndrome did show malabsorption of xylose to a significantly greater extent (p < 0.001) than adults with mental retardation of other etiologies [36]. Ninety percent of the subjects with Down syndrome had a xylose excretion below the normal range. This difference between children and adults with Down syndrome is puzzling and may be due to technical problems or unknown factors in the control population (of patients with other forms of mental retardation). In any event, much further work needs to be done to clarify these preliminary studies of xylose tolerance testing.

Celiac sprue has been reported in a number of individuals with Down syndrome [37–41]. Researchers from Finland report that celiac disease is 20 times greater in a Down syndrome than in a non–Down syndrome population [38]. Researchers from England report a figure that is 16 times more frequent in patients with Down syndrome than in those without Down syndrome [39]. On the other hand, researchers from Austria dispute this result finding no increase of celiac sprue in their population of Down syndrome patients [40]. Symptoms of this problem include recurrent diarrhea, slowing of growth, and delayed puberty. In the more retarded patients, rumination also may be a presenting sign.

There also has been a fairly extensive medical literature discussing problems in vitamin A malabsorption in patients with Down syndrome. As early as 1955, investigators have been reporting this abnormality in both institutionalized and home-reared children [42–47]. The study by Palmer [46] is particularly modern in methodology and reported a decrease in the incidence of infection related to vitamin A supplementation of 1000 IU/month.

However, a study by Barden of institutionalized children reported that individuals with Down syndrome had normal or higher levels of vitamin A in the serum than other retarded individuals and normal controls [48]. The patients also had very high carotene levels. This study raised the possibility of an inefficient mechanism for carotene-to-vitamin A conversion in this patient group. Using an oral vitamin A tolerance test, Cutress et al. also failed to find a statistical difference between mentally retarded subjects with and without Down syndrome [49]. Pueschel et al. performed a careful study of vitamin A absorption in this patient group and found no statistical difference between the patients and a control group [50]. These investigators noted that the patients had more symptoms usually seen in individuals with hypovitaminosis A than did controls; to explain these clinical findings, the possibility of decreased utilization or peripheral resistance to vitamin A was mentioned. One recent study found only hypercarotenemia and no deficiency [51].

The contradictory results of vitamin A studies published to date raise the question about whether a few children with Down syndrome may have something wrong with their handling of vitamin A and were included, for example, in the Palmer study, whereas many or most patients do not. Another possible interpretation is that there may be something wrong with the vitamin A receptor in some of this patient group so that children, even if they have normal or even high levels of this vitamin, may still show signs of deficiency. A third possibility is that many studies were done with inadequate methodology and that there simply is no more problem than in any other patient group.

Generally, the dictum in medicine is that baseline investigation of a problem such as vitamin A metabolism in a particular child makes sense only if clinical symptoms warrant it. Preventive testing techniques try to anticipate and head off problems, but such recommendations need to be based on reasonable scientific evidence in the patient group being examined. Symptoms of vitamin A deficiency can be poor growth, skin problems (dry, scaly skin, follicular hyperkeratosis, xerosis, and dry mucous membranes), blepharitis, impaired night adaption or night blindness, and photophobia. There is speculation in the medical literature that a tendency to serous otitis media and keratoconus in patients with Down syndrome may be increased by low or borderline functional levels of vitamin A. Adequate levels of zinc also are needed in vitamin A metabolism; studies of the levels of this element in patients with Down syndrome are discussed in Chapter 15.

This controversy over vitamin A in the medical literature reminds one of the century long fight in that literature about whether patients with Down syndrome did or did not have thyroid disease. Investigators were confident of their results on both sides of the controversy. Modern laboratory testing gave an answer that turned out to be both yes and no—some patients did have thyroid disease (28 times the usual rate at birth, for example), yet many of the patients were truly euthyroid.

REFERENCES

1. Smith GV, Teele RL. Delayed diagnosis of duodenal obstruction in Down syndrome. AJR 1980;134:937–940.
2. Van Dyke DC, Lang DL, Miller JD, Heide F, van Duyne S, Chang H. Common medical problems. In: Van Dyke DC, Lang DJ, Heide F, van Duyne S, Soucek MJ, eds. Clinical Perspectives in the Management of Down Syndrome. New York: Springer-Verlag, 1990:3–14.
3. Carter CO. A life table for mongols with the causes of death. J Ment Defic Res 1958;2:64.

4.   Knox GE, Bensel RW. Gastrointestinal malformations in Down syndrome. Minn Med 1972;55:542–545.
5.   Kilcoyne RF, Taybi H. Conditions associated with congenital megacolon. Am J Roentgenol Rad Therm Nucl Med 1970;108:615–620.
6.   Buchin PJ, Levy JS, Schullinger JN. Down's syndrome and the gastrointestinal tract. J Clin Gastroenterol 1986;8:111–114.
7.   Smith D. Recognizable patterns of human malformations. 3rd ed. Philadelphia: Saunders, 1982.
8.   Warkany J. Uses and misuses of syndromes in associated congenital anomalies. In: Shafie ME, Klippel CH, eds. Baltimore, Md: William & Wilkins, 1981.
9.   Lahman TH. Discussion on intestinal obstruction. Ann Surg 1949;130:509.
10. Grove L, Rasmussen E. Congenital atresia of the small intestine with report of cases. Ann Surg 1950;131:869–878.
11. Bodian M, White LLR, Carter CO, Louw JH. Congenital duodenal obstruction and mongolism. Br Med J 1952;2:77–78.
12. Wolraich ML, Siperstein GN, Reed D. Doctors' decisions and prognostications for infants with Down syndrome. Dev Med Child Neurol 1991;33:336–342.
13. Harberg F, Pokomy W, Hahn H. Congenital duodenal obstruction: A review of 65 cases. Am J Surg 1979;138:825–828.
14. Loveday BJ, Barr JA, Aitken J. The interuterine demonstrations of duodenal atresia by ultrasound. Br J Radiol 1975;48:1031–3032.
15. Balcar I, Grant DC, Miller WA, Bieber FA. Antenatal detection of Down syndrome by sonography. AJR 1984;143:29–30.
16. Clark JF, Hales E, Ma P, Rosser SB. Duodenal atresia in utero in association with Down syndrome and annular pancreas. JAMA 1984;76:190–192.
17. Puri P, O'Donnell B. Outlook after surgery for congenital intrinsic duodenal obstruction in Down syndrome. Lancet 1981;2:802.
18. Stauffer UG, Irving I. Duodenal atresia and stenosis—long term results. Progr Pediatr Surg 1977;110:49–60.
19. Oster J. Mongolism: A clinico-geneological investigation comprising 526 mongols living in Seeland and neighboring islands of Denmark. Copenhagen: Danish Science Press, 1953.
20. Gross RE. The surgery of infancy and childhood: Its principles and techniques. Philadelphia: Saunders, 1953.
21. Caplan A, Cohen CB. A history of neonatal intensive care and decision making. Hastings Cent Rep 1987;17:7–9.
22. Curtis GT, Simpson W, Lowden AGR. Intraluminal diverticulum of the duodenum in a mongol. Clin Radiol 1965;16:289–291.
23. Ashraf A. Intraluminal diverticulum of the duodenum in a two year old. Mo Med 1985;82:762–763.
24. Passarge E. Genetics of Hirschsprung's Disease. N Engl J Med 1967;276:138–143.
25. Vacher LB, Garcia WM, Palacio AG. Hirschsprung's disease in a 38-day-old mongoloid. Rev Cubana Pediatr 1956;28:473–484.

26. Cohen IT, Gadd MA. Hirschsprung's disease in a kindred: Possible clue to the genetics of the disease. J Pediatr Surg 1982;17:632–634.

27. Graivier L, Siber WK. Hirschsprung's disease and mongolism. Surgery 1966; 60:458–461.

28. Teitelbaum DH, Qualman SJ, Caniano DA. Hirschsprung's disease: identification of risk factor for enterocolitis. Ann Surg 1988; 207:240–244.

29. Emanuel B, Padoff MP, Swenson D. Mongolism associated with Hirschsprung's disease. J Pediatr 1965;66:2.

30. Aniano DA, Teitelbaum DH, Qulaman SJ. Management of Hirschsprung's disease in children with trisomy 21. Am J Surg 1990;159:402–404.

31. Lieberthal MM, Frank HD. Chronic ulcerative colitis in a mongolian idiot. Gastroenterology 1955;28:1034–1036.

32. Burgess JN, Kelly KA. Regional enteritis and Down's syndrome. Minn Med 1971; 54:793–794.

33. Cartlidge PHT, Curnock DA. Specific malabsorption of vitamin B-12 in Down's syndrome. Arch Dis Child 1986;61:514–515.

34. Tichy J, Saxl O, Hradsky M, Hrstka V. Electron microscope study of mucous membrane of the small intestine in patients with mongolism: Preliminary report. Cesk Gastroenterol Vyz 1968;22:457–462.

35. Chapman MJ, Harrison PM, Stern J. Xylose absorption in mentally retarded children. J Ment Defic Res 1966;10:19.

36. Williams CA, Quinn H, Wright EC, Sylvester PE, Gosling PJH, Dickerson JWT. Xylose absorption in Down's syndrome. J Ment Defic Res 1985;29:173–177.

37. Novak TV, Ghisan FK, Schultz-Deirieu K. Celiac sprue in Down's syndrome: Consideration of a pathogenic link. Am J Gastroenterol 1983;78:280–283.

38. Simila S, Kokkonen J. Coexistence of celiac disease and Down syndrome. Am J Ment Defic 1990;95:120–122.

39. Dias JA, Walker-Smith J. Down's syndrome and coeliac disease. J Pediatr Gastroenterol Nutr 1990;10:41–43.

40. Granditsch G, Rossipal E. Down's syndrome and celiac disease. J Pediatr Gastroenterol Nutr 1990;11:279. Letter to the Editor.

41. Levo Y, Green P. Down's syndrome and autoimmunity. Am J Med Sci 1977; 273:95–99.

42. Hirsch W, Fisher MD. Chemical examination of the blood in mentally retarded children. Harefuah 1955;48:27.

43. Sobel A, Strazzulla M, Sherman B, Elkan B, Morgenstern S, Marius N, Meisel A. Vitamin A absorption and other blood composition in mongolism. Am J Ment Defic 1958;62:642–656.

44. Auld RM, Pommer JC, Houck JC, Burke FG. Vitamin A absorption in mongoloid children. 1959;63:1010–1013.

45. Appleton MD, Haab W, Casey PJ, Castellino F, Schorr JB, Miraglia R. Role of vitamin A in gammaglobulin biosynthesis and uric acid metabolism of mongoloids. Am J Ment Defic 1964;69:324–328.

46. Palmer S. Influence of vitamin A nutriture on the immune response: Findings in children with Down syndrome. Int J Vit Nutr Res 1978;48:188–216.

47. Matin MA, Sylvester PE, Edwards D, Dickerson JWT. Vitamin and zinc status in Down syndrome. J Ment Defic Res 1981;25:121–126.

48. Barden HS. Vitamin A and carotene values of institution mentally retarded subjects with and without Down's syndrome. J Ment Defic Res 1977;21:63–74.

49. Cutress TW, Mickleson KN, Brown RN. Vitamin A absorption and periodontal disease in trisomy G. J Ment Defic Res 1976;20:17–23.

50. Pueschel SM, Hillemeier C, Caldwell M, Senft K, Mevs C, Pezzullo JC. Vitamin A gastrointestinal absorption in persons with Down's syndrome. J Ment Defic Res 1990;34:269–275.

51. Storm W, Hypercarotenaemia in children with Down's syndrome. J Ment Defic Res 1990;34:283–286.

11

The Musculoskeletal System

The possible ailments of individuals with Down syndrome are many. These individuals are susceptible to a variety of musculoskeletal disorders, including some with serious neurological sequelae. However, farsighted preventive techniques can sometimes prevent and often ameliorate the effects of these potential joint problems by identifying areas of risk in an individual in the early stages or sometimes even in advance of clinical symptoms.

Joints at risk in this patient population are the occipitoatlantal, atlantoaxial as well as the lower cervical spine, the lumbosacral fusion area, the femoral head, acetabulum, the patella, and the articulations of the bones of the feet, particularly the subtalar joint.

THE SPINE

The first and second cervical vertebrae are functionally and anatomically different from the rest of the cervical spine. The flexion and extension of the head occur at the articulation between the occipital condyles and the facets of the atlas (0-C1). No rotational movement is believed to occur at this point. Movement at the next articulation, the atlantoaxial (C1-C2), is primarily rotational. Three quarters of all the rotational movement and about 10 degrees of flexion occurs at this point [1].

The first spinal joint (0-C1), which articulates the skull with the spine, has been described as unstable in many individuals with Down syndrome [2–6]. Occipitoatlantal instability usually is asymptomatic in this patient group. There has been a recent study of occiput-C1 translation in 73 patients with Down syndrome using flexion and extension lateral cervical spine radiographs [7]. The study was limited to individuals who had no congenital cervical spine anomalies, C1-C2 instability, or previous neck surgery. Even so, only 37% of these adults showed anteroposterior translation within normal limits (1 mm or less) by the Wiesel and Rothman method [8].

The second spinal joint (C1-C2) is a joint particularly at risk in patients with Down syndrome. Atlantoaxial subluxation with neurological sequelae can be a dangerous complication. The radiographic evidence that such an abnormality might develop was first recorded in the medical literature by Tishler and Martel in 1965 who recorded that 4 of 18 patients with Down syndrome had an atlanto-odontoid interval greater than 5 mm [9] (Fig. 11.1). The following year, these two investigators evaluated 70 individuals from ages 2 to 56 years and found that 20% had atlanto-odontoid instability greater than 5 mm [10].

Since that time, hundreds of patients with Down syndrome have had their cervical spines examined by radiological methods. The largest series is by

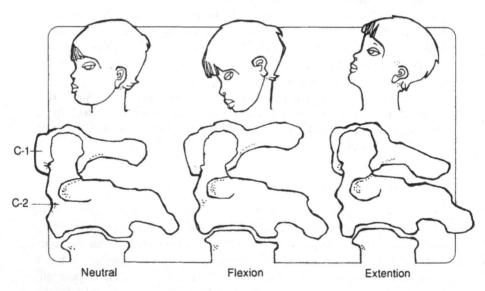

C-1

C-2

Neutral   Flexion   Extention

Figure 11.1 Atlantoaxial dislocation. When the head flexes, the dens of the axis (C-2) moves backward compressing the spinal cord behind it. The job of the transverse ligament of the atlas (C-1) is to retain the dens in its place—pathological compression of the spinal cord occurs when there is too much laxity or hypotonia of the transverse ligament. (Drawing by Johanna Vogelsang)

Pueschel and Scola who examined 404 patients and found atlantoaxial instability in 14.6% [11]. Most of the individuals with the instability were asymptomatic. However, 1.5% (6 patients) had developed symptomatic atlantoaxial subluxation and underwent surgery to prevent further injury to the spinal cord. Another large series of 130 children, aged 1–16 years, showed differing incidence rates of atlantoaxial instability with different age groups [12]. The incidence between 1 and 5 years was only 5%, whereas the figure rose to 12.8% between 6 and 10 years. In addition to the difficulty of completely visualizing cervical bones in children less than 2 years of age, there are many questions of the natural history of this disability highlighted by this study. Whether atlantoaxial instability is more common in boys [13] or girls [14] and whether the percentage of patients displaying the radiological findings increases with age is still far from clear.

Based on their extensive studies, Pueschel et al. concluded that no single assessment technique, such as cervical roentgenography was adequate for diagnosis. They suggested a combined approach using the neurological examination plus neurophysiological, roentgenographic, and imaging techniques [15].

In a recent study, the Pueschel team reported that skeletal anomalies of the cervical spine may be a contributing factor in the pathogenesis of atlantoaxial instability [16]. These anomalies reported by this group were persistent synchondrosis of the odontoid process and spina bifida occulta of C1.

Davidson, who extensively reviewed the literature [17], raised the question of whether we fully understand the natural history of atlantoaxial instability developing into atlantoaxial subluxation. He addressed the issue of how we anticipate which individuals with the dislocation are most likely to develop the subluxation. He raised a question about the value of the lateral-view roentgenograms of the upper cervical region in full flexion and extension before high-risk activities as recommended by the committee on sports medicine of the American Academy of Pediatrics in 1984 (see Appendix B). The Special Olympics committee defines high-risk activities as those involving flexion and extension of the cervical spine, gymnastics (tumbling and trampoline), diving, butterfly stroke in swimming, high jump in track and field, soccer, and any warm-up exercise that places pressure on the head or neck muscles. Davidson suggested that there is an urgent need for carefully designed longitudinal studies because his review demonstrated that *nearly all of the cases of actual dislocation were preceded by at least several weeks of readily detectable physical signs*. This led him to conclude that a physical examination with careful attention to neurological signs before participation in sports was more predictive of potential or impending dislocation than the radiological criteria currently recommended. Clinical symptoms of impending atlantoaxial dislocation have been described as neck pain, exhibited head tilt, torticollis, dyspnea, transient or progressive weakness or changes in gait pattern, increased clumsiness, changes in bowel or bladder habit, or a sudden preference for sitting. Neurological examination may show hyperactive deep tendon reflexes, ankle clonus, positive Babinski sign, increased muscle tone or spasticity, developing diparesis or quadriparesis, or sensory deficits.

In a follow up to Davidson, Roy et al. checked the relationship of cervical radiological abnormality with the neurological examination in patients with Down syndrome and concluded that there was no correlation [18a]. Selby et al. found that radiographs were unreliable and could change *within 10 minutes* from normal to abnormal or vice versa [18b]. Patients with no radiological evidence of atlantoaxial dislocation had as many neurological signs as those with a radiological finding. The investigators then suggested that symptoms might be of greater diagnostic predictive significance than signs.

So it is not clear at which age children with Down syndrome should be tested for this disability or which testing procedures are adequate for general screening or testing before sports participation. But one thing we do know. If nothing is done, there will be a small group of individuals with Down syndrome with undiagnosed atlantoaxial instability who sooner or later will progress to neurological symptoms ranging from mild spasticity to becoming wheel-chair bound to death itself. Pueschel, in his comprehensive textbook on Down syndrome [19], lists a number of patients with symptomatic spinal cord compression who were described in the medical literature. In the more recent literature, 11 additional patients and their surgical treatments have been recorded [20–22a]. The investigators emphasize the catastrophic presentation of this illness, and Aoki, who was dealing with a 4-year-old quadraplegic girl, even raised the question of the necessity of treatment for some individuals with the asymptomatic form of the disability [22a].

The most reasonable approach to the prevention of this serious disability remains to be determined. In the meantime, one consensus of recommendations is outlined in the Down Syndrome Preventive Medicine Checklists (Chapters 4 and 5) and Appendix B.

There seems to be no question that the upper cervical spine in general is at greater risk in individuals with Down syndrome. In addition to well-defined problems, a comparison of age- and sex-matched controls shows a significant increase in degenerative changes [22b].

The lower cervical spine is not only an area of subluxation but also may have degenerative changes in relatively young adults with Down syndrome. Gahagen and Van Dyke evaluated four adults from the ages of 26 to 42 years by radiographs and found all four had some degenerative changes of the cervical spine with spur formation, narrowing of foramina, narrowing of the disc inner space, and osteophyte formation [23]. Cervical myelopathy secondary to abnormalities of the lower cervical spine has been documented in a number of adults in a series that evaluated 105 cases [24]. The patients presented with ataxia, hyperreflexia, and bilateral ankle clonus. Sixty-three percent of these individuals had signs of lower cervical spondylosis. The investigators raised a question of whether this problem of the lower cervical spine (spondylosis leading to myelopathy) may pose a greater risk to adults with Down syndrome than the main problem of the upper cervical spine (atlantoaxial dislocation).

Are scoliosis and lordosis a major problem in patients with Down syndrome? Although several large series evaluating individuals with Down syndrome found evidence of these orthopedic conditions, they tend to be mild and rarely require intervention. In one survey of 265 patients in an institution, 52% had some degree of thorocolumbar scoliosis, yet only 4% needed to be admitted to acute care facilities, and only one of these patients required surgery [25]. In another series of 190 patients living at home, scoliosis was present in 11% and lordosis in 14%, yet there was no history of bracing or surgery being required [23].

Radiographic examination of the lower spine has shown a higher-than-normal evidence of incomplete fusion in the lumbosacral area [26] and an unusual configuration to the lumbar vertebrae [27].

THE LOWER EXTREMITY

Problems with hips in patients with Down syndrome spring from both the shape of the bones and the laxity of the capsules and ligaments. Before the discovery of the chromosome aberration in Down syndrome, radiography of the hips sometimes was used to confirm the diagnosis in newborns. The average iliac index (the sum of both acetabular and both iliac angles divided by two) usually is less than 60 in infants with Down syndrome compared to 81 in normal infants of less than 3 months of age [19]. The accuracy of this iliac index in determining the diagnosis of Down syndrome is about 80%. (The medical literature on this subject is summarized by Scola [19]).

However, despite these variations, there is relatively little dislocation and subluxation of the hips in children with Down syndrome. In fact, congenital dislocation of the hip does not appear to be increased above average rates [28]. However, in adolescents and adults, there does appear to be an increased incidence of dislocation of the hip [25,28]. The patients with hip problems tend to fall into two groups—one group has normal acetabula, whereas the other group has dysplastic and insufficient acetabula. Adding severe acetabular dysplasia, dislocation, subluxation, and epiphysiolysis, Diamond et al. found major hip problems in about 10% of an institutionalized population [25]. Epiphysiolysis can occur in 1% or 2% of the patients with Down syndrome and is almost always accompanied by severe aseptic necrosis of the femoral head with loss of hip function. In older persons with Down syndrome, osteoarthritis of the hip may occur and can be treated by total hip replacement if necessary [29, 30]. Other forms of surgery—capsular imbrication, acetabuloplasty, and femoral varus derotational osteotomy—have been used for subluxation [25,31].

The patella tends to be unstable in patients with Down syndrome; in the series by Diamond et al. of 265 patients, 51% had some degree of patellar hypermobility [25]. Thirty-four percent of the individuals in this series had significant problems, including frank subluxation of the patella in 19%, dislocation in 4%, and chondromalacia patella in 6%. Knee problems present as a giving away of the knee, swelling, inability to walk, and repeated falls with secondary injury. Management of knee problems may be surgical if conservative programs, such as exercise and braces, are unsuccessful.

Finally, we come down to the feet of the patient with Down syndrome—the famous flat feet (pes planus). If these feet become painful and tender, the individual may become relatively immobile. In addition, medial deviation of the first ray of the foot (metatarsus primus varus) is seen in 91% of institutionalized persons with Down syndrome [25]. This may be accompanied by hallux varus and later by hallux valgus. All of these factors interfere with the fitting of shoes, and many patients end up wearing sneakers. There is an excellent section on the feet and their care in Chapter 6 of the Gahagen and Van Dyke monograph [23] that points out that there are medical solutions (orthoses) as well as the better-known surgery for some of the feet problems hindering the gait of this patient population.

The etiology of the joint problems in Down syndrome may not be as simple as originally thought. Livingstone and Hirst go so far as to state that hypotonia and laxity does not appear to be a major etiological factor in joint problems occurring in Down syndrome [32]. Pueschel et al. postulated an intrinsic defect of connective tissue as a basis for the hyperflexibility, citing evidence of abnormal protein structure of the tendons [33], whereas another investigator speculated about the impact of the developmental delay of tonus systems stemming from the central nervous system [34].

ARTHROPATHY

Arthritis occasionally develops in children with Down syndrome. Autoimmunity may be involved; other factors may be an increased incidence of joint mobility and unusual shapes of the bones at joint surfaces.

A juvenile rheumatoid arthritislike arthropathy is described in the literature [35,36]. An adult with inflammatory polyarthritis also is reported [37]. Even psoriatic arthritis has been described [38]. Despite the elevated uric acid levels, gout is rare and is not associated with a high metabolic turnover of purines [39].

As in other systems in the body, looking ahead and anticipating problems can save function and alter the quality of activities during the lifetime of the patient. Preventive medicine is particularly important when it comes to protection of the joints. Early handling of the medical problems arising in the joints can keep an individual free from pain, mobile, and active with the prevention of the new problems that arise from an otherwise increasingly sedentary lifestyle.

REFERENCES

1. Locke GR, Gardner JI, van Epps EF. Atlas-dens interval (ADI) in children: A survey based on 200 normal cervical spines. AJR 1966;97:135–140.
2. Brooke DC, Burkus JK, Benson DR. Asymptomatic occipito-atlantal instability in Down syndrome (trisomy 21). J Bone Joint Surg [Am] 1987;69:293–295.
3. French HG, Burke SW, Roberts JM, Johnston CE 2nd, Whitecloud T, Edmunds JO. Upper cervical ossicles in Down syndrome. J Pediatr Orthop 1987;7:69–71.
4. El-Khourry GY, Clark CR, Dietz FR, Harre RG, Tozzi JE, Kathol MH. Posterior atlantooccipital subluxation in Down syndrome. Radiology 1986;159:507–509.
5. Hungerford GD, Akkaraju V, Rowe SE, Young GF. Atlanto-occipital and atlanto-axial dislocations with spinal cord compression in Down syndrome: A case report and review of the literature. Br J Radiol 1981;54:758–761.
6. Rosenbaum DM, Blumhagen JD, King HA. Atlantooccipital instability in Down syndrome. AJR 1986;146:1269–1272.
7. Gabriel KR, Mason DE, Carango P. Occipitoatlantal translation in Down syndrome. Spine 1990;15:997–1002.
8. Weisel S, Rothman RH. Occipitoatlantal hypermobility. Spine 1979;4:187–191.
9. Tishler J, Martel W. Dislocation of the atlas in mongolism. Radiology 1965; 84:904–906.
10. Martel W, Tishler JM. Observations on the spine in mongolism. AJR 1966; 97:630–638.
11. Pueschel SM, Scola FH. Epidemiologic, radiographic and clinical studies of atlantoaxial instability in individuals with Down syndrome. Pediatrics 1987; 80:555–560.
12. Cullen S, et al. Atlanto instability in Down's syndrome: Clinical and radiological screening. Ir Med J 1989;82:64–65.
13. Burke SW, French HG, Roberts JM, Johnston CE 2nd, Whitecloud TS, Edmunds JO Jr. Chronic atlanto-axial instability in Down syndrome. J Bone Joint Surg [Am] 1985;67:1356–1360.
14. Alvarez N, Rubin L. Atlantoaxial instability in adults with Down syndrome: A clinical and radiological survey. Appl Res Ment Retard 1986;7:67–78.
15. Pueschel SM, Findley TW, Furia J, Gallagher PL, Scola FH, Pezzullo JC.

Atlantoaxial instability in Down syndrome: Roentgenographic, neurologic, and somatosensory evoked potential studies. J Pediatr 1987;110:515–521.

16. Pueschel SM, Scola FH, Tupper TB, Pezzullo JC. Skeletal anomalies of the upper cervical spine in children with Down syndrome. J Pediatr Orthoped 1990;10: 607–611.

17. Davidson RG. Atlantoaxial instability in individuals with Down syndrome: A fresh look at the evidence. Pediatrics 1988;81:857–865.

18a. Roy M, Baxter M, Roy A. Atlantoaxial instability in Down syndrome— guidelines for screening and detection. J R Soc Med 1990;83:433–435.

18b. Selby KA, Newton RW, Gupta S, Hunt L. Clinical predictions and radiological reliability in atlantoaxial subluxation in Down's syndrome. Arch Dis Childhood 1991;66:876–878.

19. Scola PS. Musculoskeletal system. In: Pueschel SM, Rynders JE. Down Syndrome: Advances in Biomedicine and the Behavioral Sciences. Cambridge, Mass: Ware Press, 1982, pp. 213–219.

20. Shikata J, Yamamuro T, Mikawa Y, Lida H, Kobori M. Surgical treatment of symptomatic atlantoaxial subluxation in Down's syndrome. Clin Orthop 1987; 220:111–118.

21. Chaudhry V, Stugeon C, Gates AJ, Myers G. Symptomatic atlantoaxial dislocation in Down's syndrome. Ann Neurol 1987;21:606–609.

22a. Aoki N. Atlantoaxial dislocation presenting as sudden onset of quadriplegia in Down's syndrome. Surg Neurol 1988;30:153–155.

22b. Tangerud A, Hestnes A, Sand T, Sunndalsfoll S. Degenerative changes in the cervical spine in Down's syndrome. J Ment Defic Res 1990;34:179–185.

23. Gahagen CA, Van Dyke DC. Foot and other musculoskeletal problems. In: Van Dyke DC, Lang DJ, Heide F, van Duyne S, Soucek MJ, eds. Clinical Perspectives in the Management of Down Syndrome. New York: Springer-Verlag, 1990:80–92.

24. Olive PM, Whitecloud TS 3rd, Bennett JT. Lower cervical spondylosis and myelopathy with Down's syndrome. Spine 1988;13:781–784.

25. Diamond LS, Lynne D, Sigman B. Orthopedic disorders in patients with Down syndrome. Orthop Clin North Am 1981;12:57–71.

26. Mautner H. Abnormal findings on the spine in mongoloids. Am J Ment Defic 1950;55:105–107.

27. Rabinowitz JC, Moseley JE. The lateral lumbar spine in Down's syndrome: A new roentgen feature. Radiology 1964;83:74–79.

28. Fabia J, Drolette M. Malformations and leukemia in children with Down's syndrome. Pediatrics 1970;45:600–670.

29. Kaufmann HJ, Taillard WF. Pelvic abnormalities in mongols. Br Med J 1961; 1:948–949.

30. Skoff HD, Keggi K. Total hip replacement in Down's syndrome. Orthopedics 1987;10:485–489.

31. Aprin H, Zink WP, Hall JE. Management of dislocation of the hip in Down syndrome. J Pediatr Orthop 1984;5:428–431.

32. Livingstone B, Hirst P. Orthopedic disorders in school children with Down syndrome with special reference to the incidence of joint laxity. Clin Orthop 1986;207:74–76.
33. Pueschel SM, Scola FH, Perry CD, Pezzullo JC. Atlanto-axial subluxation in children with Down syndrome. Pediatr Radiol 1981;10:129–132.
34. Cowie V. A study of the early development of mongols. Oxford: Pergamon Press, 1970.
35. Yancey CL, Zmijewski C, Athreya BH, Doughty RA. Arthropathy of Down's syndrome. Arthritis Rheum 1984;27:929–934.
36. Olson JC, Bender JC, Levinson JE, Oestreich A, Lovell DJ. Arthropathy of Down syndrome. Pediatrics 1990;86:931–936.
37. Dacre JE, Huskisson EC. Arthritis in Down's syndrome. Ann Rheum Dis 1988; 47:254–255.
38. Tudor RB. Psoriatic arthritis in a child with Down's syndrome. Arthritis Rheum 1976;19:651. Letter to the Editor.
39. Ciompi ML, Bazzichi LM, Bertolucci D, Mazzoni MR, Barbieri P, Mencacci S, Macchia D, Mariaani G. Uric acid metabolism in two patients with coexistent Down's syndrome and gout. Clin Rheumatol 1984;3:229–233.

12

The Endocrine System

There a number of unusual aspects of the endocrine system in patients with Down syndrome. Most work to date has been on the hormones that stimulate target organs, such as the thyroid hormones and the gonadotrophins. The pituitary and its hormones, also subjects of interest and speculation for decades, are discussed in Chapter 13.

The mechanisms that underlie the abnormalities of the endocrine system are poorly understood at this time. Hormones are proteins. We are entering the age where genetic control of protein synthesis is beginning to be decoded. However, it will be some time before we will have unraveled the exact mechanisms for the endocrine disorders in Down syndrome because the path from the primary action of the genes to the final manifestation of a disorder is extremely complex; it involves many interactions along the way. The story is even more complicated when there is extra genetic material playing an additional role as occurs in so many chromosome disorders.

Yet it is not necessary to wait until the full picture of endocrine dysfunction in Down syndrome emerges from DNA probes. Already, there is medical information available that can lead to early diagnosis and rational medical care of the endocrine disorders that present in some individuals with Down syndrome. This early diagnosis and treatment is particularly important in the thyroid disorders because the thyroid hormone plays a number of important roles in human brain function.

THYROID DYSFUNCTION

Down syndrome and hypothyroidism now have come full circle. The differentiation of children with Down syndrome (a chromosome disorder) from children with cretinism (infant hypothyroidism) in 1866 was a major step forward in the ability to accurately diagnose children with mental retardation [1]. The historical confusion between the two patient groups is understandable because clinically the patients do have some resemblances to each other (Table 12.1). After Down syndrome was distinguished from cretinism, the history of Down syndrome in the late nineteenth and twentieth centuries still showed a great number of studies and trials of therapy focused on thyroid—this history is thoroughly reviewed in Pueschel and Rynders' fine textbook [2]. The idea that all Down syndrome children had a thyroid problem kept reappearing in the minds of some investigators for more than a century after the two syndromes (Down and cretinism) were distinguished [3]. The clinical resemblance between the two patient groups (Down syndrome and hypothyroidism) makes it very difficult for a physician to this day to pick up developing thyroid disease in a Down syndrome patient by clinical observation alone; for example, is that dry skin and weight gain indicative of a new endocrine complication or just part of the original Down syndrome?

Table 12.1 Comparison of Physical Characteristics of Children with Down Syndrome and Hypothyroidism

Characteristic	Down Syndrome	Hypothyroidism
Appearance	Dull, chubby	Dull, chubby
Head	Microcephalic	Normal
Tongue	Large	Large
Nasal bridge	Underdeveloped	Underdeveloped
Eyes	Slanted	Not slanted
Neck	Short	Short
Heart	Murmur (AV canal)	Murmur (thick valve and septum)
Abdomen	Protuberant umbilical hernia	Protuberant umbilical hernia
Neuromuscular	Hypotonia	Hypotonia
Skin	Dry	Dry
Extremities	Short, transverse palmar crease	Short, no transverse
Development	Retarded	Variable

AV = atrioventricular.
Source: From Ref. 20, used with permission.

In the last decade, it has become quite clear that, although some individuals with Down syndrome are born with or later develop thyroid disease, it is likely that the majority of people with the syndrome remain euthyroid throughout their lives. The studies suggest that the percentage of individuals with Down syndrome at risk for thyroid disease gradually increases with age. At birth, 0.7% of the infants with Down syndrome have persistent primary congenital hypothyroidism [4], whereas the figure for adults with hypothyroidism rises to at least 12% [5]. Other studies of adults have reported abnormalities in one or more tests of thyroid function as high as 22% [6] or 40% [7]. The problem of determining the age or ages at which children with Down syndrome have the highest level of risk for the onset of thyroid disease has not been adequately studied, but a preliminary study suggests it can occur at any age. In a clinic using the Down Syndrome Preventive Medical Checklists, previously un-suspected thyroid disease was identified by routine annual laboratory testing in ages 1–3, 6, 10, 11, 13–15, and 16 years—in short, throughout the childhood years and beyond [8] (see Figure 12.1).

This increased proclivity that individuals with Down syndrome have for developing thyroid disease, combined with the difficulties of making the diagnosis on clinical grounds alone underlies the recommendation in the Down Syndrome Preventive Medicine Checklists for routine annual thyroid screening in patients in a Down syndrome clinic (see Chapters 3–7).

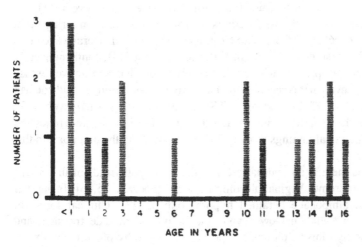

Figure 12.1 Age at onset of hypothyroidism in 16 young trisomy 21 patients who received routine follow-up in a preventive medicine clinic.

Routine screening for congenital hypothyroidism in every newborn that now exists in many countries has removed the difficulties of diagnosis in the neonatal period [9]. A report from one large screening program detected various degrees of thyroid dysfunction in 12 out of 1130 infants identified with Down syndrome [4]. One infant died, and that original test result could not be confirmed. Of the remaining 11 infants, three had only transient thyroid abnormalities. This left eight with persistent primary hypothyroidism; however, the etiology of the thyroid aberrations in these infants with Down syndrome was unclear. None had agenesis or ectopia of the thyroid gland. In this screening study, the incidence of persistent primary congenital hypothyroidism in infants with Down syndrome was 1:141, which is 28 times more frequent than found in the general population [4].

It also is of interest that maternal thyroid disease has been noted in an increased incidence in the parents of children with Down syndrome by several investigators [10,11].

In young children with Down syndrome, the problem of diagnosis of hypothyroidism by clinical criteria alone remains difficult. Goiter, which can be seen with hypothyroidism, hyperthyroidism, or even euthyroidism is one of the more obvious clues [12]. The prominent features of severe hypothyroidism include growth deviation from a previous channel of growth, increased lethargy, constipation, and eventually the development of myxedema. Growth deviation also has been reported in children who do not meet the classic laboratory criteria of hypothyroidism because they have normal thyroxine (T_4) levels in association with elevated thyroid-stimulating hormone (TSH) levels [13].

Developing thyroid disease in adults also needs careful monitoring. In a recent study of 106 adults from 20 to 67 years of age (with an average age of 38 years), 40% had test results of abnormal thyroid function [14], confirming early studies [7]. Not all patients with abnormal test results have an active disease process: Only seven in this recent study had active hypothyroidism and one had thyrotoxicosis [14]. Elevated levels of TSH combined with normal levels of T_4 accounted for the majority of abnormal test results. The investigators reiterated the point that clinical findings were of little use in making the diagnosis in this patient group.

Sometimes there is an unusual presentation of hypothyroidism in patients with Down syndrome. Vaginal bleeding has been reported [15,16]. In another case, cardiac tamponade heralded hypothyroidism [17]. Clinical forms of hypothyroidism found in Down syndrome individual include transient and primary hypothyroidism, pituitary-hypothalamic hypothyroidism, thyroxine-binding globulin (TBG) deficiency, and chronic lymphocytic thyroiditis.

Hyperthyroidism also occurs in Down syndrome. In each series reporting on the frequency of hypothyroidism in Down syndrome, one or more cases of hyperthyroidism also may be mentioned [18,19]. Exophthalmus is even rarer. In children with Down syndrome, clinical recognition of hyperthyroidism can be as difficult as diagnosing hypothyroidism because symptoms may be masked. The existing hypotonia, inactivity, and lack of subjective complaints fail to alert the examiner to the correct diagnosis [20]. Suggestive findings of hyperthyroidism include weight loss, hyperactivity, diarrhea, nervousness, and goiter. The shortness and chubbiness of the neck make it difficult to detect thyromegaly by observation. In such patients, careful palpation of the neck is necessary to detect a goiter.

One of the most interesting things about thyroid disease in Down syndrome patients is that one type of thyroid disease—autoimmune thyroid disease—found in this patient group is also found in other cytogenetic disorders [21]. Trisomy 21 is an autosomal trisomy; autoimmune thyroiditis is also found in several of the sex chromosomal abnormalities. These include Klinefelter's syndrome (XXY), Turner's syndrome (XO), and a syndrome resembling Turner's (Noonan's syndrome) that has normal chromosomes. The thyroid antibodies are frequently found and become commoner with age but are not, in themselves, guides to clinical dysfunction and the need for therapy. Regular testing of TSH and the other thyroid hormone levels remains the bedrock of accurate diagnosis in these individuals. In all patients with positive antibody titers—Down syndrome and other groups—it is assumed that these persons are at greater risk of developing thyroid disease and should be followed closely (see Chapter 15 regarding autoimmunity in Down syndrome).

There have been a number of recent clinical studies supporting the importance of regular thyroid screening in Down syndrome. In 1985, Pueschel and Pezzullo reported on the results of 151 children and their sibling controls [22]. The children with Down syndrome were 3 to 21 years old. In their series, 27% had an abnormality of TSH, T_4, or both. Ten (7%) had both increased TSH levels and decreased T_4 levels, whereas another 15 (10%) had increased TSH levels with normal T_4 levels. They noted that there were higher TSH concentrations in adolescents and decreasing T_4 levels with the advancing age of the patients. They even raised the question of whether the described decline of intelligence quotients of persons with Down syndrome over time might be, in part, due to undetected, inadequate thyroid function.

Loudon et al. also published a large series in 1985 of 116 home-based children; three were hypothyroid, one was hyperthyroid [19]. They found thyroid antibodies in 29% of the patients and also a high incidence in their normal relatives and those of controls. Transient increases in TSH levels seemed common in these children, particularly during periods of intercurrent illness [19]. In 1986, Cutler et al. studied 49 children less than 3 years of age [18]. Three had congenital hypothyroidism, two had thyroid antibodies (one each with acquired hypothyroidism and hyperthyroidism), but 27% already had mildly increased TSH levels. In 1990, Van Dyke et al. evaluated 132 children from 2 months to 19 years of age and found that 8% had some abnormality of thyroid function [23].

Thus, the medical literature is unequivocal about the increased frequency of thyroid dysfunction among a population of individuals with Down syndrome. Important investigations remain to be completed regarding the reason for this increased frequency in Down syndrome and other chromosomal disorders and, most importantly, the implications for brain function and general health in these patient groups.

Screening techniques (i.e., TSH, T_4 for children) are already in place in the Down Syndrome Preventive Medical Checklists to anticipate and thus to prevent the complications, particularly the intellectual deterioration [22], that may accompany the onset of active thyroid disease in children with Down syndrome. When there is any question, additional studies such as TBG, IRMA, and RAI uptake can be used to evaluate the status of thyroid dysfunction. The presence of thyroglobulin and antimicrosomal antibodies may be needed to determine the etiology of the thyroid dysfunction or to alert the physician that this patient may be at even higher risk than usual.

A major unsolved problem regarding endocrine studies in patients with Down syndrome is the question of why so many individuals have elevated TSH levels in the presence of normal thyroid hormone (T_4) levels. Exaggerated TSH responses to thyrotropin-releasing hormone have been recorded in these individuals who have elevated levels of TSH yet normal levels of T_4 [24]. This is an area of active current research. One hypothesis is that the deficiency in the cholinergic pathway in individuals with Down syndrome may affect central mechanisms controlling TSH secretion. Triple gene dosage creating auto-immune phenomena is another hypothesis under study.

GONADAL FUNCTION

The development of secondary sex characteristics, which heralds the onset of puberty, occurs in the usual order of appearance in children with Down syndrome. In 1987, Hsiang et al. studied 100 home-reared children with Down syndrome excluding patients with abnormal thyroid function [25]. For both males and females, they found the ages of onset and completion of puberty were normal. In a study of adolescent development in males with Down syndrome in 1985, Pueschel et al. found that the secondary sex characteristics generally to be similar to that of youngsters who do not have a chromosome disorder [26]. However, they noted that axillary hair development and the emergence of facial hair, particularly mustache development, was delayed when compared to that of normal subjects. This confirmed earlier reports of later development of axillary and pubic hair [27,28].

It is unclear whether cryptorchidism is found in boys with Down syndrome more frequently than in normal controls. Hsiang et al. found the frequency similar to that of the general population [25], whereas Oster found unilateral or bilateral cryptorchidism present in 27% of his study population of individuals with Down syndrome [29]. Thompson and Thompson's results support Oster's findings; they claim up to 50% of male patients with Down syndrome have cryptorchidism [30]. The size of the testicles is also controversial. Several studies [25,31a] have found reduced testicular volume in adult males, whereas Pueschel et al. found no statistically significant difference between the size of the genitalia of adolescents with Down syndrome and that of normal controls [26]. It may be possible to reconcile these conflicting reports if one accepts the thesis of Hsiang et al. that gonadal deficiency is often found in Down syndrome and, when present, is a progressive phenomenon with age and is most clearly manifested in adult patients [25]. Yet it should be noted that testosterone levels as measured by techniques utilizing both serum [26] and plasma [25] are reported to be normal in adolescent and adult males. One study of institutionalized adults found diminished prolactin levels in men with Down syndrome [31b].

The patterns of follicle-stimulating hormone (FSH) and luteinizing hormone (LH) levels were evaluated in age groups by Hsiang et al. [25]. FSH serum levels were greater than normal in 55% of the male infants, whereas serum LH levels were abnormally elevated in 38% of female infants. In prepubertal children, a few boys and girls had abnormally elevated FSH and LH levels. In the 23 adult men in the study, the mean serum levels of both FSH and LH were significantly elevated [25]. These data suggest that there may be partial Leydig cell deficiency consistent with the findings of Horan et al. [32], Hasen et al. [33], and Campbell et al. [34]. However, Pueschel et al. reported normal levels of these serum gonadotrophins [26]. Six out of 14 women in the study by Hsiang et al. had primary gonadal dysfunction [25].

Regarding menstruation, Pueschel et al. reported that girls with Down syndrome have regular menstrual cycles occurring, on the average, every 27 days with a menstrual flow about 4 days long [26]. However, hypoplasia of the ovaries has been reported [35]. Hojager et al. examined the ovaries of girls with Down syndrome who died before age 14 years and found that the number of small antral follicles was diminished [36]. As in the control group, the number of follicles declined with age, but there was a dramatic decrease in follicles among the girls with Down syndrome after 3 years of age.

Ovulatory patterns to date have only been reported in 13 women living mostly in residential facilities [37]. Through vaginal smears, five had evidence of normal ovarian function, whereas four had no evidence of ovulation. Results were equivocal in the remaining patients. Twenty-nine pregnancies in 26 women with Down syndrome have been reported in the literature clearly documenting that there was adequate ovarian function for these individuals (Table 12.2). There are also a number of less-well-documented pregnancies that have been reported [38].

Table 12.2 Reproduction in Females with Nonmosaic Down Syndrome

Number of Mother	Karyotype of Offspring Where Verified	Sex and Status of Offspring	Presumptive Father and Mental Status Where Known
1	—	1 Normal female	Patient's father
2	—	2 Male with DS	Mentally retarded; not DS
3*	47,XX, +21	3 Female with DS	Patient's father suspected
4*	46,XY	4 Slight MR; suspect CHD	Blind 60-year-old patient with epilepsy (not MR) (normal 46,XY)
5	—	5 Female with MR; may represent "partial trisomy"	Patient's father suspected
6*	46,XY	6 Normal male	—
7	—	7 Normal male	Mental debility?
8*	—	8 Male with DS	Mother's brother with MR (46,XY)
	47,XY, +21	9 Female with DS	Mother's brother with MR (46,XY)
9*	46,XY	10 Apparently normal monozygotic twin males	Patient's father (normal IQ)
10	—	11 Normal male	Question of father having DS but unsubstantiated

Table 12.2 Continued

Number of Mother	Karyotype of Offspring Where Verified	Sex and Status of Offspring	Presumptive Father and Mental Status Where Known
11*	—	12 Macerated female fetus, spontaneous abortion at 28 weeks; status not known	—
		13 Male with DS	—
12*	46,XX	14 Normal female	—
13*	—	15 3-month-old fetus, sex and status not known	—
	46,XX	16 Normal female	—
14*	47,XX, + 21	17 Female with DS	—
15*	47,XY, + 21	18 Male with DS	MR but may be due to brain damage
16*	46,XX	19 Normal female	—
17*	46,XX	20 Normal female	—
18*	46,XY	21 Normal male	Normal
19*	47,XX, +21	22 Female with DS	+50-year-old invalid with tuberculosis
20*	46,XX	23 Normal female	Patient's husband (IQ = 70)
21*	47XY, + 21	24 Male with DS	Patient's husband (normal IQ)
22	46,XY + additional chromosome in 4.4%	25 Normal male with some stigmata of DS; question of mosaicism	—
23*	47,XX, +21	26 Female with DS	—
24*	46,XY	27 Normal male except for hypospadias, low set ears, syndactyly of 2nd/3rd toes, and subluxed right hip	Patient's father
25*	46,XY	28 Normal male karyotype; multiple malformations	Patient's brother
26*	46,XY	29 Normal male born prematurely at 30 weeks	Patient's uncle

*Mother's karyotype verified cytogenetically.
CHD = congenital heart disease; DS = Down syndrome; IQ = intelligence quotient; MR = mental retardation.
Source: Adapted from Ref. 38.

Fertility in males is less likely. One case is well documented of a 29-year-old man with nonmosaic trisomy 21 who impregnated a mentally retarded girl who had no specific medical diagnosis and who lived in the same group home with him [38]. The fetus, lost a few weeks after a prenatal diagnosis procedure (transcervical chorionic villus sampling), had a normal male chromosomal complement (46, XY). This is the first documented case in the medical literature. Studies of spermatogenesis to date report abnormal semen quality and impaired fertility [30,39]. This is an area where further detailed studies are needed.

REFERENCES

1. Down JL. Observations on an ethnic classification of idiots. Lond Hosp Clin Lect Rep. 1866;3:259–262.
2. Pueschel SM, Rynders JE. Down Syndrome: Advances in Biomedicine and the Behavioral Sciences. Cambridge, Mass: Ware Press, 1982.
3. Benda CE. Down's Syndrome: Mongolism and Its Management. New York: Grune & Stratton, 1969:166–208.
4. Fort P, Lifshitz F, Bellisario R, Davis J, Lanes R, Pugliese M, Richmond R, Post EM, David R. Abnormalities of thyroid function in infants with Down syndrome. J Pediatr 1984;104:545–549.
5. Korsager S, Chatham EM, Ostergaard-Kristensen HP. Thyroid function tests in adults with Down syndrome. Acta Endocrinol (Copenh) 1978;88:48–54.
6. Mani C. Hypothyroidism in Down's syndrome. Br J Psychiatry 1988;153:102–104.
7. Murdoch JC, Ratcliffe WA, McLarty DG, Rodger JC. Thyroid function in adults with Down's syndrome. J Clin Endocrinol Metab 1977;44:453–458.
8. Abassi V, Coleman M. A preventive medicine report on Down's syndrome and hypothyroidism. Down's Syndrome: Papers and Abstracts for Professionals 1984;7:1–2.
9. Fisher DH, Dussault JH, Foley TP, Klein AH, LaFranchi S, Larsen PR, Mitchell ML, Murphey WH, Walfish PG. Screening for congenital hypothyroidism: Results of screening one million North American infants. J Pediatr 1979;94:700–705.
10. Myers CR. An application of the control group method to the problem of the etiology of mongolism. Proc Am Assoc Ment Defic 1938;43:142.
11. Fialkow PJ, Thuline HC, Hecht F, Bryant J. Familial predisposition to thyroid disease in Down's syndrome: Controlled immunoclinical studies. Am J Hum Genet 1971;23:67–86.
12. Hayle AB, et al. Thyroid disease among children with Down's syndrome. Pediatrics 1965;36:608.
13. Sharav T, Collins RM, Baab PJ. Growth studies in infants and children with Down's syndrome and elevated levels of thyrotropin. Am J Dis Child 1988; 142:1302–1306.

14. Dinani S, Carpenter S. Down's syndrome and thyroid disorder. J Ment Defic Res 1990;34:187–193.
15. Hubble D. Precocious menstruation in a mongoloid child with hypothyroidism-hormonal overlap. J Clin Endocrinol Metab 1963;23:1302.
16. Lund PKM. Samtidig forekomst av mongolism og hypothyreose. Tid Norsk Lsegeforen 1959;18:394.
17. Heydarian M, Kelly PJ. Radiological case of the month: Cardiac tamponade heralding hypothyroidism in Down's syndrome. Am J Dis Child 1987;141: 641–642.
18. Cutler AT, Benezra-Obeiter R, Brink SJ. Thyroid function in young children with Down syndrome. Am J Dis Child 1986;140:479–483.
19. Loudon MM, Day RE, Duke EM. Thyroid dysfunction in Down's syndrome. Arch Dis Child 1985;60:1149–1151.
20. Abassi V. Thyroid disease and Down's syndrome. Down's Syndrome: Papers and Abstracts for Professionals 1980;3:7–8.
21. Kelnar CJH. Thyroid disturbances in cytogenetic disease. Dev Med Child Neurol 1989;31:400–404.
22. Pueschel SM, Pezzullo JC. Thyroid dysfunction in Down syndrome. Am J Dis Child 1985;139:636–639.
23. Van Dyke DC, Lang DL, Miller JD, Heide F, van Duyne S, Chang H. Common medical problems. In: Van Duke DC, Lang DJ, Heide F, van Duyne S, Soucek MJ, eds. Clinical Perspectives in the Management of Down Syndrome. New York: Springer-Verlag, 1990:3–14.
24. Pozzan GB, Rigon F, Girelli ME, Rubello D, Busnardo B, Baccichetti C. Thyroid function in patients with Down syndrome: Preliminary results from non-institutionalized patients in the Veneto region. Am J Med Genet 1990;(suppl 7): 57–58.
25. Hsiang YH, Berkovitz GD, Bland GL, Migeon CJ, Warren AC. Gonadal function in patients with Down syndrome. Am J Med Genet 1987;27:449–458.
26. Pueschel SM, Orson JM, Boylan JM, Pezzullo JC. Adolescent development in males with Down syndrome. Am J Dis Child 1985;139:236–238.
27. Shelley WB, Butterworth T. The absence of apocrine glands and hair in the axilla in mongolism and idiocy. J Invest Dermatol 1955;25:165.
28. Smith GF, Warren SA, Turner DR. Hair characteristics in mongolism (Down's syndrome). Am J Ment Defic 1963;68:362.
29. Oster J. Mongolism: A clinico-geneological investigation comprising 526 mongols living in Seeland and neighboring islands of Denmark. Copenhagen: Danish Science Press, 1953.
30. Thompson IM, Thompson DD. Male fertility and the undescended testis in Down syndrome: How to counsel parents. Postgrad Med 1988;84:299–303.
31a. Rundle AT, Sylvester PE. Endocrinological aspects of mental deficiency: II. Maturational status of adult males. J Ment Defic Res 1962;6:8.
31b. Hestnes A, Stovner LJ, Husoy O, Folling I, Fougner KJ, Sjaastad O. Hormonal and

biochemical disturbances in Down's syndrome. J Ment Defic Res 1991;35: 179–193.

32. Horan RF, Beitins IZ, Bode HH. LH-RH testing in men with Down's syndrome. Acta Endocrinol 1978;88:594–600.

33. Hasen J, Boyar RM, Shapiro LR. Gonadal function in trisomy 21. Horm Res 1980; 12:345–350.

34. Campbell WA, Lowther J, McKenzie I, Price WH. Serum gonadotropins in Down's syndrome. J Med Genet 1982;19:98–99.

35. Benda CE. Down's syndrome: Mongolism and its management. New York: Grune & Stratton, 1969.

36. Hojager B, Peters H, Byskov AG, Faber M. Follicular development in ovaries of children with Down's syndrome. Acta Paediatr Scand 1978;67:637–643.

37. Tricomi V, Valenti C, Hall JE. Ovulatory patterns in Down's syndrome. Am J Obstet Gynecol 1964;89:651–656.

38. Sheridan R, Llerena J, Matkins S, Debenham P, Cawood A, Bobrow M. Fertility in a male with trisomy 21. J Med Genet 1989;26:294– 298.

39. Johannisson R, Gropp A, Winking H, Coerdt W, Rehder H, Schwinger E. Down's syndrome in the male: Reproductive pathology and meiotic studies. Hum Genet 1983;63:132–138.

13

The Central Nervous System

Like all human brains, the central nervous system of a person with Down syndrome is an incredibly complex and beautiful organ. This is often forgotten in the search to demonstrate the abnormalities that underlie the brain dysfunction in these children, abnormalities rarely demonstrated satisfactorily in 100% of the patients to date. At this time, there are a number of misconceptions about the central nervous system in people with Down syndrome. Two examples of our current misunderstandings are the concept that the brain of an infant with Down syndrome is born already so compromised at birth that innate mental retardation is inevitable and the concept that elderly individuals with Down syndrome are all demented.

In this chapter, the medical information available about the brain in the Down syndrome individual will be discussed from the point of view of many disciplines, from pathology to behavioral science. While reading over these many studies, it is important to keep in mind that our knowledge of brain function in individuals with Down syndrome is quite preliminary and subject to change.

BRAIN STRUCTURE AND FUNCTION

There is information available on the size and structure of the Down syndrome brain from fetal studies until the end of life. Anatomic differences are well documented of a smaller brain weight on average, at birth and throughout life [1,2], with the brainstem and the cerebellum particularly diminished in size compared to nonhandicapped controls. A monumental study by Wisniewski of 780 children with Down syndrome from birth to 5 years of age reported that brain shape in newborn infants was the same as in non-Down syndrome infants and that the brain weight in the neonates fell within the lower normal range [3]. However, by 3–6 months of age, the brains began to decelerate their rate of growth as measured by cranial circumference in living children and the brain weights on autopsy. This midinfancy deceleration of growth resulted in 69% of the brain weights measuring below the normal range by 7–12 months of age [3]. This deceleration was more marked in girls than in boys; it was also strongly associated with the presence of congenital cardiac disease and gastrointestinal malformations. In an autopsy study of 36 persons of many ages and Down syndrome, Solitare and Lamarche obtained a range of brain weights from 850 to 1370 g [5]. In a study limited to adults, the average brain weight in Down syndrome was determined to be 76% of normal, with an average brain stem and cerebellar weight 66% of normal [4].

Usually, microcephaly is present when the cranial circumference is measured in this patient group [6], but it should be noted that, in the Wisniewski study of children up to 5 years of age, 20% were in the lower normal range [3]. People with Down syndrome are little people, and when the head size is recalculated against body length, the cranial circumference tends to fall within the lower normal range [7].

Specific details of neuropathological studies after 5 months of age show the areas contributing to the deceleration process [8]. In the front, the frontal lobes are relatively reduced [3], and in the back, the occipital poles are flatter and there is a disproportionately smaller cerebellum and brain stem [9]. A narrowing of the superior temporal gyrus has been noted [10] in approximately one-third of this patient group. Although cerebellar hypoplasia is a consistent finding in postnatal studies, it cannot be demonstrated in second trimester fetuses by ultrasound measurements, as reported in a study of 23 fetuses whose transverse cerebellar diameters were within normal range for gestational age [11].

Myelination of the brain has been found delayed in 23% of Down syndrome brains compared to a control group with 7% delay [12]. This suggests that delayed myelination, a theoretical source for past speculation as the etiology of many findings in this patient group, is not present in more than three-quarters of these infants.

The sheer volume of neurons and glia and their axonal and dendritic branches in a human brain make it difficult to quantify them; there are conflicting reports about calculating these numbers in individuals who are mentally retarded. During the last trimester of gestation, there is some preliminary evidence of prenatal slowing of neurogenesis (neuronal migration) [3].

Most reviews of the literature tend to emphasize that most abnormalities in the growth and elaboration of neuronal networks occur after birth [9,14]. In a study trying to answer the question "Is there a decreased population of neurons?" Ross et al. found a loss of granular neurons in the cerebral cortex [13]. Wisniewski also reports some diminution in the number of granular neurons of layers II and IV in the cortex [3]; these cells are the last to migrate during brain development. They are associational neurons and play a role in local circuits.

Regarding dendritic development leading to synaptogenesis, there are four interesting contemporary studies. Marin-Padilla evaluated an 18-month-old with Down syndrome [15]. Suetsugu and Meharaein compared seven young children with Down syndrome to five older patients with nonspecific retardation [16]; there is a controlled study by Becker et al. comparing the brains of eight children with Down syndrome to the brains of eight children who died of causes other than neurological disease [17]; and Wisniewski compared five brains from Down syndrome children with five brains of age-matched controls [3]. In interpreting these studies, it is necessary to keep in mind that when children with Down syndrome die at a young age, they often are severely handicapped cardiac patients whose brains may not have the full sensory input of a normally active child and may have been affected by chronic hypoxia or cardiotrophic medications. These studies reported results on the dendritic tree and, in particular, the dendritic spines.

The study by Becker et al. concentrated on the visual cortex, and they report the surprising finding that the development of the dendritic "tree" in very young infants with Down syndrome was more advanced than in the normal infants [17]. However, by 2 years of age, the dendritic branches in the cortex were much shorter and significantly fewer in number. Wisniewski studied synaptic density in the visual cortex from ages 1 day to 18 years and found various results from 1% to 29% decrease in this density; at 9 years of age, it was 91% of the control values [3]. Both the Marin-Padilla [15] and the Suetsugu and Meharaein [16] studies agreed that there was a decrease in spines along apical dendrites in children with Down syndrome past 18 months of age. Suetsugu and Meharaein make the further point that this phenomenon may not be a common feature in mental retardation because it was not found in patients with other types of retardation. Dysgenesis of dendritic spines has also been reported. Long-necked spines, usually seen in fetal brains, are reported sometimes to persist after birth [18,19]. The speculation is either that they were formed that way and have failed to mature when expected or that they underwent trans-synaptic degeneration [15,16].

Neuronal membranes have been studied in cultured human dorsal root ganglia from Down syndrome [20] and in trisomy mice [21]. Membranes from both trisomy species share unusual features including decreased action potential after hyperpolarizations and decreased voltage thresholds for action potential generation. This is an area of important future research.

Studies have been performed on the acetylcholine pathways in the infant brain in an effort to determine to what extent they are abnormal. The cholinergic marker enzymes have normal or above-normal enzyme activity during the first year of postnatal life [22,23]. These markers are mainly presynaptic. Regarding the density of postsynaptic muscarinic receptors, normal patterns were found in the forebrain, whereas a marked reduction was counted in the midbrain (superior colliculus, substantia nigra) [24].

In living patients, a semiautomated method of analysis of data obtained by computed tomography (CT) scanning can be used to estimate brain size. Such a study has been performed that shows that the smaller brains in young adults with Down syndrome reflect their smaller body stature and smaller cranial vault. For example when looking for evidence of atrophy, these investigators found that ventricular volumes, when normalized to intracranial volume, did not differ significantly between the patients and controls [25]. Even older adults with Down syndrome, provided they do not have clinical evidence of dementia, do not show cerebral atrophy [26]. (In the case of older adults with an active Alzheimer's disease process, cerebral atrophy can be documented on quantitative CT scans; see the section on Alzheimer's disease in this chapter.)

Positron-emission tomography (PET) is a relatively new technique that allows in vivo measurement of cerebral metabolism of glucose using radiolabeled fluorodeoxyglucose as a tracer. In the first study of four young adults with Down syndrome, the right cerebral hemisphere showed significantly more uptake of glucose than did controls. This increased level was also noted in other studies [27,28a]. However, after detailed technical corrections, a new study by some of the same investigators reported regional cerebral glucose metabolism normal in young adults with Down syndrome [28a]. A second study with fluorodeoxyglucose also found marked elevations in brain metabolism in young adults with Down syndrome [28b]. This correlated with a study of the basal metabolic rate (as measured by open-circuit indirect calorimeter) of the body as a whole in healthy adults with Down syndrome which does not differ from rates in nonhandicapped controls [29]. Currently, very complicated studies comparing brain regions to each other are underway using PET scanning; results are interpreted as suggesting imbalances in the functional associations of the two brain regions being tested. One early study in adults with Down syndrome reported that the inferior frontal gyrus (which includes Broca's area—an important language center) appeared to be particularly affected by functional disassociation [30]. All this work with PET scanning needs duplication by other centers and control of many technical variables before it will be clear exactly what is being described by these provocative results.

Electroencephalography (EEG) is another tool to evaluate brain activity. There is a quite thorough review of the subject by Scola in Pueschel and Rynders' textbook [31]. Reports of abnormal EEGs range from 23% [32] to 88% [33] in this patient group; this is not very helpful. Regarding the many EEGs reported as abnormal in Down syndrome, it is important to remember to treat the patient, not the EEG. Probably the greatest value of the baseline EEG in this patient group is as an aid to diagnosis of seizure disorders.

The patterns formed from computer analysis of baseline EEG amplitudes (which appear to be somewhat different in Down syndrome children compared to their nonhandicapped controls) is an interesting finding that needs further replication and interpretation [34].

Computer-averaged click-evoked potentials (auditory, visual, and somatosensory) of the EEG that can be obtained on any child while sleeping have been studied in Down syndrome children beginning in 1967 [35]. These early studies consistently recorded abnormalities of sensory processing in this patient group up through the cortical level of functioning [36–43]. Such evoked potential studies also can be useful to detect spinal cord compression in patients with atlantoaxial dislocation [44].

The state of the peripheral sensory organ transmitting the impulse has to be taken into account in evaluating evoked potentials in any individual child with Down syndrome. Currently, auditory brain stem-evoked responses (ABERs) are used to measure peripheral auditory function in this patient group [45]. Because hearing loss is so frequent in patients with Down's syndrome, most of these ABER results reflect anatomic and inflammatory abnormalities of the ear in children with Down syndrome (see Chapter 8).

The contemporary method of using evoked potentials to measure cortical processing in patients with Down syndrome are the novelty and attention-related event potentials (ERPs) [46–48]. They require the patient to be awake with at least some focus of attention. Using these ERPs, the response amplitudes tend to be smaller and the peak latencies longer than controls. These abnormalities may be exaggerated in elderly and demented patients.

There are several examples of how evoked potentials have been used to correlate with cognitive function in children with Down syndrome. One study examined the effect of administering pyridoxine to children with Down syndrome [49]. A group of infants were given either pyridoxine or a placebo from the neonatal period through 3 years of age in an attempt to improve cognitive function. Evoked potentials at 1 year of age were not significantly different between patients and controls [50,51]. However, the data from the children at

3 years of age showed that evoked potential amplitudes of the placebo group actually increased farther from the normal range, whereas those of the children receiving pyridoxine had a decrease of their evoked potential amplitudes to within the normal range [51]. Despite the improved evoked potential amplitudes, there was no statistically significant difference in the cognitive performance on intelligence quotient tests of the pyridoxine or placebo group [50,52].

Another study of the use of a single evoked potential component, the P300 latency, failed as an assessment measure to determine cognitive ability in patients with Down syndrome even though this particular measurement was helpful for such a measurement in other patient groups [53].

SLEEP

Sleep disturbances occur with many children, and those with Down syndrome are no exception to this rule. Probably only two types of sleep disturbances occur significantly more frequently in children and young adults with Down syndrome when compared to the general population.

Sleep apnea, especially the obstructive type, may be seen in children with Down syndrome who have a tendency to obstruction of the upper airway during sleep. A number of different factors may combine to cause this disturbance, including hypotonia in pharyngeal muscles, tongue placement, and relatively undersized throat structures combined with upper respiratory infections that may enlarge the tonsils and adenoids. Apnea temporarily lowers the amount of oxygen in the blood, and this hypoxia can cause an interrupted sleep with frequent half-awakenings. If the episodes occur chronically, long-term consequences could be poor weight gain and eventually even pulmonary hypertension. Such children may need an apnea monitor and may need surgical procedures.

Noetzel has identified a sleep disturbance in children with Down syndrome that he calls the "restless sleep syndrome" [54]. It refers to an unusually high level of motor activity during sleep, particularly in the first part of the night. Polysomnographic recordings show the underlying basis of this phenomenon. Body movements during sleep are statistically more frequent during sleep in these children than in controls [55]. The disturbed sleep does not have a known medical implication and does not need evaluation or treatment.

SEIZURE DISORDERS

Seizure disorders have never been as prominent a feature in Down syndrome as in some other forms of mental retardation [56]. Special patterns of seizure disorders that can be seen in this patient group are infantile spasms in early childhood, reflex seizures in adults, and seizures associated with Alzheimer's disease in older adults.

In recent years, there have been studies with large enough groups of individuals with Down syndrome evaluated with a standard definition of convulsive disorders to allow some conclusions to be drawn (Table 13.1). There is evidence that the overall prevalence of seizure disorders increases with age. In the case of children, one study even has suggested that febrile convulsions are less prevalent in children with Down syndrome than in the general population [57]. Half of the studies suggested that less than 2% of children have seizures [57,58], whereas the other half have 5% and 8.5% figures with a heavy weighting of babies with infantile spasms [59,60]. Regarding adults, the prevalence figures are somewhere near 6% [58,60,61]. The Veall study, with a large number of patients surveyed, reported two peaks for the age of onset between ages 16 and 23 years and ages 45 and 54 years [58]. The Strafstrom et al. study also showed a seizure increase in the group from 15 to 22 years of age [56].

Infantile spasms (also known as West's syndrome) are an age-dependent epileptic encephalopathy that has a classic hypsarrhythmic pattern on the EEG. It is usually followed by developmental retardation and autisticlike symptoms even in the infants who would not otherwise be mentally affected after the seizures ceased. Infantile spasms are found in patients with many established syndromes as well as in a group of babies with no known predisposing factor— a group labeled "idiopathic" [62]. There are a number of articles reporting infantile spasms in infants with Down syndrome [57,59,60,63–65]. A seizure disorder closely resembling infantile spasms also has been induced by administration of 5-hydroxytryptophan, a precursor of serotonin, to infants with Down

Table 13.1 Seizure Frequency in Children and Adults with Down Syndrome

Author, Year (Reference)	Patients (N)	Children		Adults	
		Age (Yr)	Prevalence (%)	Age (Yr)	Prevalence (%)
Veall, 1974 [58]	1,154	1–19	1.9	20–55	6
Tansye, 1979 [61]	128	—	—	15–50	4
Tatsuno et al., 1984 [57]	844	1–14	1.4		
Van Dyke et al., 1990 [59]	190	1–20	5		
Romano et al., 1990 [60]	113	1–11	8.5	12–51	6.5

syndrome; this complication led to the termination of a research project [66]. In some children with Down syndrome, there is evidence that malformations of the brain may underlie the predisposition to the infantile spasms [67].

The traditional treatment for infantile spasms is adrenocorticotropic hormone (ACTH) or dexamethasone; other drugs available include valproic acid, clonazepam, and clobazam. In the case of infants with Down syndrome, the possible side effects of ACTH or steroids might be particularly troubling. These include suppressive action on human growth hormone secretion possibly affecting growth [44] and hypertrophic cardiomyopathy [68,69], which is not desirable in children already at risk for cardiac disease. In addition to the other drug treatments available as listed above, pharmacological doses of pyridoxine also have been used in suppressing the spasms [70–72].

Seizures beginning after 13 years of age are most often a result of head injury or the delayed sequelae of cardiac disease [63]. Most adult seizures are of the classic generalized tonic/clonic pattern. However, reflex seizures have been described as common in adults in Down syndrome and epilepsy, as high as 20% of the seizure patients in one series [73]. *Epilepsy with reflex seizures* is defined as a form of epilepsy that also has reflex seizures that occur in association with many other spontaneous seizures. In contrast, *reflex epilepsy* is defined as a form of epilepsy in which virtually all the seizures are precipitated by a triggering stimulus and spontaneous seizures rarely occur. In one case, in which seizures started at 20 years of age, a therapeutic trial of clonazepam substantially reduced the frequency of reflex-induced and spontaneous seizures [74]. Seizures in Alzheimer's disease are discussed later in this chapter.

BEHAVIOR DISORDERS

Down syndrome children are often described as affectionate and easy in temperament. Gibson reviewed the literature on this subject and noted that, if one adds obstinacy, the medical literature tends to support this stereotype [75]. In a more recent parent questionnaire, 95% of the parents described their child as happy, playful, affectionate, and liked by other children. Over 90% reported that the child was well behaved with their parents, brothers, and sisters [76].

Is this fantasy or reality? A study of the family background of children with Down syndrome reported that "Parents appeared to show a remarkable degree of tolerance toward abnormal behavior in their retarded children. Using objective measures, many more children were found with serious behavior disorders than had been identified as such by their parents. Many parents regarded the behavior difficulties as an integral part of the handicap, and their attitude was one of "resignation" [77]. In a companion article, these investigators call the concept that children with Down syndrome are easy children a "myth" [78].

It is more likely that temperament in individuals with Down syndrome is not uniform but rather that a large variety of temperamental profiles exist within this population, as in any other group of children. Although there may be some questionable evidence that these children on the whole are more passive, recent evaluations note that the organization of abilities that underlie temperament in Down syndrome is similar to that found in individuals without Down syndrome [79,80]. The personality of each child is a composite of so many factors, it is really more useful to understand each child as that special individual he or she is. To give one example of the importance of individual evaluation, the role of undiagnosed medical factors may color many studies from the past. A child reported as placid, dull, or listless could easily be suffering from undiagnosed and untreated hypothyroidism. Until this patient group as a whole has access to appropriate and comprehensive medical care, generalizations about temperament may be premature.

When this literature is reviewed, it sometimes appears that each study is about a different group of children. To compare two recent articles, by Van Dyke et al. [76] and Gath and Gumley [78], is to compare work from two centers both known for their excellence. Yet Van Dyke et al. report that only 11% of the children with Down syndrome had school problems by parent report, whereas Gath and Gumley identify 69% of children not to be well adjusted, with 38% of those having a significant behavior disorder. They report that the deviant behavior was markedly more common in the children with Down syndrome than in their siblings next in age. It may well be that the populations are different—in level of sophisticated medical care, adequacy of school placement, level of parent involvement with the child, and so on. At this time in the history of Down syndrome, generalizations about behavior should be viewed with caution. Some of the theoretical problems and interesting possibilities for research in this field are discussed by Wagner et al. [81].

As in any group of children, a small percentage of children with Down syndrome have difficulty concentrating at school, a low frustration tolerance, a high activity level, impulsivity with increased emotional lability, and are relatively unresponsive to social demands. Such children may be negativistic, irritable, and difficult for the parents, as well as for the teachers, to handle. Fortunately, in modern times, these children have been labeled "hyperactive" or "attentional deficit disorder" rather than just "bad." These children often are first identified in infant stimulation programs as infants with irritability.

There are no adequate statistics on this subgroup of children with Down syndrome; it is likely that their frequency is at least 10% and probably considerably higher. Gath and Gumley found that conduct disorders were the most common behavior problems in children with Down syndrome [78].

A truly irritable and difficult child with Down syndrome is entitled to psychological and neurological evaluation just as any other child with those symptoms would be. Among the agents available for treatment of such children are the stimulating drugs amphetamine and methylphenidate that have been shown to be effective in helping concentration and attention span [82]. A special problem in using them in children with Down syndrome is the side effect of suppression of growth by amphetamine like drugs. Shortness of stature is already a problem in children with Down syndrome. Because children with Down syndrome have a depressed whole blood serotonin level [83], they are eligible for the pyridoxine therapy of the attentional deficit disorder [84,85]. This therapy has no negative effect on growth; all therapies, including vitamins, have some side effects [49].

There is very little written about children with Down syndrome who have autistic features. Yet everyone who runs a Down syndrome clinic occasionally sees a child of this type [86]. On the other hand, physicians evaluating children with the autistic syndrome also occasionally see an individual with Down syndrome [87].

The definition of a child with Down syndrome with autistic features is one who has two or more of these criteria:

1. Significant disturbance of social relatedness to parents and peers, with poor eye contact and a sense of "aloneness."
2. Repetitive routines, such as lining up objects and insisting on the sameness of certain clothes or certain foods or certain spaces between objects, and so on. These children may have a fascination with spinning objects such as wheels of toy cars or records, bizarre attachments to certain objects such as stones, pins, pieces of plastic toys, and so on.
3. Unusual, inconstant sensory responsiveness. This can be seen in children who appear deaf at one moment and then overly sensitive to sound at another. Another example is a child who often shrinks from a touch but sometimes enjoys being tickled very forcefully.

Evaluating autistic features in a child with Down syndrome sometimes can be quite difficult. For example, deciding about hearing and sensory processing could be misleading if the auditory problem is due to recurrent otitis media (see Chapter 8), a common infection found in children with Down syndrome. A child who is irritable, withdrawn, and has poor eye contact may be developing a hidden infection, such as in the bladder (see Chapter 15). Thus, the diagnosis of autistic features should be made only if it is a consistent pattern that is well established over a period of time and after other etiologies of the symptoms have been ruled out.

Some of these children with such dual diagnoses are children with Down syndrome who developed infantile spasms as infants and who are left with subsequent autistic features. Other children may have had their dual diagnoses discovered during the original chromosome test where a fragile X site was discovered along with the supplementary material from the twenty-first chromosome. The remainder of the patients need medical evaluation for adequate diagnosis and treatment of the autistic symptoms.

In contrast to Down syndrome, in which the phenotypic symptoms all can be traced to a selective portion of one arm of a twenty-first chromosome, autism is not a single disease but a syndrome of many different etiologies. The work-up of such patients is described in full detail in the volume, *The Biology of the Autistic Syndromes* [88]. Examples of such testing include blood tests of phenylalanine, magnesium, lactic acid, and pyruvic acid; 24-hour urine tests of uric acid, calcium, HVA, and creatinine; an EEG; and an imaging test such as magnetic resonance imaging or CT. Examples of two patients with Down syndrome and autistic features who were helped by such a work-up are described in Ref. 86.

Rarely, individuals with Down syndrome may have true psychoses, indistinguishable from manic-depressive disease, schizophrenia, and so on, as seen in adults without Down syndrome [89a,89b]. They need the appropriate care as any other psychiatric patient. Perhaps the most interesting case history in the literature describes a mother with a 29-year-old son with Down syndrome. The mother developed paranoid psychosis and was treated; her son also became symptomatic. Successful therapy of the mother's illness also resulted in full recovery of the son without the need for medication; this case suggests folie à deux relationship between these two family members [90].

MOYAMOYA DISEASE

Moyamoya disease is being reported in children with Down syndrome [91]. Moyamoya refers to something hazy "just like a puff of cigarette smoke drifting in the air," referring to the impression left on viewing the arteriograms (Fig. 13.1). The arteriogram demonstrates blood vessels in the brain (the internal carotid and middle and anterior cerebral arteries) partially or completely occluded as well as prominent telangiectasia of the blood vessels in the basal ganglia. It is believed that the moyamoya vessels represent collaterals

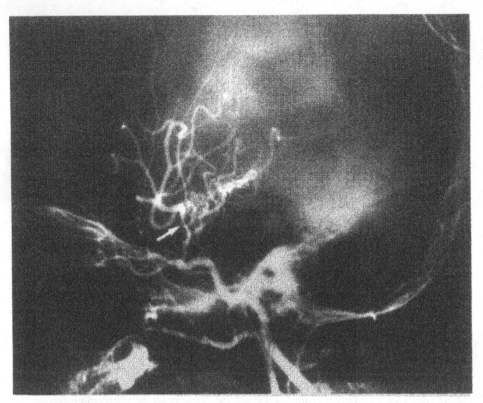

Figure 13.1 Arteriogram demonstrating moyamoya disease.

resulting from the occlusion of the carotid arteries. Down syndrome children as young as 3 years of age have been reported with this disease; however, the frequency in this patient population must be quite rare. Treatment consists of anticoagulation methods.

AGING AND ALZHEIMER'S DISEASE

One of the concerns of parents of children with Down syndrome is that their child is doomed to certain Alzheimer's disease in young adult life. It has been found that there are many biochemical and immunological abnormalities common to the brains of people with Alzheimer's disease and those with Down syndrome [92–94].

It is true that neuropathology similar to Alzheimer's disease has been found in virtually all individuals after 40 years of age (the many studies confirming this are reviewed in Ref. 95). However, it is not true that all or even most of adults with Down syndrome are going to develop Alzheimer's starting at 40 years of age. A review of the data available about the often discussed "premature aging" in individuals with Down syndrome suggests that the 50s and 60s are the age when this patient group is at risk. Even so, many individuals with Down syndrome never develop dementia when they are older.

One of the largest studies in the field is by Zigman et al. who studied 2144 individuals with Down syndrome ranging in age from 20 to 69 years of age and compared them to 4172 controls who were developmentally disabled individuals who did not have Down syndrome [96]. The diagnoses of the controls included autism, cerebral palsy, epilepsy, mental retardation, and other neurological impairments. Activities of daily living were measured in a standardized way.

At younger adult ages, individuals with Down syndrome performed better than did retarded control subjects. The pattern reversed between the two groups of retarded individuals at about 60 years of age or older. It is after 60 years of age that individuals with Down syndrome began to lose their skills at a faster rate than individuals with other forms of developmental disability. This pattern of age-associated deficits among individuals with Down syndrome was not affected by developmental level and was observed among randomly selected individuals who resided in a wide range of placements. Studies of the people with Down syndrome between 50 and 69 years of age revealed a bimodal peak that began to develop, indicating that a larger proportion of people with Down syndrome between 50 and 69 years of age had dementia compared to the other subject groups. The most significant decline in cognitive skills among the individuals with Down syndrome did not appear until the individuals reached 60 years of age. In older patients with Down syndrome, imaging studies can be helpful in differentiating those likely to develop dementia. As seen in Fig. 13.2, progressive cerebral atrophy heralds the onset of dementia; in older patients unlikely to present with dementia, the development of atrophy is much slower and less marked.

In another detailed study of 96 institutionalized individuals with Down syndrome greater than 35 years of age, Lai and Williams found that only 8% of the patients less than 49 years of age met the criteria of Alzheimer-type dementia [97]. At more than 60 years of age, however, 75% (six out of eight individuals) met these criteria. The average duration of the dementia in the individuals who died was 3.2 ± 4.6 years. (In this report, it is relevant to note that 59% of the demented patients had adequately treated hypothyroidism.) In a study of 50 adults with mild retardation living at home, Franceschi et al. reported a figure of 18% dementia—all of it starting after 30 years of age [98].

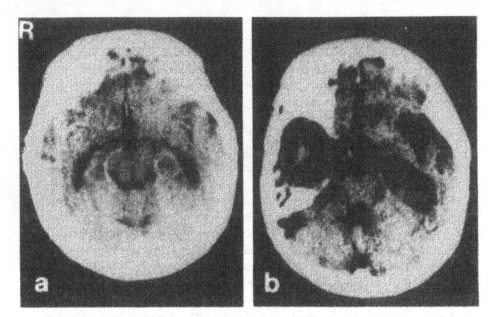

Figure 13.2 Progressive cerebral atrophy in an adult with Down syndrome. a. CT scan taken through the temporal horn. b. CT scan taken 4 years later through the temporal horns. (Reprinted with the permission of Neuroradiology)

Neuropathological studies sometimes use lipofuscin accumulation in the brain as an index of aging. In normal individuals, the proportion of lipofuscin to cell size is a linear function of age between 14 and 92 years of age. In a study performed on the brains of individuals with Down syndrome, there was no difference in the amount of lipofuscin accumulated with age compared to individuals with normal central nervous systems [99].

In contrast to lipofuscin, calcification of the basal ganglia does occur prematurely in some individuals with Down syndrome [100]. In a study of 30 living patients, 11–48 years of age and with an average age of 25 years, a CT scan revealed that 26.6% already had detectable basal ganglia calcification. Pathological studies have confirmed and expanded the CT findings. The random population frequency is 0.3–0.6%. One possible explanation of this phenomenon, because some of the individuals were relatively youthful, is that it is a manifestation of ischemic brain damage secondary to the congenital cardiac disease that is commonly found in children with Down syndrome (see Chapter 9).

There is an interesting study of the decline of visual-perceptual abilities in

44 adults with Down syndrome 14–43 years of age. At more than 25 years of age, a general decline of performance sets in—except in the visual-motor subtest [101]. The investigators note that this is the area where the ability continues to be exercised in craft work. An implication of this article is that skills not used tend to decline with age, certainly a generalization not limited to adults with Down syndrome. The importance of adult living and working lifestyles that utilize the full range of cognitive abilities of the individual with Down syndrome is again emphasized by this study.

Alzheimer's disease is the major cause of dementia in the elderly. In 1907, Alois Alzheimer described a 51-year-old woman who died after 4 years with characteristic neuropathology [102]. This led to the distinction in the medical literature between presenile dementia (onset before 65 years) or Alzheimer's disease and senile dementia of the Alzheimer type (onset after 65 years). However, there is no marker to distinguish the two groups other than age, and many investigators now prefer to conclude that all afflicted patients have Alzheimer's disease. Alzheimer's disease frequently appears first as a defect in recent memory. This is followed by a reduced visual-spatial and language function and general cognitive deterioration. Sleep, appetite, gait, and the emotions may become abnormal. The disease begins insidiously, advances in an uneven manner, and limits life expectancy.

In patients with Down syndrome, the same symptoms appear and usually are quite evident to close family members. Personality changes (100%), loss of independent living skills (100%), seizures (53%), gait deterioration (73%), sphincteric incontinence (40%), and pathological release reflexes (67%) were described in one study from a neurology clinic [103]. An even higher rate of seizures (84%) has been described in institutionalized patients [104].

It is important not to confuse peripheral and central dysfunctions in older individuals with Down syndrome. Sometimes they become unresponsive. Like other people, older people with Down syndrome show the typical presbyacusic gradual decline in auditory sensitivity, at first above 1–2 kHz and then for all frequencies. However, they have an earlier onset of presbyacusis, in some cases as early as the second decade of life [105]. Sometimes the appetite declines accompanied by weight loss and poor nutritional status; this can be a sign of an olfactory deficit [106]. In these cases, before cognitive decline or Alzheimer's disease is diagnosed, the possibility of presbyacusis or olfactory deficit needs to be considered.

Slight biochemical differences are being noted in testing between Down syndrome patients with and without Alzheimer's disease of comparable ages. Preliminary tests show lower T_3 levels and lower superoxide dismutase levels [107,108].

Family studies and detailed pedigrees have raised a question of an association between Alzheimer's disease and Down syndrome. Current new findings from the field of molecular biology suggest that many, if not most, cases of Alzheimer's disease may have a genetic basis, but in the past, people did not live long enough for genetic expression of the disease. Two chromosomes have been implicated to date in the familial Alzheimer's disease process, and it is anticipated that there may be even more genetic factors [109]. In some families, there appears to be an association with chromosome 19. However, of greater interest to Down syndrome are the families who have a mutation on a gene of the twenty-first chromosome that directs cells to produce beta amyloid, a crucial nerve cell protein. Deposits of amyloid fibers are found in large numbers in the walls of blood vessels and in neuritic plaques in the brains of patients with Alzheimer's disease and in the brains of adults past 40 years with

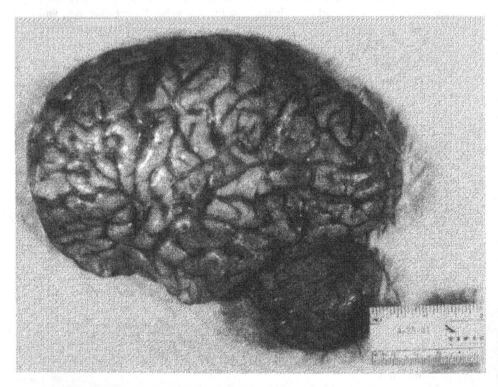

Figure 13.3 Photograph of the left cerebral hemisphere and cerebellum in a patient with dementia and Down syndrome. Note foreshortening and rounding of the cerebral hemisphere, incomplete eversion of the superior temporal gyrus, and small cerebellum. (Reprinted with the permission of Neurology)

Down syndrome. Another similarity seen in both Alzheimer's disease and Down syndrome is abnormal function of the cholinergic pathways [110] (see Appendix A).

A typical case history shows a detailed assessment of a 47-year-old man with Down syndrome and autopsy-confirmed Alzheimer's disease [111]. Clinically, dementia developed with classic symptoms. PET scanning of mean hemispheric fluorodeoxyglucose was 28% less than in younger persons with Down syndrome. CT scanning revealed prominent cortical sulci and large ventricles. Neuropsychological assessment showed very low scoring. Autopsy findings included extensive number of neuritic plaques, neurofibrillary tangles, and amyloid angiopathy. In Fig. 13.3 anatomic changes in the brain are visible.

The voluminous information in the medical literature on Down syndrome and Alzheimer's disease illustrates a reasonable connection between the two except for one fact that does not quite fit. Despite massive Alzheimer-type neuropathological changes in the central nervous system, progressive dementia is not observed in many mature and elderly persons with Down syndrome [112]. There is even a hint that the plaques may be different in the two disease entities [113]. Certainly, persons with Down syndrome appear to have a higher threshold for dementia as measured by the amount of neuritic plaques and neurofibrillary tangles they can tolerate without clinical symptoms of dementia. Until the reason for this is fully explained, the story of the relationship between Alzheimer's disease and Down syndrome remains incomplete.

REFERENCES

1. Crome I, Stern J. Pathology of Mental Retardation, 2nd ed. Edinburgh: Churchill Livingston, 1972.
2. Sylvester PE. The hippocampus in Down syndrome. J Ment Defic Res 1983; 27:227–236.
3. Wisniewski KE. Down syndrome children often have brain with maturation delay, retardation of growth, and cortical dysgenesis. Am J Med Genet 1990; (suppl 7):274–281.
4. Crome L, Cowie V. Slater E. A statistical note on cerebellar and brain stem weight in mongolism. J Ment Defic Res 1966;10:69–72.
5. Solitare GB, Lamarche JB. Brain weight in the adult mongol. J Ment Defic Res 1967;11:79–84.
6. Baer MT, Waldron J, Gumm H, Van Dyke DC, Chang H. Nutrition assessment of the child with Down syndrome. In: Van Dyke DC, Lang FH, van Duyne S, Soucek MJ, eds. Clinical Perspectives in the Management of Down Syndrome. New York: Springer-Verlag, 1990:107–125.
7. Cronk CE, Pueschel SM. Anthropometric studies. In: Pueschel SM, ed. The

Young Child with Down Syndrome. New York: Human Sciences Press, 1984: 104–141.

8. Zellweger H. Down syndrome. In: Vinken PJ, Bruyn GW, eds. Handbook of Clinical Neurology, vol. 31, part II. New York: North Holland, 1977:367–469.

9. Crome L, Cowie V, Slater E. A statistical note on cerebellar and brain-stem weight in mongolism. J Ment Defic Res 1966;10:69–72.

10. Kemper TL. Neuropathology of Down syndrome. In: Nadel L, ed. The Psychobiology of Down Syndrome. Cambridge, Mass: MIT Press, 1988:189–270.

11. Hill LM, Rivell D, Peterson C, Marchese S. The transverse cerebellar diameter in the second trimester is unaffected by Down syndrome. Am J Obstet Gynecol 1991;164:101–103.

12. Wisniewski KE, Schmidt-Sidor B. Postnatal delay of myelin formation in brains from Down syndrome infants and children. Clin Neuropathol 1989;8:55–62.

13. Ross MH, Galuburda AM, Kemper TL. Down's syndrome: Is there a decreased population of neurons? Neurology 1984;34:909–916.

14. Courchesne E. Physioanatomical considerations in Down syndrome. In: Nadel L, ed. The Psychobiology of Down Syndrome. Cambridge, Mass: MIT Press, 1988: 291–314.

15. Marin-Padilla M. Pyramidal cell abnormalities in the motor cortex of a child with Down's syndrome: A Golgi study. J Comp Neurol 1976;167:63–82.

16. Suetsugu M, Meharaein P. Spine distribution along the apical dendrites of the pyramidal neurons in Down syndrome. Acta Neuropathol 1980;50:207–210.

17. Becker LE, Armstrong DL, Chan F. Dendritic atrophy in children with Down's syndrome. Ann Neurol 1986;20:520–526.

18. Takashima S, Becker LE, Armstrong DL, Chan F. Abnormal neuronal development in the visual cortex of the human fetus and infant with Down's syndrome: A quantitative and qualitative Golgi study. Brain Res 1981;225:1–21.

19. Wisniewski KE, Laure-Kamionowska M, Wisniewski HM. Evidence of arrest of neurogenesis and synaptogenesis in brains of patients with Down's syndrome. N Engl J Med 1984;311:1187–1188.

20. Scott BS, Petit TL, Becker LE, Edwards BAV. Abnormal electric membrane properties of Down's syndrome DRG neurons in cell culture. Dev Brain Res 1982;2:257–270.

21. Epstein CJ, Cox DR, Epstein LB. Mouse trisomy 16: An animal model of human trisomy 21 (Down syndrome). Ann N Y Acad Sci 1985;450:157–168.

22. Brookbank BWL, Walker D, Balazs R, Jorgensen OS. Neuronal maturation in the foetal brain in Down syndrome. Early Hum Dev 1989;18:237–246.

23. Kish S, Karlinsky H, Becker L, Gilbert J, Rebbetoy M, Chang LJ, DiStefano L, Hornykiewicz O. Down's syndrome individuals begin life with normal levels of brain cholinergic markers. J Neurochem 1989;52:1183–1187.

24. Florez J, del Arco C, Gonzalez A, Pascual J, Pazos A. Autoradiographic studies of neurotransmitter receptors in the brain of newborn infants with Down syndrome. Am J Med Genet 1990(suppl 7):301–305.

25. Schapiro MB, Creasey H, Schwartz M, Haxby JV, White B, Moore A, Rapoport SI. Quantitative CT analysis of brain morphometry in adult Down's syndrome at different ages. Neurology 1987;37:1424–1427.

26. Schapiro MB, Luxenberg JS, Kaye JA, Haxby JV, Friedland RP, Rapoport SI. Serial quantitative CT analysis of brain morphometrics in adult Down's syndrome at different ages. Neurology 1989;39:1349–1353.

27. Schwartz M, Duara R, Haxby J, Grady C, White BJ, Kessler RM, Kay AD, Cutler NR, Rapoport SI. Down's syndrome in adults: Brain metabolism. Science 1983;221:781–783.

28a. Cutler NR. Cerebral metabolism as measured with positron emission tomography (PET) and [18F] 2-deoxy-D-glucose: Healthy aging, Alzheimer's disease and Down syndrome. Prog Neuropsychopharmacol Biol Psychiatry 1986;10:309–321.

28b. Schapiro MB, Grady CL, Kumar A, Herscovitch P, Haxby JV, Moore Am, White B, Friedland R, Rapoport SI. Regional cerebral glucose metabolism is normal in young adults with Down syndrome. J Clin Blood Flow Metab 1990;10:199–206.

29. Schapiro MB, Rapoport SI. Basal metabolic rate in healthy Down's syndrome adults. J Ment Defic Res 1989;33:211–219.

30. Horwitz B, Schapiro MB, Grady CL, Rapoport SI. Cerebral metabolic pattern in young adult Down syndrome: Altered intercorrelations between regional rates of glucose utilization. J Ment Defic Res 1990;34:237–252.

31. Scola PS. Neurology. In: Pueschel SM, Rynders JE, eds. Down Syndrome: Advances in Biomedicine and the Behavioral Sciences. Cambridge, Mass: Ware Press, 1982;219–225.

32. Ellingson RJ, Menolascino FJ, Eisen JD. Clinical EEG relationships in mongoloids confirmed by karyotype. Am J Ment Defic 1970;74:645–650.

33. Seppalainen AM, Kivalo E. EEG findings and epilepsy in Down's syndrome. J Ment Defic Res 1967;11:116–125.

34. Elul R, Henley J, Simmons JO III. Non-Gaussian behavior of the EEG in Down's syndrome suggests decreased neuronal connections. Acta Neurologica Scandinavica 1975;51:21–28.

35. Barnet A, Lodge A. Click evoked EEG responses in normal and developmentally retarded infants. Nature 1967;214:252.

36. Bigum HB, Dustman RE, Beck EC. Visual and somatosensory evoked responses from mongoloid and normal children. Electroencephalogr Clin Neurophysiol 1970;28:576.

37. Barnet A, Ohlrich E, Shanks B. EEG evoked responses to repetitive stimulation in normal and Down's syndrome infants. Dev Med Child Neurol 1971;13:321.

38. Straumanis JJ, Shagass C, Overton DA. Auditory evoked responses in young adults with Down's syndrome and idiopathic mental retardation. Biol Psychiatry 1973;6:75.

39. Gliddon JB, Busk J, Galbraith GC. Visual evoked responses as a function of light intensity in Down syndrome and nonretarded subjects. Psychophysiology 1975; 12:416.

40. Lichy J, Vesely C, Alder J, Zizka J. Auditory evoked cortical responses in Down's syndrome. Electroencephalogr Clin Neurophysiol 1975;38:440.

41. Callner DA, Dustman RE, Madsen JA, Schenkenberg T, Beck EC. Life span changes in the averaged evoked responses of Down's syndrome and nontreated persons. Am J Ment Defic 1978;82:398.

42. Dustman RE, Callner DA. Cortical evoked responses and response decrement in nonretarded and Down's syndrome individuals. Am J Ment Defic 1979;83:391.

43. Schafer EWP, Peeke HVS. Down syndrome individuals fail to habituate cortical evoked potentials. Am J Ment Def 1982;87:332–337.

44. Miyanomae Y, Yoshida A, Nomoto N, Yoshioka Y. Developmental changes of somatosensory evoked potentials and auditory brainstem responses in Down syndrome children. No To Hattatsu 1987;19:22–28.

45. Widen JE, Folsom RC, Thompson G, Wilson WR. Auditory brainstem responses in young adults with Down syndrome. Am J Ment Defic 1987;91:472–479.

46. Courchesne E. Event-related potentials: Comparison between children and adults. Science 1977;197:589–592.

47. Lincoln AJ, Courchesne E, Kilman BA, Galambos R. Neurophychological correlates of information processing by children with Down syndrome. Am J Ment Def 1985;89:403–414.

48. Muir WJ, Squire I, Blackwood DHR, Speight MD, St Clair DM, Oliver C, Dickens P. Auditory response in the assessment of Alzheimer's disease in Down's syndrome: A two year follow-up study. J Ment Defic Res 1988;32:455–463.

49. Coleman M. Studies of the administration of pyridoxine to children with Down syndrome. In: Leklem J, Reynolds R, eds. Clinical and Physiological Applications of Vitamin B-6. New York: Alan R. Liss, 1988:317–328.

50. Pueschel SM, Linuma K, Katz J, Matsumiya Y. Visual and auditory evoked potential studies. In: Pueschel SM, ed. The Young Child with Down Syndrome. New York: Human Sciences Press, 1984, pp. 319–334.

51. Frager J, Barnet A, Weiss I, Coleman M. A double blind study of vitamin B-6 in Down's syndrome infants: Part 2. Cortical evoked potentials. J Ment Defic Res 1985;29:241–246.

52. Coleman M, Sobel S, Bhagavan H, Coursin D, Marquart A, Guay M, Hunt C. A double blind study of vitamin B-6 in Down's syndrome infants: Part 1. Clinical and biochemical results. J Ment Defic Res 1985;29:233–240.

53. Shantz SL, Brown WS. P300 latency and cognitive ability. In: Van Dyke DC, Lang DJ, Heide F, van Duyne S, Soucek MJ, eds. Clinical Perspectives in the Management of Down Syndrome. New York: Springer-Verlag, 1990:139–146.

54. Noetzel MJ. Sleep disturbances in children with Down syndrome. Down Syndrome News 1989;13:48–49.

55. Hamaguchi H, Hashimoto T, Mori K, Tayama M. Sleep in Down syndrome. Brain Dev 1989;11:399–406.

56. Stafstrom CE, Patxot OF, Gilmore HE, Wisniewski KE. Seizures in children with Down syndrome: Etiology, characteristics and outcome. Dev Med Child Neurol 1991;31:191–200.

57. Tatsuno M, Hayashi M, Iwamoto H, Suzuki Y, Kuroki Y. Epilepsy in childhood Down syndrome. Brain Dev 1984;6:37–44.

58. Veall RM. The prevalence of epilepsy among mongols related to age. J Ment Defic Res 1974;18:99–106.

59. Van Dyke DC, Lang DL, Miller JD, Heide F, van Duyne S, Chang H. Common medical problems. In: Van Dyke DC, Lang DJ, Heide F, van Duyne S, Soucek MJ, eds. Clinical Perspectives in the Management of Down Syndrome. New York: Springer-Verlag, 1990:3–14.

60. Romano C, Tine A, Fazio G, Rizzo R, Colognola RM, Sorge G, Bergonzi P, Pavone L. Seizures in patients with trisomy 21. Am J Med Genet 1990;(suppl 7): 298–300.

61. Tansye SR. The EEG and the incidence of epilepsy in Down's syndrome. J Ment Defic Res 1979;23:17–24.

62. Nolte R, Christen H-J, Doerrer J. Preliminary report of a multi-center study on the West syndrome. Brain Dev 1988;10:236–242.

63. Smith GR, Berg JM. Down's Anomaly, 2nd ed. New York: Churchill Livingston, 1976.

64. Coriat LF, Fejerman N. Infantile spasms in children with trisomy 21. LaSemana Med Ed Pediatr 1963:493–500.

65. Pollack MA, Golden GS, Schmidt R, Davis JA, Leeds N. Infantile spasms in Down syndrome: A report of 5 cases and review of the literature. Ann Neurol 1978;3:406–408.

66. Coleman M. Infantile spasms induced by 5-hydroxytryptophan in patients with Down's syndrome. Neurology 1971;21:911–919.

67. Izumi T, Imaizumi C, Ashida E, Ochiai T, Wans PJ, Fukuyama Y. Suppressive action of ACTH on growth hormone secretion in patients with infantile spasms. Brain Dev 1985;7:636–639.

68. Youns RS, Fripp RR, Stern DR, Darowish C. Cardiac hypertrophy associated with ACTH therapy for childhood seizure disorder. J Child Neurol 1987;2: 311–312.

69. Apert BS. Steroid-induced hypertrophic cardiomyopathy in an infant. Pediatr Cardiol 1984;5:117–118.

70. Wolcott GJ, Chun RW. Myoclonic seizures in Down's syndrome. Dev Med Child Neurol 1973;15:805–808.

71. Blennow G, Starck L. High dose B-6 in infantile spasms. Neuropediatrics 1986; 17:7–10.

72. Ohtsuka Y, Matsuda M, Osino T, Kobayashi K, Ohtahara S. Treatment of the West syndrome with high-dose pyridoxal phosphate. Brain Dev 1987;9:418–421.

73. Guerrini R, Genton P, Bureau M, Dravet C, Roger J. Reflex seizures are frequent in patients with Down syndrome and epilepsy. Epilepsia 1990;31:406–417.

74. Gimenez-Roldan S, Martin M. Startle epilepsy complicating Down syndrome during adulthood. Ann Neurol 1980;7:78–80.

75. Gibson D. Down Syndrome: The Psychology of Mongolism. Cambridge, Engl: Cambridge University Press, 1978.

76. Van Dyke DC, Hoffman MN, van Duyne S, Heide F, Zemke R. Development and behavior. In: Van Dyke DC, Lang DJ, Heide F, van Duyne S, Soucek MJ, eds. Clinical Perspectives in the Management of Down Syndrome. New York: Springer-Verlag, 1990:171–180.

77. Gath A, Gumley D. Family background of children with Down's syndrome and of children with a similar degree of mental retardation. Br J Psychiatry 1986;149: 161–171.

78. Gath A, Gumley D. Behaviour problems in retarded children with special reference to Down's syndrome. Br J Psychiatry 1986;149:156–161.

79. Ganiban J, Wagner S, Cicchetti D. Temperament and Down syndrome. In: Cicchetti D, Beeghly M, eds. Children with Down Syndrome: A Developmental Perspective. Cambridge, Engl: Cambridge University Press, 1990.

80. Huntington GS, Simeonsson RJ. Down's syndrome and toddler temperament. Child Care Health Dev 1987;13:1–11.

81. Wagner S, Ganiban J, Cicchetti D. Attention, memory and perception in infants with Down syndrome: A review and commentary. In: Cicchetti D, Beeghly M, eds. Children with Down Syndrome: A Developmental perspective. Cambridge, Engl: Cambridge University Press, 1990.

82. Wender PH. Minimal Brain Dysfunction in Children. New York: Wiley, 1971.

83. Coleman M. Serotonin and central nervous system syndromes of childhood: A review. J Autism Child Schizophr 1973;3:27–35.

84. Bhagavan HN, Coleman M, Coursin DB. The effect of pyridoxine hydrochloride on blood serotonin and pyridoxal phosphate contents in hyperactive children. Pediatrics 1975;55:437–441.

85. Coleman M, Steinberg G, Tippett J, Bhagavan HN, Coursin DB, Gross M, Lewis C, DeVeau L. A preliminary study of the effect of pyridoxine administration in a subgroup of hyperkinetic children: A double-blind crossover comparison with methylphenidate. Biol Psychiatry 1979;14:741–751.

86. Coleman M. Down's syndrome children with autistic features. Down's Syndrome: Papers and Abstracts for Professionals 1986;9:1–2.

87. Gillberg C, Wahlstrom J. Chromosome abnormalities in infantile autism and other childhood psychoses: A population study of 66 cases. Dev Med Child Neurol 1985;27:293–304.

88. Coleman M, Gillberg C. The Biology of the Autistic Syndromes. New York: Praeger, 1985:210–212.

89a. Singh L. Down's syndrome with mania. Br J Psychiatry 1988;152:436–437. Letter to the Editor.

89b. Sovner R. Divalproex-responsive rapid cycling bipolar disorder in a patient with Down's syndrome: Implications for the Down's syndrome-mania hypothesis. J Ment Defic Res 1991;35:171–173.

90. Meakin CJ, Renvoize EB. Folie à deux in Down's syndrome: A case report. Br J Psychiatry 1987;151: 258–260.

91. Fukusima Y, Kondo Y, Kuroki Y, Miyake S, Iwamoto H, Sekido K, Yamaguchi

K. Are Down syndrome patients predisposed to moyamoya disease? Eur J Pediatry 1986;144:516–517.

92. Schweber M. Interrelation of Alzheimer disease and Down syndrome. In: Pueschel SM, Tingey C, Rynders JE, Crocker AC, Crutcher D. New Perspectives on Down syndrome. Baltimore, Md: Paul H Brookes, 1987:135–146.

93. Yates CM, Simpson J, Gordon A. Regional brain 5-hydroxytryptamine levels are reduced in senile Down's syndrome as in Alzheimer's disease. Neurosci Lett 1986;65:189–192.

94. Kay AD, Schapiro MB, Riker AK, Haxby JV, Rapoport SI. Cerebral fluid monoaminergic metabolites are elevated in adults with Down's syndrome. Ann Neurol 1987;21:408–411.

95. Friedland RP, moderator. Alzheimer Disease: Clinical and biological heterogeneity. Ann Int Med 1988;109:298–311.

96. Zigman WB, Schupf N, Lubin R, Silverman WP. Premature regression of adults with Down syndrome. Am J Ment Defic 1987;92:161–168.

97. Lai F, Williams RS. A prospective study of Alzheimer disease in Down syndrome. Arch Neurol 1989;46:849–853.

98. Franceschi M, Comola M, Piattoni F, Gualandri W, Canal N. Prevalence of dementia in adult patients with trisomy 21. Am J Med Genet 1990;(suppl 7): 306–308.

99. West CJ. A quantitative study of lipofuscin accumulation with age in normals and individuals with Down's syndrome, phenylketonuria, progeria and transneuronal atrophy. Comp Neurol 1979;186:109–116.

100. Wisniewski KE, French JH, Rosen JF, Kozlowski PB, Tenner M, Wisniewski HM. Basal ganglia calcification (BGC) in Down's syndrome (DS)—another manifestation of premature aging. Ann N Y Acad Sci 1982:179–189.

101. Saviolo-Negrin N, Soresi S, Baccichetti C, Pozzan G, Trevisan E. Observations on the visual-perceptual abilities and adaptive behavior in adults with Down syndrome. Am J Med Genet 1990;(suppl 7):309–313.

102. Alzheimer A. Uber eine eigenartige Erkrankung der Hirnrinde. Allg S Psychiatr 1907;64:146–148.

103. Lott IT, Lai F. Dementia in Down's syndrome: Observations from a neurology clinic. Appl Res Ment Retard 1982;3:233–239.

104. Miniszek NA. Development of Alzheimer disease in Down syndrome individuals. Am J Ment Defic 1983;87:377–385.

105. Buchanan LH. Early onset of presbyacusis in Down syndrome. Scand Audiol 1990;19:103–110.

106. Warner MD, Peabody CA, Berger PA. Olfactory deficits and Down's syndrome. Biol Psychiatry 1988;23:836–839.

107. Percy ME, Dalton AJ, Markovic VD, McLachlan DRC, Gera E, Hummei JT, Rusk ACM, Somerville MJ, Andrews DF, Walfish PG. Autoimmune thyroiditis associated with mild "subclinical" hypothyroidism in adults with Down syn-

drome: A comparison of patients with and without Alzheimer disease. Am J Med Genet 1990;36:148–154.

108. Percy ME, Dalton AJ, Markovic VD, McLachlan DRC, Hummei JT, Rusk ACM, Andrews DF. Red cell superoxide dismutase, glutathione peroxidase and catalase in Down syndrome patients with and without manifestations of Alzheimer disease. Am J Med Genet 1990;35:459–467.

109. Hardy J, et al. Nature. 1991.

110. McGeer PL, McGeer EG, Suzuki J, Dolman CE, Nagari T. Aging, Alzheimer's disease and the cholinergic system of the basal forebrain. Neurology 1984;34: 741–745.

111. Schapiro MB, Ball MJ, Grady CL, Haxby JV, Kaye JA, Rapoport SI. Dementia in Down's syndrome: Cerebral glucose utilization, neuropsychological assessment and neuropathology. Neurology 1988;38:938–942.

112. Wisniewski HM, Rabe A. Discrepancy between Alzheimer-type neuropathology and dementia in persons with Down's syndrome. Ann N Y Acad Sci 1986; 477:247–260.

113. Allsop D, Kidd M, Landon M, Tomlinson A. Isolated senile plaque cores in Alzheimer's disease and Down's syndrome show differences in morphology. J Neurol Neurosurg Psychiatry 1986;49:886–892.

14

The Ocular System

There are a number of ocular problems in individuals with Down syndrome that occur in a slightly greater frequency than in the general population [1] (Table 14.1). There is one relatively rare problem, acute keratoconus, that occurs more frequently in individuals with Down syndrome than in individuals with any other known syndrome [2].

Good ocular care is important to any child. This is particularly true for a child who needs all possible advantages when entering the classroom. Thus, the preventive medicine concept of routine ophthalmological examinations and thoughtful visual care can have a very realistic impact on both the health and educational performance of a child with Down syndrome.

In the old medical literature such as the Lowe article published in 1949 [3], a great deal of visual loss was noted in populations of individuals with Down syndrome and assumed to be part of the syndrome itself. Today, we try to identify the specific problem involved in the visual loss and often find that it can be corrected. Cataracts that impair vision are relatively rare; keratoconus is rare; and optic nerve hypoplasia does not cause serious vision loss in most cases [4]. Nystagmus is usually mild, and strabismus is correctable with binocularity preserved when such correction is tended to at a very early age. Retinal detachment can cause serious visual loss but is quite rare.

So what is the major problem that causes vision loss in so many children with Down syndrome? Apparently, it is an avoidable loss; it is old-fashioned, ordinary refractive error—not checked for and not corrected. Alas, there was more interest in Brushfield spots than in helping these children see well.

Table 14.1   Ocular Problems in Down Syndrome

1. Refractive error
2. Strabismus
3. Nystagmus
4. Blepharoconjunctivitis
5. Cataracts
6. Keratoconus
7. Retinal pathology
8. Optic nerve hypoplasia

REFRACTIVE ERRORS

The single most important ophthalmological test in a child with Down syndrome, in most cases, may be a check for refractive errors, measured easily under cycloplegia with appropriate fixation conditions. It is likely that if they have adequate preventive medical care, the single most frequent ocular prescription in children with Down syndrome will be glasses.

Gaynon and Schimek found refractive errors in 70% of the individuals with Down syndrome that they studied [5]. Gardiner found 73% of the patients had a refractive error that "ordinarily" would lead to the prescription of glasses [6]. Regarding the type of refractive errors, Caputo et al. evaluated 187 cases and reported that 22.5% had myopia, 20.9% had hyperopia, and 22% had astigmatism [1]. Fierson did detailed ophthalmological evaluations on 150 children and adolescents with Down syndrome [4]. He found 12% of the patients had myopia, 18% had hyperopia and 35% astigmatic refractive errors. Because it appears that astigmatism in the general population is approximately 15%, the patients with Down syndrome had this error at a rate about twice that of the general population. In fact, in this study, astigmatism was the most characteristic refractive error in Down syndrome. Fierson gives a detailed description of the type of astigmatism seen in the Down syndrome patients in his clinic [4]. As with other refractive errors, astigmatism is most appropriately corrected by prescription of glasses in patients with Down syndrome.

STRABISMUS

Strabismus is a constant or intermittent deviation of the visual axis of the eyes. The direction may be inward (esotropia), outward (exotropia), upward (hypertropia), or a combination of these. Approximately 1–2% of the general population has strabismus in some form.

In the case of children with Down syndrome, one has to distinguish between true esotropia and pseudoesotropia. Because of the presence of epicanthic folds combined with the flat nasal bridge, many Down syndrome eyes give an esotropic appearance. Any trained ophthalmologist can easily distinguish between the two possibilities.

The incidence of strabismus in Down syndrome has been reported as 33% [3], 34% [7], 34% [8], 36% [9], 37% [4], 43% [10] and 44% [11]. Cowie noted in her study that young infants less than 2 weeks of age had less strabismus (23%) than infants older than 2 weeks (36%) [9].

When strabismus begins at an early age, esotropia predominates over all the other types. In the case of Down syndrome children, strabismus is almost always of early onset and usually of the primary, central type. As can be anticipated by an age of onset less than 6 months, the vast majority of Down syndrome children with strabismus have esotropia. In the unusual child with Down syndrome and a unilateral congenital cataract, corneal opacity, or a unilateral large refractive error, the strabismus may be secondary. Exotropia and hypertropia combined are usually less than 10% in any published series [4,8,9,12,13].

If left untreated, strabismus may result in the loss of binocular fusion, of binocular depth perception, and eventually, vision in one eye when that eye is subjected to continuous suppression. The treatment options include glasses for refractive errors (especially hyperopia in children with esotropia), surgery, and, on rare occasions, prisms.

NYSTAGMUS

Nystagmus, a rhythmical oscillation of the eyes, can be either pendular (movement in each direction of the same velocity), jerky (slow movement in one direction coupled with rapid correction in the other direction), or rotary. It is usually bilateral but can be unilateral. Pendular nystagmus is associated with severe visual loss, infantile cataract, or extreme refractive error [4]. Other forms of nystagmus (jerky and rotary) are thought to have a central origin.

There have been many reports in the medical literature since the beginning of the twentieth century of patients with Down syndrome having nystagmus [14]. Pueschel, in his fine textbook, sums up the literature and concludes that nystagmus in Down syndrome is more often secondary to lens opacities or refractive errors [15]. This certainly seems reasonable in view of what we know about the frequency of refractive errors in this patient group. However, in the 1990 study by Fierson, 15 out of 150 (10%) children had nystagmus, and one had the pendular form. Fourteen children had jerky nystagmus, and one had the rotary type [4].

The prevalence of nystagmus in patients with Down syndrome as reported in the literature varies from 4.5% [16] to 20% [8]. Some investigators have reported cases where the nystagmus improved or even disappeared with increasing age.

BLEPHAROCONJUNCTIVITIS

Marginal blepharitis, infection of the eyelids, often can lead to conjunctival vascular infection and inflammation termed "blepharoconjunctivitis." Symptoms include discharge and morning eyelid margin crusting. This condition can become chronic or reoccur intermittently. Studies have shown a frequency rate of 2% [16], 33% [13], 41% [17] and 46% [10]. Treatment is standard; usually, eyelid scrubs followed by a topical antibiotic ointment are recommended.

CATARACTS

Cataract formation, the clouding of the usually clear lens of the eye, can be found in a significant percentage of even young children with Down syndrome if these opacities are searched for systematically. The literature on cataracts is divided between investigators who count any clouding of the lens as evidence of cataract and those who count only clouding that is dense enough to affect visual acuity. For the purpose of this discussion, the term *cataract* refers to any changes in opacity in the lens, whether or not they affect visual acuity. Cataracts that occur in the central (visual) axis of the lens usually are the ones that impair vision. Opacities in the periphery often have little or no visual significance.

In the detailed examination by Fierson of 150 children with Down syndrome, a combination of slit lamp examination and direct ophthalmoscopy with retroillumination was used after pupillary dilatation [4]. Although the average age was only 4–5 years, 42% of the patients were found to have some lenticular opacities including minor ones. Other investigators, with somewhat older populations, report that more than 50% of their patients have detectable opacities [12,18]. Some studies have reported percentages as high as 86% [19].

Are there particular patterns of cataract opacities seen in patients with Down syndrome (Fig. 14.1)? Falls thought so [12]. He described dense arcuate opacities that arc about the fetal nucleus combined with polychromatic crystalline deposits in the lens as a combination of opacities that is highly suggestive of Down syndrome. A number of variations of arcuate, sutural, and flake opacities have been described by several investigators [3,19,20]. There does

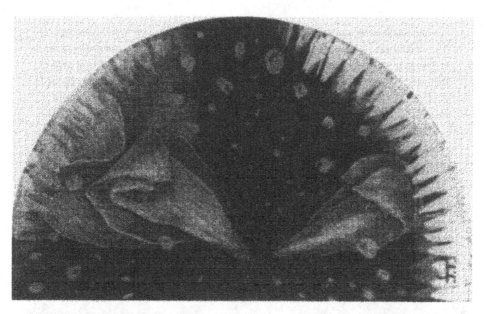

Figure 14.1 Cataract changes showing arcuate and flakelike opacities. (Reprinted with the permission of the British Journal of Ophthalmology.)

seem to be general agreement that, although cataracts frequently are found in children and adults, they usually are peripheral and are visually debilitating in only a very small percentage of cases.

On the other hand, congenital cataracts often interfere with vision. Relatively rare in Down syndrome, there are few reports [3,12,13,21,22]. MacGillivray suggested that the congenital cataracts found in infants with Down syndrome may be due to an infectious process during pregnancy [21].

Modern surgical techniques for cataract removal, with shortened postoperative times, have created a practical procedure for patients with Down syndrome who have impaired vision due to cataracts. Fierson recommends intraocular lens implantation as a good choice for this patient group because it requires the least postoperative cooperation for visual rehabilitation [4].

KERATOCONUS

Like the lens, the cornea also can have opacities usually due to trauma, infection, or developmental anomaly. These complications, however, are rarely seen in patients with Down syndrome [15].

The most common corneal problem in this patient group is keratoconus. In this condition, a progressive thinning and stretching of the corneal stromal lamellae develops, and the generally spherical curvature of the cornea instead becomes a conical curvature. As this process progresses, the irregular conical cornea creates an irregular refraction of the incoming light rays that cannot be resolved to a coherent image on the retina with any known spectacle lens [4].

Acute keratoconus (acute hydrops) is the further development of this stretching of the basement membrane (Descement's membrane) until it ruptures [23]. At that point, aqueous humor from the anterior chamber rushes into the stroma of the cornea disrupting its lamellar organization and resulting in a milky opacity at the apex of the cone. Vision becomes greatly impaired. Munson's sign, distortion of the lower lid on downward gaze, can be seen (Fig. 14.2).

Acute keratoconus is a rare occurrence; however, it occurs more frequently in Down syndrome than in any other known disorder [2]. The patient can

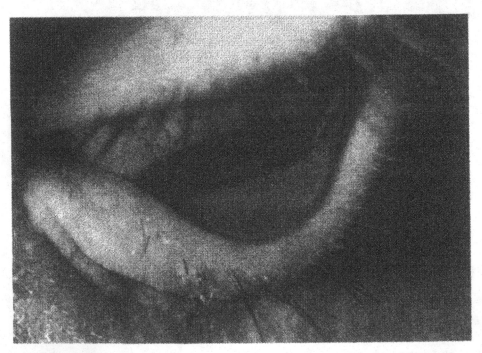

Figure 14.2 Keratoconus with hydrops producing a prominent distortion of the lower lid on downward gaze (Munson's sign). (Reprinted with the permission of the Archives of Ophthalmology.)

present with decreased vision, tearing, and redness of the affected eye. Sometimes both eyes are affected, and the problem can reoccur.

Keratoconus is estimated to occur in about 0.1% of the general population. The incidence in Down syndrome has been reported as high as 15% [10,16,17]. At one institution for individuals with mental retardation, it was found as high as 30% [24]. In normal populations it is a disease of older patients, but in Down syndrome, it has been seen in children and adolescents. The etiology is unknown; speculations about the cause include mechanical trauma from rubbing the eyes to an error in vitamin A metabolism. The present treatment of keratoconus is the surgical replacement of the cornea by penetrating keratoplasty and usually is successful [25].

RETINAL PATHOLOGY

It is unclear whether the serious retinal pathology that occasionally is reported in patients with Down syndrome is a chance occurrence or an indication of increased prevalence in Down syndrome, a relatively common chromosomal disorder. Six patients have been reported with retinal detachment; trauma was said to be a predisposing factor [26]. Also, retinoblastoma has occurred in six individuals with Down syndrome and has been reported in the literature [27,28].

A number of clinically insignificant variations have been reported in the retina in patients with Down syndrome. Decreased pigmentation has been noted by a number of investigators, and an increase in the number of retinal vessels that radiate like spokes (instead of arching temporally around the macular region) has been documented.

OPTIC NERVE HYPOPLASIA

Optic nerve hypoplasia is a congenital anomaly of the optic nerve in which there are a diminished number of axons. The condition is nonprogressive, representing a true absence of fibers at birth rather than an acquired optic atrophy. In the 1990 study of 150 children and adolescents with Down syndrome, Fierson reported that 10.1% had optic nerve hypoplasia [4]. Before this project, there had been only a single case report [29].

Because visual acuity can be quite variable in cases of optic nerve hypoplasia, this recent finding raised an area of concern regarding vision in children with Down syndrome. In Fierson's series, 14 patients had bilateral optic nerve hypoplasia; in two individuals, it was unilateral. Three patients also had esotropia. Regarding visual loss, most patients were too young for standard testing, but in six patients, Allen symbol testing was accomplished. Fortunately, no evidence of visual loss was documented in these six patients.

CONCLUSION

Starting with the infant learning programs, continuous education at a level of excellence is one major factor in the later quality of life of a child with Down syndrome. Maximization of visual potential of each child is necessary so that full benefit from the educational programming is achieved. In the past, children with Down syndrome have been allowed to function, or try to function, with forms of visual loss that could have been remediated. Refractive error, strabismus, or cataracts must not be allowed to impede learning in any child with Down syndrome.

REFERENCES

1. Caputo AH, Wagner RS, Reynolds DR, Guo S, Goel AK. Down syndrome: Clinical review of ocular features. Clin Pediatr 1989;28:365–368.
2. Pierse D, Eustace P. Acute keratoconus in mongolism. Br J Ophthalmol 1971; 55:50.
3. Lowe RF. The eyes in mongolism. Br J Ophthalmol 1949;33:131–174.
4. Fierson WM. Ophthalmological aspects. In: Van Dyke DC, Lang DJ, Heide F, van Duyne S, Soucek MJ, eds. Clinical Perspectives in the Management of Down Syndrome. New York: Springer-Verlag, 1990:26–54.
5. Gaynon MW, Schimek RA. Down's syndrome: A ten-year study. Ann Ophthalmol 1977;9:1493–1497.
6. Gardiner PA. Visual defects in cases of Down's syndrome and in other mentally handicapped children. Br J Ophthalmol 1967;51:469–474.
7. Sheller E, Oster J. Eye symptoms in mongolism. Acta Ophthalmol 1951;29:149–161.
8. Hiles DA, Hoyme SH, McFarlane F. Down's syndrome and strabismus. Am Orthoptom J 1974;24:63–68.
9. Cowie VA. A Study of the Early Development of Mongols. Oxford, Engl: Pergamon Press, 1970.
10. Shapiro MB, France TD. The ocular features of Down syndrome. Am J Ophthalmol 1985;99:659–663.
11. Eissler R, Langenecker LP. The common eye findings in mongolism. Am J Ophthalmol 1962;54:398–406.
12. Falls HF. Ocular changes in mongolism. Ann N Y Acad Sci 1970;171:627–636.
13. Petersen RA. Ophthalmological manifestations. In: Pueschel SM, ed. The Young Child with Down Syndrome. New York: Human Sciences Press, 1984:343–350.
14. Sutherland GA. Differential diagnosis of mongolism and cretinism. Lancet 1900; i:23.
15. Pueschel SM. Ophthalmology. In: Pueschel SM, Rynders JE. Down Syndrome: Advances in Biomedicine and the Behavioral Sciences. Cambridge, Mass: Ware Press, 1982:190–196.

16. Cullen JF, Butler HG. Mongolism (Down's syndrome) and keratoconus. Br J Ophthalmol 1963;47:321–330.
17. Lyle WM, Woodruff ME, Zuccaro VS. A review of the literature on Down's syndrome and an optometrical survey of 44 patients with this syndrome. Am J Optom 1972;49:715–727.
18. Francois J. Les Cataractes Congenitales. Paris: Masson, 1963.
19. Spitzer R, Rabinowitch JY, Wybar KC. A study of the abnormalities of the skull, teeth and lenses in mongolism. Can Med Assoc J 1961;84:567–572.
20. Robb RM, Marchevsky A. Pathology of the lens in Down's syndrome. Arch Ophthalmol 1978;96:1039–1042.
21. MacGillivray RC. Congenital cataract and mongolism. Am J Ment Defic 1968;72: 631–633.
22. Ingersheimer J. The relationship of lenticular changes to mongolism. Trans Am Ophthalmol Soc 1952;49:595–624.
23. Kenyon K, Kidwell E. Corneal hydrops and keratoconus. Arch Ophthalmol 1976; 94:494–495.
24. Hestnes A, Sand T, Fostad K. Ocular findings in Down syndrome. J Ment Defic Res 1991;35:194–203.
25. Frantz JM, Insler MS, Hagenah M, McDonald MB, Kaufman HE. Penetrating keroplasty for keratoconus in Down's syndrome. Am J Ophthalmol 1990;109: 143–147.
26. Ahmad A, Pruett RG. The fundus in mongolism. Arch Ophthalmol 1976;94: 772–776.
27. Day RW, Wright SW, Koons A, Quigley M. XXX, 21 trisomy and retinoblastoma. Lancet 1965;ii:154.
28. Bentley D. A case of Down's syndrome complicated by retinoblastoma and celiac disease. Pediatrics 1975;56:131–133.
29. Awan KJ. Uncommon ocular changes in Down syndrome (mongolism). J Pediatr Ophthalmol 1977;14:215–216.

15

The Immune System

"Infection is the leading cause of death in individuals with Down syndrome of all ages," wrote two highly knowledgeable specialists in Down syndrome in 1987 [1]. As we end the twentieth century, much progress has been made in improved medical care of people with Down syndrome, yet the cause of death has not altered since the syndrome was first described. Life tables, such as the one by Oster et al., emphasize the great susceptibility to infections [2]. In addition to infections, there also is increased risk for the leukemias and autoimmune disease, which suggests that problems in immunodeficiency frequently can be found in individuals with Down syndrome [3]. This chapter discusses the consequences of that immunodeficiency in individuals with Down syndrome.

THE IMMUNE SYSTEM

Infections

Young children with Down syndrome are quite susceptible to respiratory infections. The mortality rate resulting from such infections is high during the first year of life [4,5] and remains elevated through the first 5 years [6]. Comparing a Down syndrome population to an age- and sex-matched non-Down syndrome population from 1960 to 1971 disclosed an increase of respiratory diseases 62 times greater and of infectious disease in general 12 times greater in the Down syndrome patient group [2]. The reason for these striking figures is not fully understood, but a good start has been made in the studies that document abnormalities of the immune response to influenza antigen in children with Down syndrome [7]. In a home-based program of children receiving modern medical care, 30% came down with pneumonia [8].

Institutionalized patients with Down syndrome have been shown in many studies to have a high incidence of hepatitis A and B; chronic carriers of hepatitis B occur at a higher rate among those with Down syndrome than other mentally retarded patients in such institutions [9]. In a study designed to minimize the environmental influences of living in an institution, studies of serological markers were performed on individuals with Down syndrome living at home with their families [10]. In this study, there was no evidence that patients with Down syndrome had a higher frequency of a previous hepatitis A infection, but the data suggested that hepatitis B virus infection was hyperendemic even in noninstitutionalized individuals with Down syndrome. Fortunately, patients with Down syndrome respond normally to hepatitis B surface antigen vaccination and need not be considered a special group regarding guidelines for vaccination [11]. Hepatitis B vaccine is highly advisable in this patient group because of the risk of becoming a chronic carrier once the individual is infected [12].

Patients with Down syndrome also are at risk for infections of the middle ear (see Chapter 8). In fact, the occurrence of otitis media is among the highest of any population who are at risk for this disease [13]. Anatomic defects of the ear may contribute to this high rate of infection, but the cause is thought to be primarily related to immunological defects. Other infectious problems seen in this patient group include blepharoconjunctivitis, bladder infections in girls, and skin infections in individuals past childhood.

However, at this time, there is no solid evidence that patients with Down syndrome on the whole are more prone to pyrogenic or fungal infections [14].

General Principles of Immunity

For a full and detailed account of the often-conflicting laboratory studies that have been published regarding the immunology of Down syndrome, see a thoughtful and comprehensive review by Levin [14]. This chapter highlights some of the clinically relevant material by reviewing information about the major subdivisions of the immune system.

The immune system can be arbitrarily divided into four main components:

1. The polymorphonuclear-phagocytic system
2. B cells or plasma cells, produced and secreted by a subpopulation of lymphocytes. They are antibody mediated.

3. T cells, other lymphocytes that function with the aid of lymphokines or mediators. They are cell mediated.
4. The complement system that acts together with other systems.

The thymus is the organ that controls these mechanisms, particularly the first three.

The Polymorphonuclear-Phagocytic System

In an effort to explain the increased infection rate in patients with Down syndrome, many studies have evaluated the polymorphonuclear-phagocytic system. It has been established that the number of neutrophils responding to an infection was normal. Nevertheless, some of the details of the process do not function well as seen in Table 15.1. It is possible that alterations found in these cell functions are due to intrinsic cellular defects, which would help explain why these patients tend to undergo repetitive infective processes [15]. One report noted that after zinc therapy in patients with Down syndrome, depressed neutrophil chemotaxis, defective skin hypersensitivity, and low lymphocyte responsiveness to phytohemagglutinin (PHA) stimulation returned to normal, indicating that zinc deficiency may partially explain some poor immune

Table 15.1 Polymorphonuclear-Phagocytic System Studies in Down Syndrome

1.	Number of PMN neutrophils	Normal
2.	Neutrophil and monocyte chemotaxis	Impaired
3.	Phagocytosis	Diminished
4.	Digestion and killing of candida and staphylococcus	Diminished
5.	Intracellular oxidative metabolism (killing)	Impaired
	Superoxide levels in phagocytosis	Low
6.	NBT test (oxidative metabolism)	Normal
7.	Neutrophil chemiluminescence	Normal
8.	Zinc levels in blood	Low
	After zinc therapy—chemotaxis returns to	Normal
9.	Leukocyte enzymes (catalase, myeloperoxidase)	Normal
	CuZn dismutase (on chromosome 21)	Increased
	Acid + alkaline phosphatase; *G6PD*	Increased
	Galacto-1-phosphate-uridyl transferase	Increased
10.	Ultrastructure—6× increased number of leukemia-like nuclear abnormalities	

PMN = polymorphonuclear; NBT = nitro blue tetrazolium.
Source: From Ref. 14.

functioning in this patient group [16]. However, it is difficult to be certain that all these variations, often minor, found in the phagocytes of individuals with Down syndrome can explain the increased incidence of respiratory infections [14].

The B-Lymphocyte System

Regarding the B-lymphocyte system, most studies have found the number of B cells circulating in the peripheral blood within the normal range [17] (Table 15.2). The function of B cells can be evaluated by estimating immunoglobulin (Ig) and specific antibody production. A summary of these studies shows a tendency toward higher-than-normal IgG and lower-than-normal IgM levels. Minor variations have been reported in other immunoglobulins. Studies of specific antibody production suggest some deficiencies, and there is variation with age in several studies, but the pattern is not consistent [14]. Antibody

Table 15.2 B-System Studies in Down Syndrome

1.	B-cell numbers	Normal (may be diminished in older patients)
2.	IgG, IgA, IgM, IgE, and IgD B cells	Normal
3.	Immunoglobulins	
	IgG	Normal or high
	IgG in newborns	Normal or increased
	IgM	Normal or low
	IgA + IgG in children >6 years	Normal or increased
	IgE	Varies—low or high
4.	Genetic (GM) markers—4, 5, 10, and 11	Higher than normal
5.	Antibodies to O × 174 in older people with DS	Impaired
6.	Natural antibodies to *E. coli*	Low or normal
7.	Antibody response to several bacterial and viral antigens	Normal
8.	HBs antigenemia	Increased
9.	Antibody to HBsAg	×6 lower
10.	Seroconversion after HBV vaccination	Normal
11.	Autoantibodies—low titer (including ANF)	Commoner
12.	Milk precipitins in blood	Commoner
13.	HLA phenotypes 1, 2, and 3	Diminished
14.	HLA allele frequency	Normal

IgG = immunoglobulin G, etc.; DS = Down syndrome; HB = hepatitis B; ANF = atrial natriuretic factor; HLA = human leukocyte antigen.
Source: From Ref. 12.

responses to the viral antigens commonly found in the respiratory tract infections such as adenovirus, influenza A and B, parainfluenza 1, 2, and 3, respiratory syncytial virus, reovirus, and mycoplasma pneumoniae were similar to those of controls [18].

Levin has summarized the information about B cells by stating that there are no significant abnormalities in the number of B cells in Down syndrome, and there are no major abnormalities in their ability to produce immunoglobulins, although he noted that there are marked discrepancies between different studies [14].

The T-Lymphocyte System

The T-lymphocyte system seems to be a different story (Table 15.3). In this system, some of the abnormalities may even affect some of the regulation of the B cells. A defect in T-cell regulation of B-cell function may explain why, in some limited cases, the lymphocytes of individuals with Down syndrome respond less well to selected antigens than do controls without Down syndrome.

The T cells in the peripheral blood of patients with Down syndrome, even in the newborn period, have been described as diminished in number and proportions [18]. More importantly, when one looks at their functional ability, it is apparent from almost every study that they are defective [14]. The in vitro response to PHA of lymphocytes from adult and infant patients is markedly less than normal [19]. There is evidence that these defects in cellular immunity relate only to specific antigens, such as viral influenza antigens and tetanus toxoid. Also, both B- and T-cell responses to antigens are regulated by subpopulations of T cells, of which the helper and suppressor T cells are the main components; the helper T cells are reported as diminished [20], and the suppressor T cells are reported as increased in this patient group [21].

Humoral factors, such as interferons, interleuken-2, and migration inhibition factor, determine some functions of T cells. (The gene for the interferon-alpha/beta receptor is located on chromosome 21, see chapter 1.) It has been shown that Down syndrome children produce less interferons in vivo compared to non-Down syndrome children at the onset of a viral infection [22], yet lymphocytes from Down syndrome patients have three times more binding sites per cell for interferons [23]. Enhanced sensitivity to the antiviral effects of interferon has been demonstrated [24]. Delayed hypersensitivity skin tests are further in vivo evidence of defective T-lymphocyte function in patients with Down syndrome.

Levin summarizes the T-cell story by stating that the majority of studies

Table 15.3 T-system Studies in Down Syndrome

T-cell numbers and proportion (T3) generally	Diminished
T-helper cells (T4)	Diminished
T-suppressor cells (T8)	Increased
Thymidine uptake (blast transformation)	Decreased
Proliferative response to PHA, Con-A, and PWM	Normal or decreased
Proliferative response to antigens (tetanus virus)	Decreased
Proliferative response to staphylococcus, streptococcus, sendai	Normal
Proliferative response (early protein synthesis)	Normal
Mixed leukocyte reaction	High or low
Delayed skin sensitivity (PHA, PPD)	Diminished
Delayed skin sensitivity improved after zinc therapy	
IFN in vivo (during viral infections)	Diminished
IFN-alpha and IFN-gamma production in vitro	Normal or diminished
IFN binding sites per cell	Increased
Sensitivity to antiviral effects of IFN	Enhanced
IFN effects of defective lymphoblastogenesis	Enhanced
IFN-dependent natural killer cell activity (adults)	Enhanced
IFN-dependent natural killer cell activity (children)	Decreased
MIF production in newborns and children	Diminished
IL-2 production by lymphs, stimulated with PHA	Normal
IL-2 production, stimulated by bacteria or viruses	Decreased
IL-2 production in mixed lymphocyte culture	Normal

PHA = phytohemagglutinin; PWM = pokeweed mitogen; PPD = purified protein derivative; IFN = interferon; MIF = migration inhibition factor; IL = interleuken.
Source: From Ref. 14.

seem to indicate a quantitative and qualitative deficiency of the T-lymphocyte system in patients with Down syndrome. Methodological discrepancies, however, continue to produce conflicting results [14].

The Complement System

The complement system in patients with Down syndrome has been evaluated in only a few studies; if there are any abnormalities, they are only minor [15,17].

The Thymus

The thymus has been known since 1965 to have unusually large and often calcified Hassall corpuscles in autopsy studies in Down syndrome [25]. The

Table 15.4 The Thymus in Down Syndrome

Smaller than in matched patients without Down syndrome
T-cell depleted, with contraction and diminution of cortex
Blurring of corticomedullary boundaries
Hassall's corpuscles—increased in number
Hassall's corpuscles—many giant sized (mean size ×8 normal)
Hassall's corpuscles—cystic, hyalinized, or calcified
T-cell zones in glands and spleen diminished
Thymic hormone (FTS) reduced
Zinc therapy increased FTS to normal
Zinc therapy prevented appearance of inhibiting factor
THF in vivo increased T-cell proportion and function
THF in vitro induced competency in T cells

FTS = facteur thymique serique; THF = thymic humoral factor.
Source: From Ref. 14.

thymuses of patients with Down syndrome are generally smaller than those of matched controls without Down syndrome [26]. A number of abnormalities of this organ, which are particularly marked in young children, have been documented in the literature (Table 15.4). Larocca et al. studied thymus fragments and thymocyte suspensions in an effort to correlate the histologically observed thymic abnormalities with the cellular immunodeficiency of this patient group. Their work suggested that Down syndrome thymuses have a deficient expansion of immature T cells resulting in a reduction of the various thymocyte subpopulations—including the thymocyte pool able to differentiate into functionally mature T cells [27–29]. There is evidence of aberrant T-cell maturation [30].

Levin summarizes the thymus as histopathologically and functionally abnormal and giving rise to deficiencies of the cells and functions that are thymic dependent [14].

Thus, the basis for the immunodeficiency that underlies the infections in patients with Down syndrome is slowly being unraveled. Information from molecular biology about chromosome 21 (see Introduction) may have a unique role in helping to advance this understanding.

HEMATOLOGICAL DISEASES

Children with Down syndrome occasionally manifest extensive defects in bone marrow function. Often the course of the patient's disease has some unusual aspect to it. For example, in a case of a 26-month-old child with fatal aplastic anemia (which began as a severe persistent neutropenia at the age of 9 months), the existence of a suppressor activity in both the serum and the peripheral blood mononuclear cells was demonstrated [31]. In addition to aplastic anemia, there are several unusual features of the leukemias in this patient group. These include the transient leukemoid reaction of newborns and myelofibrosis, the preleukemias, the young age of diagnosis in acute nonlymphocytic leukemia, and the relatively high frequency of certain chromosomal defects.

The Leukemias and Related Disorders

Acute leukemia is the most common malignancy in persons less than 15 years of age in the United States [32]. Although the association between Down syndrome and acute leukemia is well established and has been known since 1930 [33], the magnitude of risk to Down syndrome patients has not been precisely determined. Given all the information available, it appears that individuals with Down syndrome are 10–20 times more likely to manifest acute leukemia than are individuals in the general population [34]. Of the acute leukemias, 83% of all cases in the childhood age group are generally classified as acute lympho-cytic leukemia (ALL), with the remaining 17% classified as acute nonlympho-cytic leukemia (ANLL) [32]. The proportion of ALL and ANLL in patients with Down syndrome is similar to patients without Down syndrome matched for age. This statistic comes from a review by Robinson et al. of 5406 children with ALL or ANLL registered with the Children's Cancer Study Group between 1972 and 1982 [35]. One hundred fifteen (2.1%) of these children were found to have Down syndrome. Also, the proportion of patients with Down syndrome was the same for ALL (2.1%) and ANLL (2.1%).

In Down syndrome, the age of onset for leukemia is bimodal, peaking first in the newborn period and again at 3–6 years. The increased risk extends into adulthood [36]. Congenital leukemia also occurs with increased frequency in Down syndrome patients and is characterized by a preponderance of acute nonlymphoblastic leukemia, which is similar to non-Down syndrome patients. In both Down syndrome and non-Down syndrome patients, the age of diagnosis for ALL appears very similar. However, the age for diagnosis of ANLL showed a significant difference between these two groups. The Down syndrome children with ANLL were significantly younger than their non-Down syndrome counterparts with ANLL.

Although there was no difference in age at diagnosis, there were a number of other factors that differentiated ALL patients with Down syndrome from those without Down syndrome. The children with Down syndrome had a significantly lower rate of remission (81% vs. 94%), a higher mortality during induction therapy (14% vs. 3%), and a poorer overall survival rate at 5 years (50% vs. 65%) [35].

All cytogenetic types of Down syndrome apparently predispose to leukemia. Besides trisomy 21, there is no other specific cytogenetic abnormality that is characteristic of the leukemia cells in patients with Down syndrome [36]. It is interesting that 19% of phenotypically normal children with leukemia have an extra chromosome 21 in their blast cells in association with aneuploidy and hyperdiploidy [37]. Chromosome 21 also can be involved in 8;21 translocation in certain cases of acute myelogenous leukemia (M_2 in the Fab system), and this has been shown to be of prognostic significance [38].

Transient leukemoid reaction of the newborn or transient leukemia is a process that disappears during the first 1–3 months of life in neonates with Down syndrome [39–41]. In most of these cases, the leukemia does not return. However, in about one-fourth of the patients, acute leukemia "develops" or "reoccurs." Zipursky et al. suggest, in a not unreasonable argument, that this transient reaction really is the first sign of acute megakaryoblastic leukemia (AMKL) developing in a child. They point out that this transient leukemia is a disorder that occurs in patients with Down syndrome or sometimes in other children with abnormalities of the twenty-first chromosome [39]. These investigators note the association of the twenty-first chromosome to AMKL, including a ring twenty-first chromosome. Dewald et al. raise a question about this generalization because, in their series, patients with acquired trisomy 21 tended to have granulocytic and monocytic lineages rather than the lymphocytic and megakaryocytic leukemias seen in patients born with Down syndrome [42].

Zipursky et al. also relate the preleukemic phase with thrombocytopenia, a virtually unique phenomenon found in patients with Down syndrome, to AMKL [39]. Based on their extensive experience and review, they conclude that approximately 20% of leukemia in Down syndrome may actually be AMKL, whereas the incidence in normal children is probably less than 1%. Although most investigators agree that transient leukemia can become a full-fledged disease, the specific diagnosis of AMKL and the percentage quoted is still under discussion.

Another unusual aspect of leukemia, particularly ALL, in children with Down syndrome is their poor tolerance of antineoplastic drugs, including methotrexate [43,44]. Their tolerance to maintenance chemotherapy is poor; often they only tolerate 30–50% of the standard doses. Gastrointestinal and hematological toxicities occur more frequently in patients with Down syndrome. Ulcers of the mouth can be particularly painful. Pneumonitis often is a problem. Kalwinsky et al. in a study of 28 ALL patients, state, "Intolerance to the antifolate methotrexate with severe gastrointestinal and skin toxicities was universal" [45].

There are several theories about the reason for this intolerance; they include altered pharmacokinetics of the agents used and increased tetrahydrofolic acid demands in this patient group from their increased purine synthesis making them sensitive to antifolate agents.

Drug and radiation preparations for bone marrow transplant therapy also induce toxicities [46]. However, it appears that survival after bone marrow transplantation is comparable in children with Down syndrome to that in patients without Down syndrome. Arenson and Forde reviewed the medical literature on bone marrow transplants in this patient group and concluded that there is no justification for denial of bone marrow therapy to otherwise appropriate candidates with Down syndrome and leukemia [47]. Others concur [48].

AUTOIMMUNITY

Problems with the immune system and autoimmune phenomena are correlated, so it is no surprise that there is evidence of autoimmunity of persons with Down syndrome. The increase of thyroid antibodies in individuals with Down syndrome is well documented [49,50]. However, thyroid dysfunction in patients with Down syndrome most likely is a heterogeneous disorder that cannot be solely explained on the basis of autoimmunity [51]. Inflammatory disease of the joints is also reported in children with Down syndrome [52]. Both alopecia areata and vitiligo occur and are quite difficult to treat (see Chapter 18). Studies of autoimmunity need to be an active area of research for this patient group.

PURINE METABOLISM

It has long been noted that the end product of purine metabolism, uric acid, is elevated in the plasma of patients with Down syndrome, yet they have surprisingly little gout. The clinical relevance of this finding may well be related to the fact that purine metabolizing enzymes have an important role in immune function, a fact first documented by the discovery of adenosine deaminase (ADA) deficiency in some children with severe combined immune deficiency. Studies show that ADA and purine nucleoside phosphorylase (NP) activity is elevated in the lymphocytes of both children and adults with Down syndrome [53].

Other children with severe combined deficiency disease and variable immunodeficiency disease share with Down syndrome children the characteristic of elevated levels of ADA in their lymphocytes. The T lymphoblasts exhibit increased ADA activity in patients with acute lymphoid and myeloid leuke-mias. Deficiency of NP in the lymphocytes is associated with defective T-lymphocyte function [54].

With this information in mind, it is possible to speculate that the increased ADA and NP activity found in patients with Down syndrome may be related to their immunological dysfunction. However, it should be noted that the various changes of purine enzyme activity patterns demonstrated in patients with Down syndrome all have a tendency to decrease the toxic purine nucleotide level within the cells—a finding that may reflect a mechanism for preserving homeostasis [53].

AT RISK IMMUNOLOGICALLY

It is reasonable to anticipate immunological problems among some children with Down syndrome; progress is now underway in both diagnostic and therapeutic approaches for such patients. The question that arises is whether anything can be done to prevent or at least ameliorate such inevitable infections and leukemias. The long-term answer lies in molecular biology; as one example, the ets-2 oncogene (a cancer-related gene) is now known to be located on chromosome 21 (see Chapter 1). In the meantime, the medical literature raises some questions possibly worth further investigation.

Palmer studied the effect of water miscible vitamin A on two groups of patients with Down syndrome who had increased respiratory and gastrointesti-nal infections as well as a high frequency of clinical symptoms of vitamin A deficiency (see Chapter 10) and reduced plasma vitamin A levels [55]. They also had increased levels of serum IgG. One group of patients received the water miscible vitamin A; the other group received placebo. The group treated with the vitamin A had a decrease in infections, a reduction of serum IgG and an increase in plasma vitamin A levels. Clearly, these were a selected group of patients chosen by clinical symptoms and plasma vitamin A levels. This work needs double-blind replication to determine whether it is relevant to the immunological handicaps found in children with Down syndrome with reduced plasma vitamin A levels. Because vitamin A is a fat soluble vitamin that can cause serious side effects if prescribed when it is not indicated, such research must be strictly limited to qualified investigators.

One cofactor of vitamin A is zinc. Zinc also is involved in many other enzyme reactions as well as cellular processes such as membrane phenomena and messenger RNA metabolism. There is a growing body of literature regarding the role of zinc in the immunological abnormalities found in patients with Down syndrome. It is very difficult to accurately measure zinc, but a consensus has developed about normal ranges for some blood analysis techniques. In patients with Down syndrome, zinc has been reported to be decreased in serum [16,56–58], plasma [59], and whole blood [60]. One study by Noble and Warren [61] failed to confirm this decrease. There is even speculation that one factor in the so-called precocious aging of the immune system in patients with Down syndrome is due to zinc deficiency [62].

Trials of zinc therapy have begun in Down syndrome patients. In an open trial without controls, Franceschi et al. reported a reduction of recurrent infections and an improvement in school attendance [63]. They report a significant increase in circulating T lymphocytes. They note that the clinical benefits of zinc supplementation were also seen in children who did not show an abnormal plasma zinc level. Bjorksten et al. report that 2 months of zinc therapy lead to improvement of delayed hypersensitivity skin tests [16], whereas a trial of levamizole failed [64]. Stabile et al. reported normalization of the lymphocyte response to PHA, a significant increase in DNA synthesis, after 2 months of zinc therapy [59]. Zinc sulphate also is reported to have induced normal amounts of the circulating thymic hormone, facteur thymique serique (FTS), and prevented FTS-inhibitory activity in young persons with Down syndrome [65]. In fact, Napolitano et al. report that the zinc supplements alter serum levels of growth hormone and somatomedin and that some children reached a higher growth percentile during 6–9 months of zinc therapy [66]. These are virtually all open trials, and, until double-blind studies are undertaken, their significance is unknown.

At this time, the main lesson to be drawn from this extensive research underway in the immunological differences in patients with Down syndrome is that increasing knowledge may lead to increasing opportunities for intervention. Any new therapeutic advances must be based on solid scientific studies. In the meantime, the care of the children always must be the best we have to offer.

REFERENCES

1. McCoy EE, Epstein CJ. Preface. In: McCoy EE, Epstein CJ, eds. Oncology and Immunology of Down Syndrome. New York: Liss, 1987. pp. xi, xii.
2. Oster J, Mikkelsen M, Nielsen A. Mortality and life-table in Down's syndrome. Acta Paediatr Scand 1975;64:322.
3. Burgio GR, Ugazio A, Nespoli L, Maccario R. Down syndrome: A model of immunodeficiency. Birth Defects 1983;19:325–237.
4. Sever JL, Gilkeson MR, Chen TC, Ley AC, Edmonds D. Epidemiology of mongolism in the collaborative project. Ann N Y Acad Sci 1970;171:328–340.
5. Wahrman J, Fried K. The Jerusalem prospective newborn survey of mongolism. Ann N Y Acad Sci 1970;171:341–360.

6. Deaton JG. The mortality rate and causes of death among institutionalized mongols in Texas. J Ment Defic Res 1973;17:117–122.

7. Epstein LB, Philip R. Abnormalities of the immune response to influenza antigen in Down syndrome (trisomy 21). In: McCoy EE, Epstein CJ, eds. Oncology and Immunology of Down Syndrome. New York: Liss, 1987:163–182.

8. Van Dyke DC, Lang DL, Miller JD, Heide F, van Duyne S, Chang H. Common medical problems. In: Van Dyke DC, Lang DL, Heide F, van Duyne S, Soucek MJ. Clinical Perspectives in the Management of Down Syndrome. New York: Springer-Verlag 1990:3–14.

9. Madden DL, Matthew EB, Dietzman DE, Purcell RH. Hepatitis and Down's syndrome. Am J Ment Defic 1976;80:401–406.

10. Renner F, Andrie M, Horak W, Rett A. Hepatitis A and B in non-institutionalized mentally retarded patients. Hepatogastroenterology 1985;32:175–177.

11. Troisi CL, Heiberg DA, Hollinger FB. Normal immune response to hepatitis B vaccine in patients with Down's syndrome. JAMA 1985;254:3196–3199.

12. Ugazio AG, Maccario R, Notarangelo LD, Burgio GR. Immunology of Down syndrome: A review. Am J Med Genet 1990;(suppl 7):204–212.

13. Downs MP, Balkany TJ. Otologic problems and hearing impairment in Down syndrome. In: Dmitriev V, Oelwein PL, eds. Advances in Down Syndrome. Seattle, Wash: Special Child Publications, 1988:19–34.

14. Levin S. The immune system and susceptibility to infections in Down's syndrome. In: McCoy EE, Epstein CJ, eds. Oncology and Immunology of Down Syndrome. New York: Liss, 1987:143–162.

15. Rascon-Trincado MV, Lorente-Toledano F, Villalobos VS. A study of the functions of polymorphonuclear neutrophil in patients with Down's syndrome. Allergol Immunopathol (Madr) 1988;16:339–345.

16. Bjorksten B, Back O, Gustavson KH, et al. Zinc and immune function in Down's syndrome. Acta Paediatr Scand 1980;73:97–101.

17. Levin S, Nir E, Mogilner BM. T-system immune deficiency in Down's syndrome. Pediatrics 1975;56:123.

18. Jacobs PF, Burdash NM, Manos JP, Duncan RC. Immunological parameters in Down's syndrome. Ann Clin Lab Sci 1978;8:17.

19. Gershwin ME, Grinella FM, Castles JJ, Trent JKT. Immunological characteristics of Down's syndrome. J Ment Defic Res 1977;21:237.

20. Noble RL, Warren RP. Altered T-cell subsets and defective T-cell function in young children with Down syndrome (trisomy 21). Immunol Invest 1987;16:371–382.

21. Philip R, Berger AC, McManus NH, et al. Abnormalities of the in vitro cellular and humoral responses to tetanus and influenza antigens with concomitant numerical alterations in lymphocyte subsets in Down syndrome. J Immunol 1986;136:1661–1667.

22. Boyer JM, Fontes AK. Interferon levels in Down's syndrome. J Am Osteopath Assoc 1975;755:437.

23. Morgensen KE, Vignaux F, Gresser I. Enhanced expression of cellular receptors

for human interferon alpha on peripheral lymphocytes from patients with Down's syndrome. FEBS Lett 1982;140:285.

24. Epstein LB, Epstein CJ. T-lymphocyte function and sensitivity to IFN in trisomy 21. Cell Immunol 1980;51:303–318.

25. Benda CE, Strassmann GS. The thymus in mongolism. J Ment Defic Res 1965; 9:109.

26. Levin S. Schlesinger M, Handzel ZT, et al. Thymic deficiency in Down's syndrome. Pediatrics 1979;63:80–83.

27. Larocca LM, Piantelli M, Valitutti S, Castellino F, Maggiano N, Musiani P. Alterations in thymocyte subpopulations in Down's syndrome (trisomy 21). Clin Immunol Immunopathol 1988;49:175–186.

28. Larocca LM, Lauriola L, Ranelletti FO. Piantelli M, Maggiano N, Ricci R, Capelli A. Morphological and Immunohistochemical study of Down syndrome thymus. Am J Med Genet 1990;(suppl 7):225–230.

29. Musiani P, Valitutti S, Castellino F, Larocca LM, Maggiano N, Piantelli M. Intrathymic deficient expansion of T cell precursors in Down syndrome. Am J Med Genet 1990;(suppl 7):219–224.

30. Murphy M, Lempert MJ, Epstein LB. Decreased level of T cell receptor expression by Down syndrome (trisomy 21) thymocytes. Am J Med Genet 1990;(suppl 7):234–237.

31. Hanukoglu A, Meytes D, Fried A, Rosen N, Shacked N. Fatal aplastic anemia in a child with Down's syndrome. Acta Paediatr Scand 1987;76:539–543.

32. National Cancer Institute. Surveillance, Epidemiology and End Results: Incidence and Mortality Data 1973–1977. Young JL, Constance PL, Asire AJ, eds. Nat Cancer Inst Monogr, no. 57, 1982.

33. Brewster HF, Cannon HE. Acute lymphatic leukemia: Report of a case in an 11 month mongolian idiot. New Orleans Med Surg J 1930;82:872–876.

34. Robinson LL, Neglia JP. Epidemiology of Down syndrome and childhood acute leukemia. In: McCoy EE, Epstein CJ, eds. Oncology and Immunology of Down Syndrome. New York: Liss, 1987:19–32.

35. Robinson LI, Nesbit ME, Sather HN, et al. Down syndrome and acute leukemia in children: A 10-year retrospective survey from Children's Cancer Study Group. J Pediatr 1984;105:235.

36. Fong CT, Brodeur GM. Down's syndrome and leukemia: Epidemiology, genetics, cytogenetics and mechanisms of leukemogenesis. Cancer Genet Cytogenet 1987; 28:55–76.

37. Rowley JD. Down's syndrome and acute leukemia: Increased risk may be due to trisomy 21. Lancet 1981;ii:1020–1022.

38. Golomb HM, Rowley JD. Significance of cytogenetic abnormalities in acute leukemia. Hum Pathol 1981;12:515–522.

39. Zipursky A, Peeters M, Poon A. Megakaryoblastic leukemia and Down's syndrome—a review. In: McCoy EE, Epstein CJ, eds. Oncology and Immunology of Down Syndrome. New York: Liss, 1987:33–56.

40. Koide R, Takahashi H, Tsunematsu Y, Sasaki M, Sugita K, Nakazawa S, Enomoto Y, Watanabe Y, Kaneko Y. Megakaryocyte proliferative disorder in neonates with Down's syndrome. Keio J Med 1987;36:57–61.

41. Coulombel L, Derycke M, Villeval JL, Leonard C, Breton-Gorius J, Vial M, Bourgeois P, Tchernia G. Characterization of the blast cell population in two neonates with Down's syndrome and transient myeloproliferative disorder. Br J Haematol 1987;66:69–76.

42. Dewald GW, Diez-Martin JL, Steffen SL, Jenkins RB, Stupca PJ, Burgert Jr EO. Hematologic disorders in 13 patients with acquired trisomy 21 and 13 individuals with Down syndrome. Am J Med Genet 1990;(suppl 7):247–250.

43. Garre ML, Relling MV, Kalwinsky D, Dodge R, Crom WR, Abromowitch M, Pui C-H, Evans WE. Pharmacokinetics and toxicity of methotrexate in children with Down syndrome and acute lymphocytic leukemia. J Pediatr 1987;111:606–612.

44. Peetes M, Poon A. Down syndrome and leukemia: unusual clinical aspects and unexpected methrotrexate sensitivity. Eur J Pediatr 1987; 146:416–422.

45. Kalwinsky DK, Raimondi SC, Bunin NJ, Fairclough D, Pui C-H, Relling MV, Ribeiro R, Rivera GK. Clinical and biological characteristics of acute lymphocytic leukemia in children with Down syndrome. Am J Med Genet 1990;(suppl 7): 267–271.

46. Rubin CM, O'Leary M, Koch PA, Nesbit ME Jr. Bone marrow transplantation for children with acute leukemia and Down syndrome. Pediatrics 1986;78: 688–691.

47. Arenson EB Jr, Forde MD. Bone marrow transplantation for acute leukemia and Down syndrome: Report of a successful case and results of a national survey. J Pediatr 1989;114:69–72.

48. Churchill LR. Bone marrow transplantation, physician bias and Down syndrome: Ethical considerations. J Pediatr 1989;114:87–88. Editorial.

49. Mellon JP, Pay BY, Greene DM. Mongolism and thyroid antibodies. J Ment Defic Res 1963;7:31.

50. Ugazio AG, Jayakar SD, Burgio GR, et al. Immunodeficiency in Down's syndrome: Relationship between presence of human thyroglobulin antibodies and HBsAG carrier status. Eur J Pediatr 1977;126:139.

51. Zori RT, Schatz DA, Ostrer H, Williams CA, Spillar R, Riley WJ. Relationship of autoimmunity to thyroid dysfunction in children and adults with Down syndrome. Am J Med Genet 1990;(suppl 7):238–241.

52. Olson JC, Bender JC, Levinson JE, Oestreich A, Lovell DJ. Arthropathy of Down syndrome. Pediatrics 1990;86:931–936.

53. Puukka R, Puukka M, Perkkila L, Kouvalainen K. Levels of some purine metabolizing enzymes in lymphocytes from patients with Down's syndrome. Biochem Med Metab Biol 1986;36:45–50.

54. Giblett ER, Amman AJ, Wara DW, Sandman R, Diamond LK. Nucleoside-phosphorylase efficiency in a child with severely defective T cell immunity and normal B cell immunity. Lancet 1975;i:1010.

55. Palmer S. Influence of vitamin A nutriture on the immune response: Findings in children with Down's syndrome. Inter J Vit Nutr Res 1978;48:188–216.
56. Anneren G, Gebre-Medhin M. Trace elements and transport proteins in serum of children with Down syndrome and of healthy siblings living in the same environment. Hum Nutr Clin Nutr 1987;4:291–299.
57. Kanavin O, Scott H, Fausa O, Ek J, Gaarder Pl, Brandtzaeg P. Immunological studies of patients with Down syndrome: Measurements of autoantibodies and serum antibodies to dietary antigens in relation to zinc levels. Acta Med Scand 1988;244:473–477.
58. Lockitch G, Singh VK, Puterman ML, Godolphin WJ, Sheps S, Tingle AJ, Wong F, Quigley G. Age-related changes in humoral and cell-mediated immunity in Down syndrome children living at home. Pediatr Res 1987;22:536–540.
59. Stabile A, Pesaresi MA, Stabile AM, Pastore M, Sopo SM, Ricci R, Celestini E, Segni G. Immunodeficiency and plasma zinc levels in children with Down's syndrome. A long-term follow-up of oral zinc supplementation. Clin Immunol Immunopathol 1991;58:207–216.
60. Colombo ML, Givrardo E, Ricci BM, Maina D. La zinchemia plasmatica nei soggetti Down e sua relazione con la loro situazione immunitaria. Minerva Pediatr 1989;41:71–75.
61. Nobel RL, Warren RP. Analysis of blood cell populations, plasma zinc and natural killer cell activity in young children with Down's syndrome. J Ment Defic Res 1988;32:193–201.
62. Cossarizza A, Monti D, Montagnani G, Ortolani C, Masi M, Zannotti M, Franceschi C. Precocious aging of the immune system in Down syndrome: Alteration of B lymphocytes, T-lymphocyte subsets and cells with natural killer markers. Am J Med Genet 1990;(suppl 7):213–218.
63. Franceschi C, Chiricolo M, Licastro F, Zannotti M, Masi M, Mocchegiani E, Fabris N. Oral zinc supplementation in Down syndrome: Restoration of thymic endocrine activity and of some immune defects. J Ment Defic Res 1988;32: 169–181.
64. Whittingham S, Pitt DB, Sharma DLB, Mackay IR. Stress deficiency of the T-lymphocyte system exemplified by Down's syndrome. Lancet 1977;i:163.
65. Fabris N, Mocchegiani E, Amadio L, et al. Thymic hormone deficiency in normal aging and Down's syndrome: Is there a primary failure of the thymus? Lancet 1984;i:983–986.
66. Napolitano G, Palka G, Grimaldi S, Giuliani C, Laglia G, Calabrese G, Satta MA, Neri G, Monaco F. Growth delay in Down syndrome and zinc sulphate supplementation. Am J Med Genet 1990;(suppl 7):63–65.

16

Dental Care

There is both good new and bad news regarding dental care in individuals with Down syndrome. Most of us want to hear the bad news first, and the bad news is that periodontal disease is a more difficult problem in individuals with Down syndrome than in other people [1]. There are also teeth problems such as malocclusions, missing incisors, delayed eruptions, and unusual shapes of teeth. On the other hand, the good news is that several studies have shown that caries is less of a problem in children and adults with Down syndrome than in a population without Down syndrome [2]. This chapter reviews these areas and provides recommendations regarding dental management.

PERIODONTAL DISEASE

It has been pointed out in the literature that in children with Down syndrome, periodontal disease can become a problem by the time of deciduous dentation [3]. A study by Lowe of 118 children and adolescents living at home and between the ages of 2 and 19 years revealed that they had a great variety of dental problems but that "gingivitis was perhaps the most widespread oral problem evidenced by these individuals" [4]. In this study, accumulations of food, plaque, and calculus produced inflammation of the gingiva and caused the tissues to become red, swollen, and hemorrhagic. The teeth most commonly affected by the periodontal disease were the lower incisors, followed by the upper incisors, and then the upper and lower first permanent molars. The cuspids were generally the last teeth to be affected.

Institutionalized patients with Down syndrome do not fare well either. In a 5-year study of alveolar bone loss comparing Down syndrome individuals to mentally retarded controls, the percentage of affected teeth was 47% in the Down syndrome group and was 6.8% in the control group [5]. Another study of persons with an average age in the late 20s found a bone loss in 60% of sites in patients with Down syndrome and a loss in 9.3% of sites in the controls [6]. Dental plaque is the primary causative agent of the periodontal disease [7]. Bacterial populations in the plaque have been studied, and a question has been raised whether their bacterial flora may be different in a population of individuals with Down syndrome [8].

In an effort to identify factors causing the early problem of periodontal disease in deciduous teeth, a study of experimental gingivitis (induced by a 21-day discontinuation of all teeth cleaning) was conducted on children with Down syndrome and controls [9]. Although the amount of plaque increased at a similar rate in both groups, in the children with Down syndrome, the developmental gingival inflammation started earlier and was more extensive. The immunological response (crevicular leukocytes) differed between the two groups—in the control group, the leukocytes increased significantly from day 0 to day 21, which contrasted with the results in the Down syndrome group. These findings correlate with the immunological abnormalities already documented in patients with Down syndrome (see Chapter 15). Other contributory factors to periodontal disease appear to be abnormal capillary morphology, disorders in connective tissue, and some of the anatomic variations in teeth [3].

DENTAL ANOMALIES

There are numerous dental abnormalities described in patients with Down syndrome [10]. Missing incisors, delayed eruptions, and prolonged retentions are reported. In a study of tooth size, permanent tooth dimensions were significantly smaller, whereas in deciduous dentition, some dimensions were significantly larger [11]. Pointed incisors and canines have been noted. The Lowe study found malocclusion in 40% of the children and adolescents [4]. A detailed study of craniofacial development (1896 patients compared to 1154 controls) suggests that the anterior open bite and Class III malocclusion are related to the proclination of the incisors, underdevelopment of the maxilla, and a more anterior position of the hypoplastic but normally shaped mandible [12].

DENTAL CARIES

With regard to dental caries, a comparison of individuals with and without Down syndrome shows opposite results. In Down syndrome, a lower overall

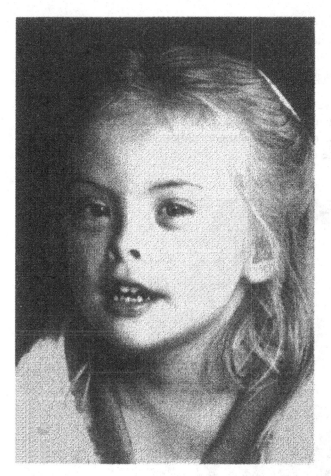

Figure 16.1 Dental anomalies cannot interfere with the loveliness of this girl with the trisomy 21 form of Down syndrome.

rate of prevalence exists. For example, in one study, seven patients with Down syndrome older than 15 years were caries free, whereas this was true of only one of the control patients [6]. Another study also showed that subjects with Down syndrome had less caries within all age groups [2]. Institutionalized subjects have a lower caries prevalence than those living at home, probably as a result of differences in environment. Within all age groups, Down syndrome subjects have less caries, especially approximal caries, mainly due to the fact that Down syndrome children have more spacing. Hypotheses to explain this finding include less sweet intake, greater spacing of the teeth, a decreased number of teeth to have caries, lower salivary pH, and characteristics not yet understood of the dentation itself.

DENTAL MANAGEMENT

Everyone should have individualized dental care appropriate for his or her specific unique problems. If malocclusion can be corrected, it is a good idea to do so. Unusual shape of the teeth or abnormalities developing from bruxism may need appropriate care.

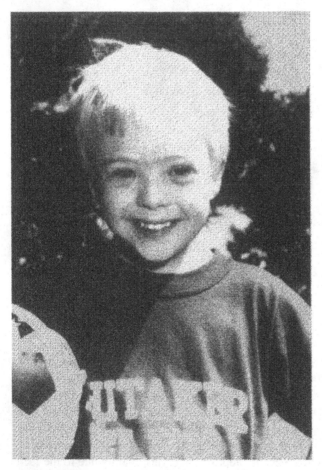

Figure 16.2   A bright smile often discloses good tooth structure in many children with Down syndrome.

But in addition to this general principle of individual care, there are two aspects of dental care in Down syndrome that need special focus. One is a preventive program for periodontal disease. From early childhood, patients with Down syndrome need to be instructed in oral hygiene and have it performed under good supervision daily. Failure of children with Down syndrome to brush and floss their teeth may have more serious consequences such as severe gingivitis and unnecessary loss of teeth than for other children their age. The program needs to be continued throughout life.

The second special concern in Down syndrome relates to preparation for dental therapy if the person with Down syndrome has cardiac disease. Patients with serious cardiac disease are usually already identified and the customary antibiotic prophylaxis prescribed before dental procedures. However, not all patients have auscultatory findings of their cardiac disease (see Chapter 9). An article in a dental journal reports that a random echocardiographic study of 83 patients with Down syndrome, 9–55 years old, revealed findings of mitral valve prolapse in 41 patients (49% of the sample) [13]. In 15 of these patients, the associated cardiac murmur could not be detected. The investigators expressed their concern that patients with Down syndrome at risk for endocarditis may not be identified if clinical auscultation is the only means used to identify cardiac disease in this patient group.

Again, we see the role of good preventive medicine in the care of persons with Down syndrome. Good dental hygiene may prevent needless tooth loss; early and thorough evaluation of each individual to determine whether cardiac disease is present can prevent later complications arising from dental intervention.

REFERENCES

1. Cohen MM, Winer RA. Dental and facial characteristics in Down's syndrome. Bull Acad Dent Handicap 1965;3:18–27.
2. Vigild M. Dental caries experience among children with Down syndrome. J Ment Defic Res 1986;30:371–376.
3. Reuland-Bosma W, van Dijk LJ. Periodontal disease in Down's syndrome: A review. J Clin Periodontol 1986;13:64–73.
4. Lowe O. Dental problems. In: Van Dyke DC, Lang DJ, Heide F, van Duyne S, Soucek MJ, eds. Clinical Perspectives in the Management of Down Syndrome. New York: Springer-Verlag, 1990:72–79.
5. Saxen L, Aula S. Periodontal bone loss in patients with Down's syndrome: A follow-up study. J Periodontol 1982;53:158–162.
6. Barnett ML, Press KP, Friedman D, Sonnenberg EM. The prevalence of periodontitis and dental caries in a Down's syndrome population. J Periodontol 1986; 57:288–293.

7. Keyes PH, Bellock G, Jordan HV. Studies on the pathogenesis of destructive lesions of the gums and teeth in mentally retarded children: I. Dentobacterial plaque infection in children with Down's syndrome. Clin Pediatr 1971;10:711–718.

8. Cutress TW, Brown RH, Guy EM. Occurrence of some bacterial species in the dental plaque of trisomy 21 (mongoloid), other mentally retarded and normal subjects. N Z Dent J 1970;66:153–161.

9. Reuland-Bosma W, van Dijk LJ, van der Weele L. Experimental gingivitis around deciduous teeth in children with Down's syndrome. J Clin Periodontol 1986; 13:294–300.

10. Lentz Jr GA. Dental care in Down's syndrome: Is it adequate? Down's Syndrome: Papers and Abstracts for Professionals 1987;10:1–2.

11. Townsend GC. Tooth size in children and young adults with trisomy 21 (Down syndrome). Arch Oral Biol 1983;28:159–166.

12. Fischer-Brandies H. Cephalometric comparison between children with and without Down's syndrome. Eur J Orthod 1988;10:255–263.

13. Barnett ML, Friedman D, Kastner T. The prevalence of mitral valve prolapse in patients with Down's syndrome: Implications for dental management. Oral Surg Oral Med Oral Pathol 1988;66:445–447.

17

Is Obesity Inevitable?

The physical appearance of anyone is an important factor in how a person is viewed by others, and this is especially true in the case of obese handicapped people [1,2]. There is a social stigma attached to obesity even in normal individuals [3]. In individuals with mental retardation, it may be one factor limiting recreational activities and many other opportunities in life. Obesity also has many negative consequences for health [4]. For example, individuals with Down syndrome who have cardiac disease should avoid obesity.

This chapter looks at what is known in the medical literature at this time regarding obese individuals with Down syndrome. The problem of defining obesity and determining how it is measured is a technical one that varies from investigator to investigator. In some centers, skinfold measurements currently are being used to determine whether a child who appears overweight is really "overfat." Studies are underway to analyze the possibility of different body-fat distribution in individuals with Down syndrome. Rather than become involved in this technical and controversial subject, this chapter accepts each investigator's own definition of obesity.

There are many known causes of obesity. Family traits, for example, can be important variables. In addition to the causes of obesity in normal populations, there may be etiologies of obesity that are more likely in children with Down syndrome. In this overview, an attempt is made to answer four questions regarding obesity and Down syndrome. They are *who*? (which persons with Down syndrome are at highest risk for obesity), *when*? (what are the ages when this problem develops), *why*? (what are the factors causing obesity), and *what can be done?* None of these questions has been fully answered, and much research remains to be done. However, there are some data on which to base preliminary observations.

WHO?

The etiology of obesity in Down syndrome is multifactorial, so it is difficult to predict the specific factors in any single individual. Some general trends suggested by the information gathered to date suggest that if a person with Down syndrome is relatively tall, has good muscle tone, and lives at home with excellent preventive medical care, he or she may be at the least risk for obesity. Conversely, a short child living in an institution, somewhat hypotonic, and with the minimum of conventional medical care may be at greatest risk.

In a longitudinal assessment of overweight children with Down syndrome, Cronk et al. studied children living in institutions and at home, including children from a variety of ages from birth to 18 years [5]. The institutions that were studied included one in Australia and one in the United States. The comparison data came from groups without mental retardation. These investigators report that children with trisomy 21 living in institutions tended to have larger mean weights for each stature interval than did those reared at home.

Whether males or females with Down syndrome are more likely to be obese is not clear. The study by Cronk et al. reported a greater tendency for obesity in girls than boys [5]. These investigators raised questions about whether females were constitutionally disposed to greater overweight or whether their greater lack of opportunity for activity caused them to be relatively more overweight than the males. The study comprised 124 girls and 138 boys and is the largest study available. Another study of very young children by Cronk and Pueschel, in 63 boys and 51 girls, reported that the difference between control and Down syndrome children's mean weight was greater for boys, particularly past early infancy [6]. A third study by Baer et al. of 190 children, ranging in age from birth to 18 years, found that 18% of the boys and 14% of the girls had a weight for height ratio greater than the 95 percentile [7]. Apparently, both boys and girls are at considerable risk for obesity.

WHEN?

The key to treatment of obesity is the prevention of it in the first place. In the field in general, it has been shown that childhood obesity tends to be related to adult obesity; this is a consideration in patients with Down syndrome. Thus, an important question that needs to be considered is when does obesity first

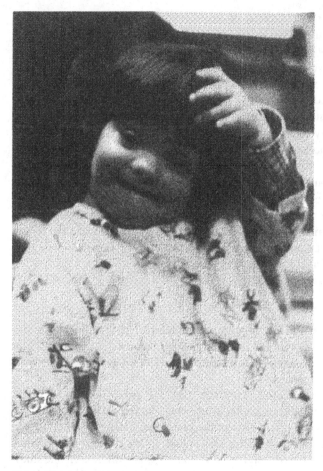

Figure 17.1 Obesity is apparent early.

begin to show up in a population of children with Down syndrome. Apparently, the answer is very early indeed.

In the Cronk and Pueschel study, approximately one-third of the children were classified as being overweight at some time during the course of the 3-year study as follows: 22% became overweight during the first year of life, 55% between 13 and 24 months, and 23% in the third year [6]. In other studies by Cronk et al., two different indicators were plotted out on the same raw data [5,8]. By one calculation, obesity began approximately between 30 and 37 months; by the other calculations, obesity became evident between 4 and 7 years. In another study, Baer et al. reported an increased risk for obesity between 25 and 48 months of age (10% were already above the 95th percentile), and they reported a tendency to gain weight with age [7].

So no matter what method of calculation is used or which study one looks at, it is clear that the tendency to obesity is present from early childhood in Down syndrome. Understanding that reality will help the development of preventive strategies in the early intervention programs.

Adolescence is another period when children in this patient group appear to be at risk for developing obesity. Children with Down syndrome have a pubescent growth spurt but the magnitude of the growth spurt is often smaller than in normal children (see Chapter 12). It is possible that these children have a normal pubescent fat spurt but that it occurs with a deficient pubescent spurt in stature [8]. This combination could result in excessive weight relative to the limited increase in stature and lead to adolescent obesity. Detailed studies of this problem in this age group are not yet available.

WHY?

Why are individuals with Down syndrome often fat? The first thought is that they consume excess calories and that they need to be on a diet. However, it is interesting to note that a careful examination of the studies available in the field does not confirm this concept.

To start with institutionalized children (i.e., the group that Cronk et al. found most likely to be obese), Culler et al. analyzed the caloric intake of 23 children 5–12 years old [9]. Each child consumed adequate calories per centimeter of stature, and each child's total caloric intake was *less* than normal for that age. There also have been studies of home-reared children. In one study of children between 1 and 12 years of age, again more than half of these children had a caloric intake less than that of normal children [10]. However, in this study, a small percentage of the children did exceed the recommended daily caloric intake by more than 50%. In another study of home-reared infants from 3 to 26 months of age, caloric intake was reported to be similar to control data [11]. So it does appear that excessive appetite or overeating is not a major problem in the age groups in Down syndrome at which obesity begins.

Another approach to losing weight is to increase one's activity level. This raises the question of whether underactivity is a factor in the obesity found in Down syndrome individuals. In normal children, a reduced level of physical activity has been shown to be associated with excess weight [12,13]. In the case of children with Down syndrome, specific studies of the question of physical

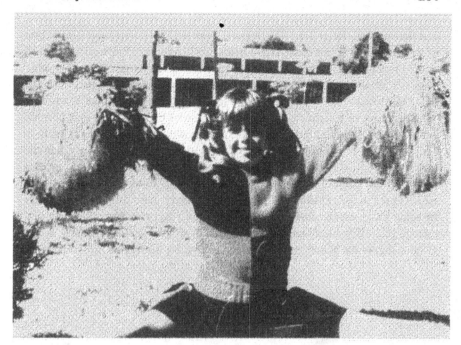

Figure 17.2 Hypotonia is not all bad.

activity have not been done. However, the hypotonia characteristics of young children with Down syndrome could have several effects. Delay in the achievement of motor milestones may limit physical activity during infancy. Later in childhood, poor gross motor performance may limit the amount of sports activity and organized play. There may be an element of the vicious cycle at which decreased physical activity results in excess weight, which then leads to an even further decrease of activity. Hypotonia even is reported to result in decreased levels of physical activity that can affect later psychological evaluations [14].

Based on what is known so far, one culprit in the development of obesity in Down syndrome is the retardation of growth resulting in short stature. It is the relationship of weight to stature that reveals a disproportion in this patient group. Length in the newborn period is normal or very close to normal if one takes into account the age of gestation [6,15].

However, the velocity of growth in stature shows the greatest deficiency between 6 and 24 months of age (24% less than normal) [16,17]. If one includes total time from birth until 3 years of age, velocity of growth in stature is 14%

less than normal. Regarding weight gain, there is also a comparable diminution of weight gain 20% less than normal from 6 to 18 months. However, between 18 and 36 months, weight gain does not differ from a comparison group. In other words, after 18 months, weight gain occurs at a normal (faster) pace than the delayed (slower) rate of height gain in young children with Down syndrome. This disparity of weight versus height percentiles can predispose to obesity. The study by Baer et al. also confirmed that growth retardation occurs early in life, with 59% of the boys and 63% of the girls having a height less than the normal percentile by 4 years of age [7]. Skeletal age, or bone age, appears not to provide relevant information on this particular problem because the bone age in children with Down syndrome differs little from normal children or may in some cases exceed that of normal children [18]. However, that does not change the reality of the height percentiles. A simple way of summing up the relationship of the height and weight percentiles for this patient group is that if

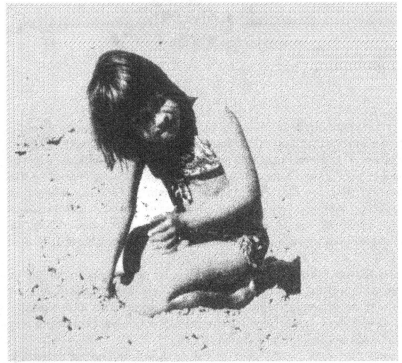

Figure 17.3 A bathing beauty.

many of the children with Down syndrome were not so short, they would not be so overweight.

A number of metabolic abnormalities, associated with obesity in normal individuals, have been reported in studies of Down syndrome. These include abnormal carbohydrate tolerance [19] and elevated blood lipid levels [20]. Their relevance to the problem of obesity in Down syndrome is not yet defined. A study of resting metabolic rate in 18 home-reared children with Down syndrome is not definitive because it did not have matched controls, but the data indicate that the rate may be depressed [21]. These investigators suggested that if energy expenditure is lower, a regular exercise program incorporated into the child's lifestyle would be the best antidote.

Serotonin, a neurotransmitter that has been linked to appetite control, is known to be low in the platelets (and probably functionally in the brain) of individuals with Down syndrome [22]. It can be elevated by pharmacological doses of pyridoxine [23], a vitamin found diminished in the whole blood of children with Down syndrome living at home compared to normal age- and sex-matched controls [24]. Again, the effect on obesity is not defined.

Finally, there is the problem of undiagnosed hypothyroidism in some dull, obese patients (see Chapter 12). This form of obesity is preventable and should not occur in any child with Down syndrome in a program conscientiously following the Down Syndrome Preventive Medicine Checklists.

WHAT CAN BE DONE?

There are no final answers regarding the underlying etiologies of obesity in children and adults with Down syndrome. However, it is already clear that there are things that can be done to make a difference in any individual child.

Above all, the importance of prevention cannot be stressed too much. Children with Down syndrome are no different than normal children; it is far easier to prevent obesity rather than struggle to take off the pounds once they are there.

There are many reasons why an infant should never go to an institution, and it is desirable that no person with Down syndrome ever live in an institution. In addition to these other reasons, home-rearing reduces the chances of obesity. This is one preventive measure that should be able to be accomplished.

Also, exercise is important to children with Down syndrome, especially those who have a lot of hypotonia. Whether it is the hypotonia, the shortness of stature, or the possibility of a depressed metabolic rate, it is exercise, more than dieting, that is likely to eliminate tendencies to obesity based on present

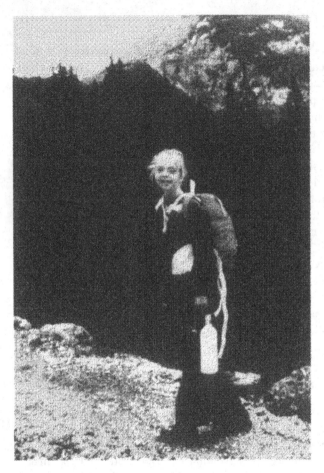

Figure 17.4 A mountain climber.

knowledge. The types of playing that involve a lot of physical exercise are both fun and healthy for these children.

Exercise is part of any infant learning program (see Chapter 2). The fight against obesity may need to start as early as 18 months of age. It is *not* a good idea to place very young children on diets; they need the fat in the whole milk for crucial myelinization of the central nervous system and elsewhere in the body. This dictum is particularly true of infants with Down syndrome in whom there is no evidence that excessive caloric intake is a factor in potential obesity.

In patients with cardiac disease, any exercise program may need medical supervision.

Another essential part of an antiobesity strategy is an excellent preventive medical program. Today, no individual with Down syndrome should suffer from hypothyroidism untreated.

For the sake of both health and attractiveness, the amelioration of the development of obesity in persons with Down syndrome is a priority.

REFERENCES

1. Romer D, Berkson G. Social ecology of supervised communal facilities for mentally disabled adults: II. Predictors of affiliation. Am J Ment Defic 1980; 85:229–242.
2. Hull JT, Thompson TC. Predicting adaptive functioning of mentally retarded persons in community settings. Am J Ment Defic 1980;85:253–261.
3. Cahnman WT. The stigma of obesity. Sociol Q 1968;283–299.
4. Bray GA. The Obese Patient: Major Problems of Internal Medicine IX. Philadelphia: Saunders, 1976.
5. Cronk CE, Chumlea WC, Roche AF. Assessment of overweight children with trisomy 21. Am J Ment Defic 1985;89:433–436.
6. Cronk CE, Pueschel SM. Anthropometric studies. In: Pueschel MS, ed. The Young Child with Down Syndrome. New York: Human Sciences Press, 1984:105–141.
7. Baer MT, Waldron J, Gumm H, van Dyke DC, Chang H. Nutritional assessment of the child with Down syndrome. In: Van Dyke DC, Lang DJ, Heide F, van Duyne S, Soucek MJ, eds. Clinical Perspectives in the Management of Down Syndrome. New York: Springer-Verlag, 1990:107–125.
8. Cronk CE, Chumlea WC. Is obesity a problem in trisomy 21? Trisomy 21 1985; 1:19–26.
9. Culler WJ, Goyal K, Jolly DH, Mertz ET. Calorie intake of children with Down's syndrome (mongolism). J Pediatr 1965;66:772–775.
10. Calvert SD, Vivian VM, Calvert GP. Dietary adequacy, feeding practices and eating and behavior of children with Down's syndrome. J Am Diet Assoc 1976; 69:152–156.
11. Madsen AL. Height, Weight and Nutritional Intake of Young Children with Down's Syndrome. Amherst, Ma: University of Massachusetts, 1979. Doctoral Dissertation.
12. Bullen B, Reed RB, Mayer J. Physical activity of obese and nonobese adolescent girls appraised by motion picture sampling. Am J Clin Nutr 1964;4:211–223.
13. Mayer J. Inactivity as a major factor in adolescent obesity. Ann N Y Acad Sci 1965; 131:502–506.
14. Cowie V. A Study of Early Development of Mongols. New York: Pergamon Press, 1970.

15. Polani PE. Chromosomal and other genetic influences on birth weight variation. In: Dawes GS, ed. Size at Birth. Ciba Foundation Symposium 27 (new series). New York: Elsevier/Excerpta Medica, 1974:127–164.

16. Cronk CE. Growth of children with Down's syndrome: Birth to age 3 years. Pediatrics 1978;61:564–568.

17. Cronk CE, Reed RB. Canalization of growth in children with Down syndrome. Human Biol 1981;53:383–398.

18. Pozsonyi T, Gibson D, Zarfas DE. Skeletal maturation in mongolism (Down's syndrome). J Pediatr 1964;64:75–78.

19. Yasuda K, Sakurda T, Yamamato M, Kikuchi M, Okuyama M, Miura K. Carbohydrate metabolism in Down's syndrome. Tohoko J Exp Med 1979;129:367–372.

20. Salo MK, Solakivi-Jaakkolo T, Kivimaki T, Nikkari T. Plasma lipids and lipoproteins in Down's syndrome. Scand J Clin Invest 1979;39:485–490.

21. Chad K, Jobling A, Frail H. Metabolic rate: A factor in developing obesity in children with Down syndrome? Am J Ment Retard 1990;95:228–235.

22. Coleman M. Serotonin in Down's Syndrome. New York: North-Holland Publishing, 1973.

23. Coleman M. Studies of the administration of pyridoxine to children with Down's syndrome. In: Leklem J, Reynolds R, eds. Clinical and Physiological Applications of Vitamin B-6. New York: Liss, 1988:317–328.

24. Bhagavan HN, Coleman M, Coursin DB, Rosenfeld P. Pyridoxal 5-phosphate levels in whole blood in home-reared patients with trisomy 21. Lancet 1973;i:889–890.

18

Miscellaneous Medical Problems

In this chapter, medical problems are discussed that are not covered elsewhere in this textbook. Diseases of the skin and genitourinary tract that occur in persons with Down syndrome are reviewed. There is a look at liver function tests. In addition, there is a discussion of individuals with Down syndrome who also suffer from a second disease entity.

DERMATOLOGICAL DISEASES

Clinicians who work with adults with Down syndrome sometimes note that they appear to be "older than their years" judged by dryness of the skin, premature loss of hair, or premature grayness. In children, also, dryness of the skin was noted to be a common medical problem in 39% of a group of 1–20 year olds [1].

Murdoch and Evans made a serious effort to address this problem by using an objective measure of the relative inextensibility of aged skin called the limit strain [2]. They performed a pilot study on the skin of five individuals with Down syndrome compared to 30 controls. Using this objective criterion, these investigators found no evidence of premature aging in the skin of individuals with Down syndrome and did not go forward into a planned full study of this problem.

A great variety of skin conditions have been reported in the literature in surveys of adults living in institutions. It is hard to sort out what is due to extra chromosomal material and what is due to the living conditions. Patchy lichenification, seborrheic dermatitis, syringomata, and elastosis perforans are described. Apparently, there is a particular tendency to disorders of keratinization, such as xerosis, keratoderma, and keratosis pilaris. A thorough review of the literature is provided in Pueschel and Rynders' comprehensive textbook [3]. The study by Carter and Jegasothy of patients living in an institution reported very high levels of xerosis, atopic dermatitis, and fungal infections [4].

Infections of the skin also can be seen in home-living adults. Mycosis can be difficult to treat [1]. The follicular papular skin eruptions, often staphaloccal in origin, also need aggressive treatment. The crusted (Norwegian) scabies is highly contagious, even on casual contact because of the vast number of mites in the exfoliating scales. It is characterized by extensive, heavily crusted skin lesions on the scalp, ears, elbows, knees, palms, soles, and buttocks. There is a special predilection of this disease for the immunologically deficient, including patients with Down syndrome (see Chapter 15 regarding susceptibility to infections).

Autoimmunity may be responsible for some of the skin problems seen at higher frequency in this patient group. Both alopecia areata [1,4,5] and vitiligo [6,7] occur in patients with Down syndrome and are difficult to treat. Regarding individuals with alopecia areata and Down syndrome, in 40% of them the partial baldness proceeds to alopecia totalis [3]. An increased incidence of antithyroid antibodies has been reported in the parents of children with Down syndrome, raising the spectrum of autoimmunity as a factor even in the etiology of this syndrome [8].

GENITOURINARY DISEASE

Although there is a general increased tendency to infection found in many children with Down syndrome (see Chapter 15), the genitourinary system is not thought to be at unusual risk in patients with Down syndrome. One outpatient survey of individuals 1–20 years old showed an incidence of 4% for urinary tract and kidney infections [1]. Pyelonephritis, reported at 6.2% in an outpatient population with Down syndrome, is similar in frequency to that in non-Down syndrome populations at that clinic [9].

Malformations of the kidneys have been reported in single cases of Down syndrome. These include stricture of the ureteropelvic junction, hydronephrosis, and focal cystic malformation of the collecting tubules with immature glomeruli [10]. Abnormalities also have been reported in the nephrogenic zone of the cortex [11], the glomerular basement membrane [12], and the renal arteries [13]. In a 14-year-old girl with Down syndrome who had primary intimal fibroplasia of the renal and other arteries, the presenting symptoms were weight loss and abdominal pain rather than the more classic symptom of hypertension [13]. Hypertension did not appear until 4 months after the onset of her illness.

Cyanotic congenital cardiac disease can result in glomerulomegaly, but there appears to be few such reports in patients with Down syndrome in the literature [12]. Membranous nephropathy secondary to hepatitis B virus infection in adults also is rarely reported. Considering the frequency of cardiac disease and hepatitis B virus infection in this patient group, the medical literature has a sparsity of kidney-related complications.

ENZYME LEVELS

Enzyme determinations have been performed on many tissues in patients with Down syndrome, including leukocytes, erythrocytes, and fibroblasts. Many of these studies have demonstrated significantly elevated levels of enzymes, including alkaline phosphatase, galactose-1-phosphate hydrogenase, galactose-1-phosphate uridyl transferase, phosphofructokinase, pyruvate kinase, 6-P-glucodehydrogenase, and glutamic oxaloacetic transaminase [14]. Physicians in clinical practice rarely meet these phenomena. However, this background of research studies might need to be kept in mind when trying to evaluate an elevation of alkaline phosphatase, for example. Not all enzyme levels are elevated, and even the elevated ones are not necessarily elevated in all tissues. This is one of a number of medically relevant factors to consider when evaluating an abnormal test result in this patient group.

DUAL DIAGNOSIS

When a child has Down syndrome, other diagnoses are not necessarily precluded. Other syndromes have been described as occurring in the same person together with the presence of extra twenty-first chromosomal material. The question that has to be asked about these dual diagnoses is whether they are mere coincidence or whether there is some etiological relationship between the two syndromes.

Another chromosomal syndrome, the fragile X syndrome, has been reported in two people who also have Down syndrome [15] (Fig. 18.1). The phenotype of these individuals has components of both syndromes. Profound mental retardation is reported. Because both Down syndrome and the fragile X syndrome are relatively common chromosomal syndromes, it is likely that the presence of these two chromosomal syndromes in one individual is coincidental.

The fetal alcohol syndrome, another relatively common etiology of mental retardation, has been described in association with five cases of Down syn-

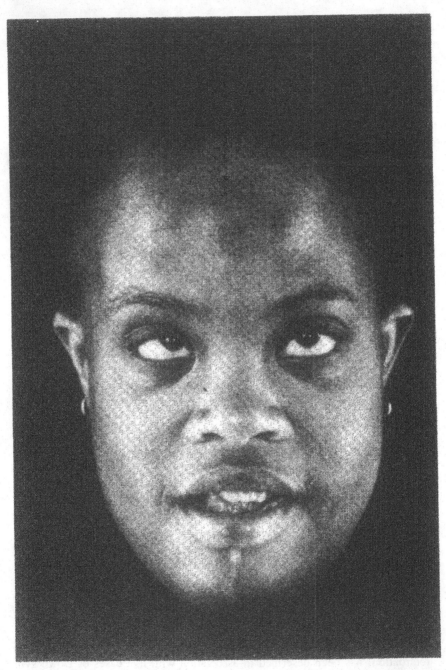

Figure 18.1   Child with a dual diagnosis—trisomy 21 and fragile X syndrome.

drome [16]. Phenotypically, these infants had manifestations of both Down syndrome and the fetal alcohol syndrome. Growth deficiency was more pronounced than is expected in Down syndrome.

The investigators in that study believe that, for their institution, there was an increase over statistical chance of these two conditions occurring in the same person. All the children had chronic alcoholic mothers as well as chronic alcoholic grandmothers, so the question was raised of a possible increased incidence of trisomy 21 in children of a second generation of alcoholic mothers. Like trisomy 21, the fetal alcohol syndrome occurs at greater frequency with the advancing age of the mother—this was true in these reported cases of dual diagnosis.

Several central nervous syndromes have been reported in patients with Down syndrome. The autistic syndrome is reviewed in Chapter 13. The Gilles de la Tourette's syndrome has also been reported in persons with Down syndrome [17]. All the patients had characteristic features of multiple motor and vocal tics. The investigators noted that basal ganglia dysfunction and neurotransmitter abnormalities are thought to underlie the development of tics. The premature calcification of the basal ganglia and the documented abnormalities of the neurotransmitters in Down syndrome (reviewed in Chapter 13) are thought by these investigators to possibly predispose this patient group to Tourette's syndrome.

REFERENCES

1. Van Dyke DC, Lang DL, Miller JD, Heide F, van Duyne S, Chang H. Common medical problems. In: Van Dyke DC, Lang DJ, Heide F, van Duyne S, Soucek MJ, eds. Clinical Perspectives in the Management of Down Syndrome. New York: Springer-Verlag, 1990:3–14.
2. Murdoch JC, Evans JH. An objective in vitro study of aging in the skin of patients with Down's syndrome. J Ment Defic Res 1978;22:131–135.
3. Pueschel SM. Dermatology. In: Pueschel SM, Rynders JE. Down Syndrome: Advances in Biomedicine and the Behavioral Sciences. Cambridge, Mass: Ware Press, 1982.
4. Carter DM, Jegasothy BV. Alopecia areata and Down syndrome. Arch Dermatol 1976;112:1397–1399.
5. DuVivier A, Munro DD. Alopecia areata, autoimmunity and Down's syndrome. Br Med J 1975;1:191–192.
6. Brown AC, Olkowski ZL, McLaren JR, Kutner MH. Alopecia areata and vitiligo associated with Down's syndrome (mongolism). Arch Dermatol 1977;113:1296.
7. Hazini AR, Rongioletti F, Rebora A. Pityriasis rubra pilaris and vitiligo in Down's syndrome. Clin Exp Dermatol 1988;13:334–335.
8. Fialkow PJ, Thuline HC, Hecht F, Bryant J. Familial predisposition to thyroid

disease in Down's syndrome: Controlled immunoclinical studies. Am J Hum Genet 1971;23:67–86.

9. Walczynski Z. Incidence of urinary tract infections in children with Down's syndrome. Pol Tyg Lek 1966;21:1479–1480.

10. Ozer FL. Kidney malformations in mongolism. Birth Defects 1974;10:189.

11. Gilbert E, Opitz J. Renal involvement in genetic hereditary malformation syndromes. In: Hamburger J, Crosnier J, Grunfeld J, eds. Nephrology. New York: Wiley, 1979.

12. Martin SA, Kissane JM. Polypoid change of the glomerular basement membrane. Arch Pathol 1975;99:249–252.

13. Fleisher GR, Buck BE, Cornfeld D. Primary intimal fibroplasia in a child with Down's syndrome. Am J Dis Child 1978;132:700–703.

14. Pueschel SM. Endocrinology. In: Pueschel SM, Rynders JE. Down's Syndrome: Advances in Biomedicine and the Behavioral Sciences. Cambridge, Mass: Ware Press, 1982:241–248.

15. Callacott RA, Duckett DP, Mathews D, Warrington JS, Young ID. Down's syndrome and fragile X syndrome in a single patient. J Ment Defic Res 1990; 34:81–86.

16. Bingol N, Fuchs M, Kosub S, Kumar S, Stone RK, Gromisch DS. Fetal alcohol syndrome associated with trisomy 21. Alcoholism 1987;11:42–44.

17. Barabas G, Wardell B, Sapiro M, Matthews WS. Coincident Down's syndrome and Tourette's syndromes: three case reports. J Child Neurol 1986;1:358–360.

19

Controversial Therapies

The birth of a baby with Down syndrome is a tremendous challenge to the parents, their family, and the professionals involved in the child's care. There is a desire by everyone to "fix" the problem—if only it could be done. A parent thinks, "If only there was a magical way to make my child normal." Such thinking, which is entirely understandable at one level, may lead to an unthinking embrace of controversial therapies.

In reality, many gains have been made in the care of these children. See Chapter 2 regarding infant learning programs and their effect on later cognitive performance. See the medical chapters (Chapters 8 and 14) on enhancing the ability of the child to see and hear well and thus be able to take advantage of these educational programs. See Chapter 12 to learn about safeguarding the precious central nervous system from further insult by the development of hypothyroidism. This entire book is a testament to how different our expectations are today regarding the health and performance of individuals with Down syndrome. Children who receive good educational and medical care have their natural intelligence and attractiveness even further enhanced.

There also is the job of the parents and everyone around the child to accept this little person and to learn to enjoy the child as the child is. Is it necessary or even desirable to force every single human being into the "usual" category regarding appearance, behavior, and patterns of thought? It could be argued that a better goal might be to help all children be fully accepted as they are, even if they look "different."

FACIAL SURGERY

In the last decade, lively discussion and debate concerning facial surgery as an active modification approach for children with Down syndrome has started [1]. It has been hoped that such surgery could improve speech, social development, and even cognitive performance. It is based on the premise that the facial features of Down syndrome are unattractive or immediately label the child as deviant.

This surgical program developed because value judgments about physical appearance are deeply embedded in our culture. For example, in the intelligence testing of any child in the United States, a long-standing Stanford-Binet Intelligence Scale item at year IV-6 credit the child for choosing the picture of the better-looking man and woman [2]. And what is "better looking?" In Shanghai, China, 100 beautiful, normal young women each day are having operations on their eyelids to achieve rounder-looking eyes of the caucasian type [3]. In the case of children with Down syndrome, originally called "mongoloid" because of the shape of their eyes, a correlation has sometimes been assumed between the total number of stigmata and or specific stigmata and IQ scores, yet objective studies have long been known to be negative regarding that correlation [4].

A study by Pueschel et al. investigated both physicians' and parents' attitudes regarding Down syndrome and reported that 72% of parents of Down syndrome children do not believe that the children's facial features affect their social development [5]. Cunningham et al. performed an elaborate evaluation by the classroom teachers of children with Down syndrome and found no significant associations between the appearance of the child and the child's development, communication, independent functioning, social life, behavior problems, parental stress, parent-child relationships, or the quality of family life [6]. Thus, this group of investigators found "no support to justify routine cosmetic surgery aimed at ameliorating such features."

Many ethical questions have been raised about this surgery as reviewed by Judith Mearig [7]. They include questions such as what message does this give the children about themselves and their natural appearance? how realistic is the availability to all children of this elective surgery? how safe is the surgery? and how effective are the procedures in terms of the stated goals?

Plastic surgery for children with Down syndrome includes tongue resection, silicone implants for the saddle nose, and silicone implant for micrognathia [8]. Much of the debate has settled on the effectiveness of tongue resection in helping speech articulation; the literature is divided on this point: Yes, it helped [9,10]; no, the effect was not different from controls [11,12].

Complications of these surgical procedures include resorption in the mandibular symphysis [13], suture dehiscence at the tip of the tongue [9], infected nasal implants [10], and the need for relengthening procedures for the tongue [9]. One group investigating these procedures even reported that the children's faces were less attractive after surgery than before [14]. Beauty is indeed in the culture-saturated eye of the beholder.

MEGAVITAMINS

Megavitamins, often combined with minerals, enzymes, and hormones, have been advocated as treatment for Down syndrome in various sections of Europe, Japan, and the United States. Haubold et al. recommended such a mixture as "basis" therapy [15]; Turkel developed a U series of nearly 50 different substances [16]; Harrell et al. recommended a high-dosage vitamin and mineral preparation [17].

These therapies often included fat-soluble vitamins, such as vitamin E. Sooner or later all vitamins given in continuous, inappropriate overdoses will have side effects that can be dangerous to the patient; this is particularly true of the fat-soluble vitamins. To take fat-soluble vitamin E (α-tocopherol) as an example), in one study samples of cortex were taken from fetuses with Down syndrome, patients with Alzheimer's disease, and a group of centenarians. The results indicated that neither the normal aging processes, Alzheimer's disease, nor the increased in vitro lipid peroxidation reported in fetuses with Down syndrome result from a gross lack of α-tocopherol or cause a significant depletion of the vitamin [18].

Independent attempts to confirm the claims of Haubold et al., Turkel, and Harrell et al. with studies using patients and controls have not been positive [19–24]. A great deal of time and energy using double-blind studies and other scientific techniques has been spent by a number of university research centers in an effort to check these claims. Confirmation of these multiple high-dosage vitamin studies was not forthcoming. In fact, an attempt to replicate the Harrell et al. therapy by Bidder et al. resulted in a great frequency of side effects, as even reported by the parents themselves [24]. The investigators noted with interest that most of the parents remain motivated despite the immediate and obvious side effects.

DMSO

Dimethylsulfoxide (DMSO) has been used to try to improve mental functioning in children with Down syndrome [25]. Again, the results reported could not be confirmed by independent study [26].

SICCACELL THERAPY

Lyophilized animal cells from various organs (siccacells) have been injected into patients with Down syndrome [27]. This therapy cannot be independently shown to be of value, and furthermore, the injection of animal cells into human patients can be dangerous and even life threatening because of actual and potential allergic and immunological reactions [28]. Because the death rate from infections among patients with Down syndrome is high, it cannot be stated with certainty exactly what the cause of death is in children who die from infections after receiving siccacell therapy. However, case histories report serious problems, such as an encephalitic immunological reaction to siccacell [28]. A recent, detailed independent study in the United States of patients treated in or from other countries with siccacells compared to untreated controls failed to support the continuing claims of improved functioning [29]. In fact, based on our current scientific knowledge, prolonged stimulation with such siccacells can lay the foundation for the development of autoimmune or even malignant processes in the future.

BENDA'S THYROID/PITUITARY THERAPIES

Because of the close resemblance of hypothyroid infants (cretins) to Down syndrome neonates (a differentiation made by Down in 1866), many investigators have attempted to treat children with Down syndrome by giving them thyroid [30]. The most recent researcher to recommend the administration of thyroid to all patients with Down syndrome was Clemens E. Benda. In 1969, he wrote, "thyroid therapy is indicated to activate the growth potentialities and stimulate general cell metabolism" [31]. He suggested a daily dose of .5–1.5 grains of thyroid. Benda also noted that the pituitary powder gained from young animals had some "definite beneficial effects on the somatic development of the mongoloid child" [32]. He raised the questions whether the powder might contain some effective somatotropin. All his recommendations grew out of detailed autopsy studies of this patient group.

As seen in Chapter 12, a small minority of children with Down syndrome do, in fact, have thyroid dysfunction, and need treatment of this endocrine system. However, even if one includes all patients with elevated thyroid-stimulating hormone levels and normal thyroxine levels, it is still a minority of the patients. To administer thyroid to patients who have no need of it is detrimental to those individuals. Regarding pituitary dysfunction, a clinical research project is currently ongoing regarding the use of somatomedins in unusually short children with Down syndrome (Chapter 21). These researchers are studying some of the same clinical questions that interested Benda but have available much more sophisticated laboratory techniques. The safety and efficacy of these programs are not established.

SUMMARY

The abandonment of infants with Down syndrome to institutions used to be recommended by physicians to the parents of these children. The medical profession has been slow in offering appropriate and aggressive therapy to these gentle little patients. As a result, many well-meaning parents have turned to unproven, even dangerous, therapies in an attempt to help the child they love. The elimination of controversial therapies may never totally occur. However, children born with Down syndrome in the future may be spared most of these negative experiences if more professionals enter this field to focus on rational and scientific approaches to enhance the health and well being of these children. A start has been made with the infant learning programs, the clinics practicing preventive medical care, research programs mapping the genes on the twenty-first chromosome, and a handful of clinical research projects using double-blind techniques. This is only the beginning.

REFERENCES

1. Feuerstein R. Down's syndrome surgery as part of an active modification program approach. Presented at a symposium: The Future of Seriously Impaired Infants: Where Do Professionals and Society Stand? Annual Meeting of the American Orthopsychiatric Association, Boston, March 24, 1983.
2. Stanford-Binet Intelligence Scale, Form L-M. Boston, Mass: Houghton-Mifflin.
3. Kristoff ND. Changing face of China, but one face at a time. New York Times, June 19, 1991, A6.
4. Domino G, Newman D. Relationship of physical stigmata to intellectual subnormality in mongoloids. Am J Ment Defic 1965;69:541–547.
5. Pueschel SM, Monteiro LA, Erickson M. Parents and physicians perceptions of facial plastic surgery in children with Down's syndrome. J Ment Defic Res 1986; 30:71–79.
6. Cunningham C, Turner S, Sloper P, Knussen C. Is the appearance of children with Down syndrome associated with their development and social functioning? Dev Med Child Neurol 1991;33:285–295.
7. Mearig J. Facial surgery and an active modification approach for children with Down syndrome: Some psychological and ethical issues. Rehabil Lit 1985;46:72–77.
8. Lemperle G. Plastic surgery. In: Lane D, Statford B, eds. Current Approaches to Down's Syndrome. Sydney, Australia: Holt, Rinehart & Winston, 1985:131–145.

9. Lemperle G, Radu D. Facial plastic surgery in children with Down's syndrome. Plast Reconstr Surg 1980;66:337–342.

10. Olbrisch RR. Plastic surgical management of children with Down's syndrome: Indications and results. Br J Plast Surg 1982;35:195–200.

11. Parson CL, Lacono TA, Rozner L. Effect of tongue reduction on articulation in children with Down syndrome. Am J Ment Defic 1987;91:328–332.

12. Margar-Bacal F, Witzel MA, Munro IR. Speech intelligibility after partial glossectomy in children with Down's syndrome. Plast Reconstr Surg 1987;79:44–47.

13. Peled IJ, Wexler MR, Ticher S, Lax EE. Mandibular resorption from silicone chin implants in children. J Oral Maxillofacial Surg 1986;44:346–348.

14. Arndt EM, Lefebvre A, Travis F, Munro IR. Fact and fantasy: Psychosocial consequences of facial surgery in 24 Down syndrome children. Br J Plast Surg 1986;39:498–504.

15. Haubold H, Wunderlich CH, Loew W. Grundzuge der therapeutischen Beeinflussbarkeit von entwicklungsgehemmten mongoloiden Kindern in sinne einer Nachreifungsbehandlung. Med Klin 1963;58:991.

16. Turkel H. Medical amelioration of Down's syndrome incorporating the orthomolecular approach. J Orthomol Psychiatry 1975;4:102–115.

17. Harrell RF, Capp LR, Davis DR, Peerless J, Ravitz LR. Can nutritional supplements help mentally retarded children? An exploratory study. Proc Natl Acad Sci U S A 1981;78:574–578.

18. Metcalfe T, Bowen DM, Muller DPR. Vitamin E concentrations in human brain of patients with Alzheimer's disease, fetuses with Down's syndrome, centenarians and controls. Neurochem Res 1989;14:1209–1212.

19. White D, Kaplitz SE. Treatment of Down's syndrome with a vitamin-mineral-hormonal preparation. Int Congr Stud Ment Retard 1964;3:224.

20. Bremer HJ. Stellungnahme zur Zelltherapie bei Kindern unter besonderer Berucksichtigung padiatrisch-metaboloscher Fragen. Mschr Kinderheilk 1975;123:674–675.

21. Hitzig WH. Stellungnahme zur Frischzellenbehandlung bei Kindern unter besonderer Berucksichtigung des Down-Syndroms und andersartiger cerebraler Schadigungen. Mschr Kinderheilk 1975;123:676–678.

22. Bumbalo TS, Morelewicz HV, Berens DL. Treatment of Down syndrome with the "U" series of drugs. JAMA 1964;187:125.

23. Smith GF, Spiker D, Peterson CP, Cicchetti D, Justice P. Use of megadoses of vitamins with minerals in Down syndrome. J Pediatr 1984;105:228–312.

24. Bidder RT, Gray P, Newcombe RG, Evans BK, Hughes M. The effects of multivitamins and minerals on children with Down syndrome. Dev Med Child Neurol 1989;31:532–537.

25. Aspillaga MJ, Morizon G, Avendano I. Dimethyl sulfoxide therapy in severe retardation in mongoloid children. In: Jacob S, Herschler R, eds. Biological Actions of Dimethyl Sulfoxide. New York: New York Academy of Sciences, 1975: 421–431.

26. Gabourie J, Becker J, Bateman B. Oral dimethyl sulfoxide in mental retardation, Part I: Preliminary behavior and psychometric data. In: Jacob S, Herschler R, eds. Biological Actions of Dimethylsulfoxide. New York: New York Academy of Sciences, 1975:449–459.

27. Schmid F. Cell-therapy—experimental basis and clinics. Cytobiol Rev 1980;2:1.

28. Levin S, Armoni M, Schlesinger M. Cell-therapy (siccacell) in Down's syndrome. Pediatric Rev Commun 1989;3:211–226.

29. Van Dyke DC, Lang DL, van Duyne S, Heide F, Chang H. Cell therapy in children with Down syndrome: A retrospective study. Pediatrics 1990;85:79–84.

30. Brousseau K. Mongolism: A study of the Physical and Mental Characteristics of the Mongolian Idiot. Baltimore: Williams & Wilkins, 1928:12–46.

31. Benda CE. Down's Syndrome: Mongolism and Its Management. New York: Grune & Stratton, 1969:240.

32. Benda CE. Down's Syndrome: Mongolism and Its Management. New York: Grune & Stratton, 1969:245.

20

Legal and Financial Advice

One of the greatest worries of parents of children with Down syndrome is what will happen to the child after their death. Most adults with Down syndrome will not be entirely self-sufficient economically; it may be important for parents to plan for their child's needs when he or she is an adult. This chapter briefly presents some of the formal mechanisms for parents to make suitable reserves available for their child in the event of their untimely death when the child is under 18 years of age and to plan for the child's adult years.

This information is relevant to parents in the United States. Similar information needs to be made available to parents in other countries. As in so many other aspects of their child's life, parents often look to the physician to steer them toward help for realistic problems concerning their child.

The information presented here may be out of date by the time it is needed. Updating of current information is a minimum for intelligent counseling and support.

A resource for parents in the United States is the booklet, *How to Provide for Their Future*, published by the Association for Retarded Citizens, National Headquarters, P.O. Box 6109, Arlington, TX 76011.

I. Guardianship
   A. Definition: A court-approved legal relationship between an adult or guardian and a child or adult who is handicapped (ward) that gives the guardian the right to act on behalf of the ward in making decisions.

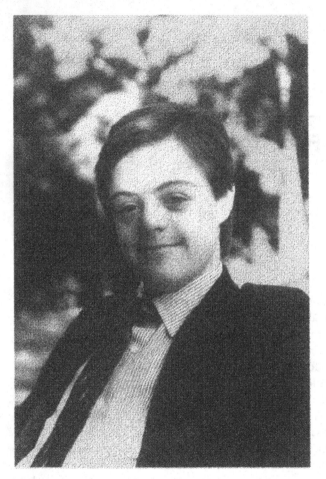

Figure 20.1 A handsome young man with Down syndrome.

B. Types
1. Total guardianship gives the guardian power over all decisions for the person with Down syndrome and results in his or her loss of certain rights such as to vote, contract, and consent to surgery or other medical procedures.
2. Partial guardianship is available in some states and limits the areas that the guardian may act and allows the person to retain rights in other areas to act.

3. Collective guardianship refers to a public agency or nonprofit organization that serves as guardians and advocates for persons.

4. Testamentary guardian is one named in a parent's will for a minor child. This guardianship begins after the death of both parents and terminates after the child reaches 18 years of age.

C. Conclusion: Guardianship may help provide some security for adults with handicaps but must be investigated very closely by the parents to make sure these options are best for their child.

II. General Estate Planning

A. The purpose of estate planning is to make sure that assets will be distributed fairly after the death of the parents and to make sure that their child will have an advocate or protector.

B. The importance of an estate plan is to make sure that the child with mental retardation will have an income for his or her entire life that will not make him or her ineligible for other governmental assistance programs such as Supplementary Security Income.

C. Each parent should have a will drafted by an attorney familiar with the state's laws and regulations for governmental benefits and federal and state tax laws.

D. This estate plan needs review frequently.

E. Making a child with mental retardation beneficiary of an insurance policy or giving legal title to property or money may make that child ineligible for governmental benefits and will be a source of funds for the government to draw on to provide services to that child.

III. Life Insurance

A. The parents of a child with mental retardation need extra life insurance if it can be afforded.

B. It is important to obtain the advice of a good insurance counselor about the amount of insurance to purchase.

C. The child should be insured to provide money for obligations left behind by the death of parents. Often, it is difficult to obtain life, as well as medical, insurance for the person with mental retardation, but programs are available through the Association for Retarded Citizens.

IV. Government Benefits

A. Social insurance programs

1. These programs return money that someone paid into a public trust fund such as Social Security mandatory payroll deductions.

2. The benefits from these programs are not affected by a person's other income.

3. Social Security benefits may be available to an adult with mental retardation by two mechanisms.
   a. An adult may have been able to work enough to meet criteria as a worker and then claim a disability due to a medical impairment or mental impairment.
   b. An adult may qualify for benefits as the dependent of an insured parent when that parent retires, dies, or becomes disabled.
4. Medicare
   a. A person who receives Social Security because of a disability will be covered by Medicare after 2 years of receiving benefits.
   b. This covers hospitalization up to 90 days and some outpatient rehabilitation services. Physician services can be covered for a premium charged by a deduction from the Social Security check.

B. Public assistance programs
   1. These programs support the needy and come from general tax revenues.
   2. The benefits from these programs will be reduced if the person has significant income or assets, earned or unearned.
   3. Supplementary Security Income
      a. The basic Supplementary Security Income is administered by the Social Security Administration, and states may choose to supplement the basic federal payments.
      b. Assets, as well as living arrangements, may affect the income from Supplementary Security Income.
      c. Most adults become eligible at the age of 18 because of their mental disability.
      d. Families may receive Supplementary Security Income benefits for their child with a mental disability if they meet an income test. A mental disability is defined usually as mental retardation in the moderate, severe, or profound range.
   4. Medicaid
      a. Each state sets up its own Medicaid program.
      b. This plan usually covers most persons eligible for Supplementary Security Income benefits.
      c. Pays for physician expenses and some costs of hospitalization.
C. Because of differences between states and frequent changes in

programs, it is very important to contact the local Association for Retarded Citizens office or district office of the Social Security Administration or state office of mental retardation.

D. Other programs
1. Benefits in kind refers to services that have a cash value such as food stamps provided by states and rent subsidies provided under section 8 of the Housing and Community Development Act.
2. Veterans who are totally disabled are entitled to certain benefits and services for their dependents.

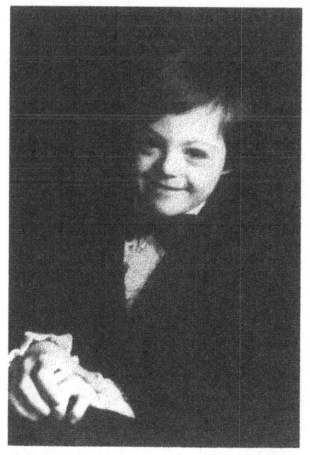

Figure 20.2 A boy with trisomy 21 out on the town.

IV

THE FUTURE

21

The Future in Down Syndrome Research

More than a century after Down syndrome was first described, new attitudes toward medical care and research are beginning to have an impact on the lives of the individuals with this syndrome. Considerably more progress can be anticipated in the next decade. An area where further improvement reasonably can be anticipated is the development of educational and medical interventions designed to improve the life of the individual with Down syndrome starting in the neonatal period and continuing through adult life. It is even possible that the laboratory studies involving the genetic mapping of chromosome 21 of humans and research utilizing the experimental mouse model may begin to have definitive clinical implications before the decade is over.

HUMAN CHROMOSOME 21 AND MURINE TRISOMY 16

Molecular biologists and other research scientists studying the twenty-first chromosome have set themselves an impressive task. They are trying to learn which genes in triple dose are responsible for each aspect of the phenotype of an individual with Down syndrome. As seen in the Introduction, some important beginnings of this task are already underway.

Unfortunately, nature often does not work in a simple way. Some genes appear to be inactive; the active genes have their effects modified in several different ways by other genes; and the mechanism of how triple dosing distorts the phenotype is yet to be understood. Studies of the difference between the effect of an entire extra chromosome in contrast to partial trisomies is an important and fruitful area for research, particularly regarding mental retardation. The technical challenges are many. If successful, this project may become a model for studying other chromosomal syndromes.

Another laboratory tool for understanding mechanisms in Down syndrome is an animal model, murine trisomy 16, which has a surprising amount of genetic homology with the human genotype [1,2]. Although the mouse chromosomes are different in number, the human twenty-first chromosome and the mouse sixteenth chromosome both code for the free radical scavenging enzyme, superoxide dismutase-1 (SOD-1), the purine biosynthetic enzyme phosphoribosylglycinamide synthetase (PRGS), the protooncogene ETS-2, the interferon alpha and beta receptors, and the gene APP coding for the precursor protein for amyloid. Phenotypic features of human and murine trisomy 16 also are similar, such as flat face, shortened neck, ear abnormalities, congenital cardiac disease, fetal edema, and thymic hypoplasia. Even some of the unusual electrical membrane properties of cultured dorsal root ganglia neurons in human Down syndrome are found in murine trisomy 16 [3].

Murine trisomy 16 may be useful for studying factors that produce immunodeficiency, leukemia, and Alzheimer's disease in individuals with Down syndrome. The finding of this animal is a marvelous bit of luck for researchers.

The ultimate goal of silencing the effect of the additional chromosomal material may still be quite far away. The one thing that can be definitely anticipated is that many new findings and surprises await the scientists.

IMPROVING THE QUALITY OF LIFE

The future is likely to bring many new clinical programs designed to enhance the life of individuals with Down syndrome.

In infants with other forms of potential mental retardation, such as infant hypothyroidism, phenylketonuria (PKU), or maple syrup urine disease, identification of the disease entity occurs in the newborn period through an infant screening program using heel stick blood tests [4]. As a result of this early identification, therapeutic intervention occurs immediately, and often the child is spared a life of mental retardation. After the infant is born, there is a limited, short time period available for identification and the beginning of appropriate therapy. This is because the protective effect of the placenta rapidly ceases and irreversible changes begin in the central nervous system. The time period for each disease and each child differ. For example, in maple syrup urine disease, it may be a matter of 2 or 3 days, whereas it is more a matter of 4–6 weeks in the case of infant hypothyroidism.

The infant with potential mental retardation most easily identified in the neonatal period is the baby with Down syndrome. The information available on the neonatal brain of such a child is reviewed in Chapter 13. There is evidence in Down syndrome (as there is in some cases of PKU and infant hypothyroidism) that the brain is already compromised in utero to some extent by the trisomic chromosomal disease process. However, there also is evidence in Down syndrome in newborns, as in other neonatally identified diseases, that the placenta has postponed at least some of the effects on the brain. For example, the pattern of the auditory evoked potential may still be within two standard deviations after birth for 10–20 days after birth [5]. (There is much less time in twins who shared a placenta.)

Because the infant with Down syndrome is quickly identified in medical centers and because it cannot be definitely said at this time that the neonatal brain is already compromised to the point of mental retardation, it is theoretically possible that a medical therapy could be developed to prevent or ameliorate the mental handicap. Such therapies are based on the finding of biochemical abnormalities in the tissues of these children. Two such trials of therapy initiated in infancy have failed [6,7], but this does not mean that more sophisticated future trials will do so. At the moment, researchers are studying the effects of the administration of selenium in this patient group [8]. Initially, their project was started to enhance glutathione peroxidase (GSH-Px) activity, which possibly protects brain damage caused by lipid peroxidation. Because selenium also affects the immune system, the four immunoglobulin (IgG) subclasses were additionally studied, and the investigators reported that selenium administration in children with Down syndrome enhanced the levels of IgG2 and IgG4, the two subclasses depressed in children with Down syndrome according to these investigators [9]. These interesting reports await future double-blind evaluation.

In childhood, one promising area of clinical research is the studies of the somatomedins in patients with Down syndrome [10]. The somatomedins are a family of polypeptide hormones that regulate growth and metabolism, and there is evidence they may be an important factor regulating brain growth [11]. Insulinlike growth factors (IGF) are deficient in fetuses with Down syndrome; growth hormone-regulated IGF-1 fails to increase during childhood and remains at a low level throughout life. (This selective deficiency of IGF-1 is also present in pygmies.) Present research suggests that there may be delayed maturation with incomplete switching from production of the fetal form of IGF to production of IGF-1 in patients with Down syndrome [12]. It has already been reported that children with Down syndrome are responders to parenteral human growth hormone therapy with increase of growth velocity during treatment [13]. Double-blind studies and the long-term implications have yet to be worked out [14]. This is only one of a number of promising medical projects in various stages of development to help children with Down syndrome.

Regarding adolescents and adults with Down syndrome, a new emphasis and commitment in vocational and other appropriate education may be the highlight of the next decade. Immense effort has been directed toward very young children in early intervention programs and toward children in the medical clinics that this book is designed to serve. All of this work is directed

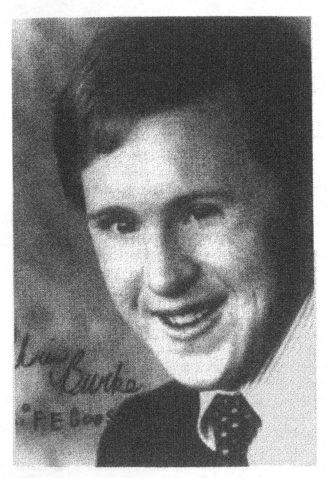

Figure 21.1 A successful television star.

toward making it possible for people with Down syndrome to achieve and maintain their potential.

In the coming decade, the actual abilities of these young adults need to be adequately utilized. Of course, not everyone can become a television star (Fig. 21.1). A new approach to vocational education and preparation for all persons with Down syndrome is needed that opens up limitless opportunities restricted only by the individual's ultimate ability. A commitment by the community needs to be made to create vocational training for wage-competitive work and appropriate and attractive housing options for these young adults.

Of course, they need to continue to have access to excellent medical care (see Chapter 7). The development of case managers and other team members will help make sure that this access is never denied.

Above all, we have to live in a society where everyone with Down syndrome is accepted as an individual person who can be interesting and productive. As one young man said, "my problem isn't how I look; it is how you see me."

REFERENCES

1. Epstein CJ, Cox DR, Epstein LB. Mouse trisomy 16: An animal model for human trisomy 21 (Down syndrome). Ann N Y Acad Sci 1985;450:157–168.
2. Reeves RH, Gearhart JD, Littlefield JW. Genetic basis for a mouse model of Down syndrome. Brain Res Bull 1986;16:803–814.
3. Orozco CB, Smith SA, Epstein CJ, Rapoport SI. Electrophysiologic properties of cultured dorsal root ganglion and spinal cord neurons of normal and trisomy 16 mice. Dev Brain Res 1987;32:111–122.
4. Infant Screening Newsletter. Vol. I–II, 1978–1988.
5. Coleman M, Barnet A. The change in evoked potentials during the neonatal period in Down syndrome. Unpublished manuscript, 1991.
6. Bazelon M, Paine RS, Cowie V, Hunt P, Houck JC, Mahanand D. Reversal of hypotonia in infants with Down's syndrome by administration of 5-hydroxytryptophan. Lancet 1967;i:1130.
7. Coleman M. Studies of the administration of pyridoxine to children with Down's syndrome. In: Leklem J, Reynolds R, eds. Clinical and Physiological Applications of Vitamin B-6. New York: Liss, 1988:317–328.
8. Anneren G, Gebre-Medhin M, Gustavson K-H. Selenium supplementation in children with Down syndrome. Acta Paediatr Scand 1989;78:879.
9. Anneren G, Magnusson CGM, Nordvall SL. Increase in serum concentrations of IgG2 and IgG4 by selenium supplementation in children with Down's syndrome. Arch Dis Child 1990;65:1353–1355.
10. Sara VR, Gustavson K-H, Anneren G, Hall K, Wetterberg L. Somatomedins in Down's syndrome. Biol Psychiatry 1983;18:803–811.

11. Sara VR, Hall K, Wetterberg L. Fetal brain growth: A proposed model for regulation by embryonic somatomedin. In: Ritzen M, Aperia A, Hall K, Larsson A, Zetterberg A, Zetterstrom R, eds. The Biology of Normal Human Growth. New York: Raven Press 1981:241–253.
12. Anneren G, Sara VR, Hall K, Tuvemo T. Growth and somatomedin responses to growth hormone in Down's syndrome. Arch Dis Child 1986;61:48–52.
13. Anneren G, Gustavson K-H, Sara VR, Tuvemo T. Growth retardation in Down syndrome in relation to insulin-like growth factors and growth hormone. Am J Med Genet 1990;(suppl 7):59–62.

Appendix A

Growth Charts for Down Syndrome

Figs. A.1 through A.4 are from Cronk C, Crocker AC, Pueschel SM, Shea AM, Zackai E, Pickens G, Reed RB. Growth charts for children with Down syndrome—one month to 18 years of age. Pediatrics 1988;18:102–110.

Figs. A.5 through A.6 are from Cross R, Rogers P, Chamberlain J, Patterson B, Holan J, Clark M. Head circumference of children with Down syndrome (in press).

Other growth charts are available in the literature. For children 0 through 14 years, refer to American Journal of Medical Genetics Supplement 7, pages 66–70, and for neonatal growth patterns, see also Supplement 7, pages 71–74.

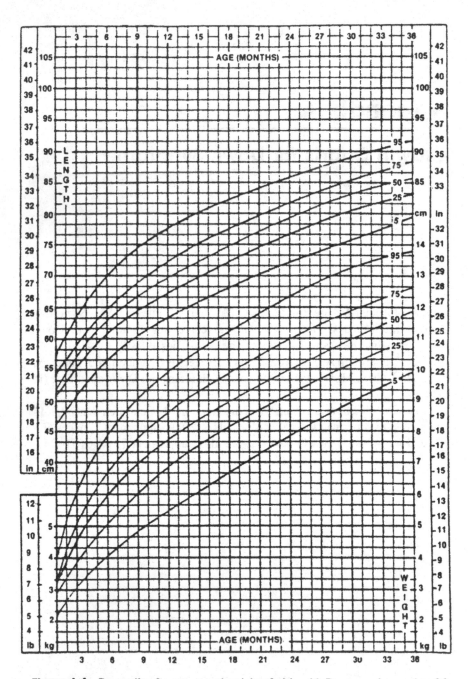

Figure A.1 Percentiles for stature and weight of girls with Down syndrome, 1 to 36 months of age. (Reproduced by permission of *Pediatrics*.)

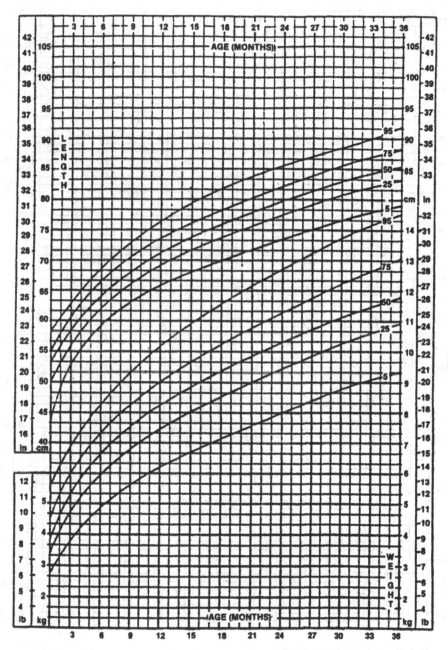

Figure A.2 Percentiles for stature and weight of boys with Down syndrome, 1 to 36 months of age. (Reproduced by permission of *Pediatrics*.)

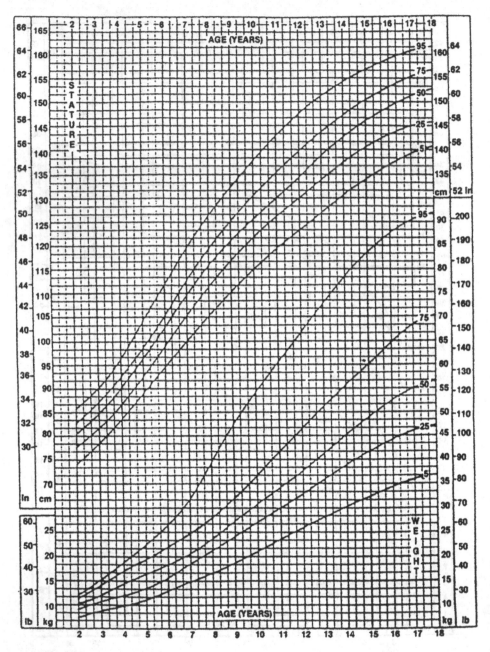

Figure A.3 Percentiles for stature and weight of girls with Down syndrome, 2 to 18 years of age. (Reproduced by permission of *Pediatrics*.)

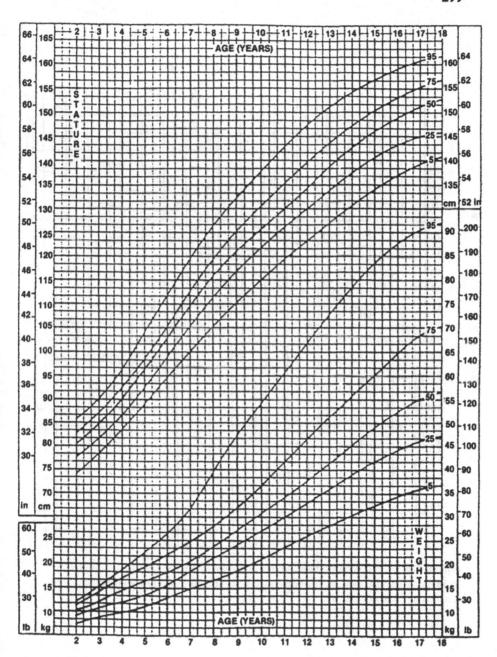

Figure A.4 Percentiles for stature and weight of boys with Down syndrome, 2 to 18 years of age. (Reproduced by permission of *Pediatrics*.)

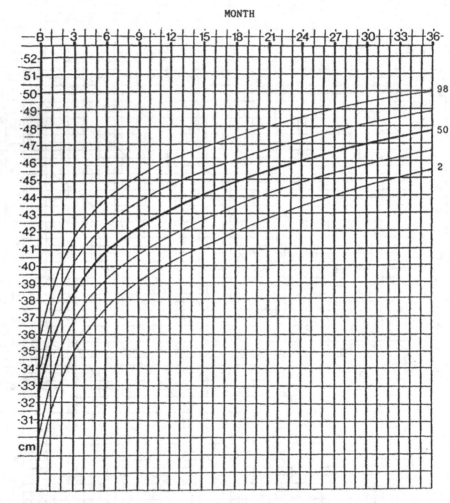

Figure A.5 Percentiles for male and female Down syndrome cranial circumference, 1 to 36 months of age; ages are pooled estimates. Sample included 174 children: males, 63; females 44; unspecified, 67.

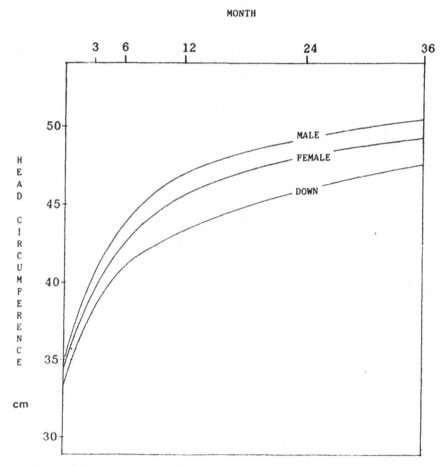

Figure A.6 NCHS male, NCHS female and down syndrome head circumference by age.

Appendix B

Specific Medical Recommendations

RECOMMENDATIONS REGARDING ANESTHESIA

Patients with Down syndrome usually can tolerate local and general anesthetics well, except for drugs in the cholinergic or anticholinergic category. Hypersensitivity to atropine was documented in 1959. In response to 1% atropine, pupils of children with Down syndrome were noted to dilate faster and to remain dilated longer than those of control subjects [1]. This initial finding has since been confirmed by two additional studies [2,3]. There is, however, some overlap with the normal population.

As seen in Fig. B.1, eyedrops of 0.01% tropicamide also produce rapid dilation of the pupils, and the dilation also remains longer [4]. In this study, pupillary responses to tropicamide exceeded those of nonhandicapped controls with statistical significance at all three observation times—20, 30–35, and 45–60 minutes. This study is based on 13 individuals with Down syndrome, 12–50 years of age and controls of similar age groupings.

Two studies have examined whether there is an abnormal tachycardiac effect of intravenous atropine in patients with Down syndrome. In the initial study of this phenomenon, Harris and Goodman found that at a low dose (0.24 mg) there was no difference between persons with Down syndrome and the control group in bradycardiac effect [5]. At increased dosages (0.48–0.96 mg), these investigators recorded a tachycardiac effect [5]. Mir and Cumming then carried out similar studies and found no difference at any dosage between individuals with Down syndrome and those without Down syndrome [6]. Thus, the initial

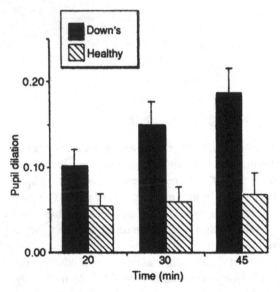

Figure B.1 Mydriatic responses mean (SEM) of those with Down's syndrome and healthy subjects following instillation of tropicamide 0.01%. Pupil dilation = increase in pupil/iris diameter ratio. (Reproduced with permission).

report could not be confirmed by a second study. So it is unclear whether there is sensitivity to intravenous atropine in any, some or all patients with Down syndrome.

Based on present knowledge, it is reasonable to assume that there may be some hypersensitivity to anticholinergic drugs in patients with Down syndrome, and caution should be used in either prescribing such agents or in selecting a dosage level of such drugs.

REFERENCES

1. Berg JM, Brandon MWG, Kirman BH. Atropine in mongolism. Lancet 1959;ii:441–442.
2. Priest JH. Atropine response of the eyes in mongolism. Am J Dis Child 1960;100:869–872.
3. O'Brien D, Haake MW, Braid B. Atropine sensitivity and serotonin in mongolism. Am J Dis Child 1960;100:873–874.
4. Sacks B, Smith S. People with Down's syndrome can be distinguished on the basis of cholinergic dysfunction. J Neurol Neurosurg Psychiatry 1989;52:1294–1295.
5. Harris WS, Goodman RM. Hyper-reactivity to atropine in Down's syndrome. N Engl J Med 1968;279:407–410.
6. Mir GH, Cumming GR. Response to atropine in Down's syndrome. Arch Dis Child 1971;46:61.

STATEMENT/COMMITTEE ON SPORTS MEDICINE OF THE AMERICAN ACADEMY OF PEDIATRICS, 1984
Atlantoaxial Instability in Down Syndrome

Some issues related to participation in certain sports by persons with Down syndrome require clarification.

Since 1965 there have been occasional reports about a condition described at various times as instability, subluxation, or dislocation of the articulation of the first and second cervical vertebrae (atlantoaxial joint) among persons with Down syndrome [1–15]. This condition has also been found in patients with rheumatoid arthritis [16,17], abnormalities of the odontoid process of the second cervical vertebra [4,5,12,13,15], and various forms of dwarfism [18]. Atlantoaxial (C-1, C-2) instability has not attracted general attention because clinical manifestations are rare and the condition is limited to a small portion of the population. The incidence of atlantoaxial instability among persons with Down syndrome has been reported by various observers to be 10% to 20% [2,9,15]. When atlantoaxial instability results in subluxation or dislocation of C-1 and C-2, the spinal cord also may be injured. This is a rare but serious complication.

In March 1983, the Special Olympics, Inc., sponsors of a nationwide competitive program for developmentally disabled persons, without prior announcement, mandated for participants with Down syndrome special precautions to prevent serious neurologic consequences from stress on the head and neck in sports competition [19]. Although thousands of persons with Down syndrome have taken part in sports events during the 15-year history of the Special Olympics without a known occurrence of neurologic complications due to participation, the new directive requires that all persons with Down syndrome who wish to participate in certain sports that might involve stress on the head and neck (gymnastics, diving, pentathlon, butterfly stroke in swimming, diving start in swimming, high jump, soccer, and warm-up exercises that place undue stress on the head and neck muscles) have a medical examination, lateral-view roentgenograms of the upper cervical region in full flexion and extension, and certification by a physician that the examination did not reveal atlantoaxial instability or neurologic disorder. Failure either to comply or to have medical certification would result in exclusion from the above-specified sports.

Parents, physicians, and sports authorities were understandably surprised by the immediacy of the edict. Many parents were resentful because of the short time for screening, the cost of the examinations, and discovery that most physicians did not know about the directive or were not aware of the atlantoaxial syndrome. Some radiologists were not familiar with exact procedures for screening. In general, physicians were perplexed by the sudden concern about a condition that had never been a problem among the largest group of disabled participants during 15 seasons of the Special Olympics.

There are no national statistics to confirm the extent of screening in 1983, but valiant efforts were made to comply with the directive during the 6-week interval allowed for the procedures. It has been stated that there were no reported casualties due to atlantoaxial instability in the Special Olympics last year. However, some participants were barred from the specified events.

Atlantoaxial (C-1, C-2) instability is a manifestation of the generalized poor muscle tone and joint laxity commonly found in persons with Down syndrome. The instability is due to (1) laxity of the transverse ligament that holds the odontoid process of the axis (C-2) in place against the inner aspect of the anterior arch of the atlas (C-1), maintaining integrity of the C-1, C-2 articulation; or (2) abnormalities of the odontoid, such as hypoplasia, malformation, or complete absence [4,5,9,13,15]. These conditions allow some leeway between the odontoid and the atlas, especially during flexion and extension of the neck. This results in a "loose joint." In extreme cases, the first cervical vertebra slips forward and the spinal cord is vulnerable to compression by the odontoid process of C-2 anteriorly or by the arch of C-1 posteriorly.

Measurement of the distance between the odontoid process and the anterior arch of the atlas on lateral roentgenograms in the neutral, flexion, and extension positions is the only way to detect atlantoaxial instability [9,14,20].

Although simple laxity and instability seldom lead to subluxation or dislocation, it has become apparent, as physicians learn more about atlantoaxial instability, that the latent condition must be viewed as a factor predisposing to neurologic complications. Detection of an abnormal space between the odontoid and the anterior arch of the atlas is a signal for precautionary measures to avoid hyperflexion or hyperextension of the neck and extreme rotation of the head.

The neurologic manifestations of spinal compression from the above causes include fatigue in walking, gait disturbance, progressive clumsiness and incoordination, spasticity, hyperreflexia, clonus, toe-extensor reflex, and other upper motor neuron and posterior column signs and symptoms from compression of the spinal cord. Onset of neck pain, head tilt, and torticollis in Down syndrome are indicative of malposition of the odontoid. Development, and particularly, progression of these neurologic signs or symptoms in a person with Down syndrome suggest atlantoaxial subluxation. Strenuous activity should be curtailed and diagnosis and management undertaken promptly.

It is very likely that many schools, recreation and rehabilitation programs, and camps in which developmentally disabled persons are enrolled will follow the example of the Special Olympics in requiring careful screening of all persons with Down syndrome before participation is permitted in activities that could result in flexion and hyperextension. Undoubtedly, pediatricians, other primary care physicians, and radiologists will be called upon to screen and authorize participation.

Recommendations

The Committee on Sport Medicine, after consultation with the Sections on Neurology, Orthopaedics, and Radiology, recommends the following guidelines:

1. All children with Down syndrome who wish to participate in sports that involve possible trauma to the head and neck should have lateral-view roentgenograms of the cervical region in neutral, flexion, and extension position within the patient's tolerance before beginning training or competition. This recommendation applies to all participants in the high-risk sports who have not previously had normal findings on cervical roentgenograms.

    Some physicians may prefer to screen all patients with Down

syndrome routinely at 5 to 6 years of age to rule out atlantoaxial instability.

2. When the distance between the odontoid process of the axis and the anterior arch of the atlas exceeds 4.5 mm, or the odontoid is abnormal, there should be restrictions on sports that involve trauma to the head and neck, and the patient should be followed up at regular intervals.

3. At the present time, repeated roentgenograms are not indicated for those who have previously had normal findings. Indications for repeated roentgenograms will be defined by research.

4. Persons with atlantoaxial subluxation or dislocation and neurologic signs or symptoms should be restricted in all strenuous activities, and operative stabilization of the cervical spine should be considered [21–23].

5. Persons with Down syndrome who have no evidence of atlantoaxial instability may participate in all sports. Follow-up is not required unless musculoskeletal or neurologic signs or symptoms develop.

Committee on Sports Medicine, 1983–1984
Thomas E. Schaffer, MD, *Chair*
Paul G. Dyment, MD
Eugene F. Luckstead, MD
John J. Murray, MD
Nathan J. Smith, MD

Liaison Representatives
James H. Moller, MD
    Section on Cardiology
David M. Orenstein, MD
    Section on Disease of the
    Chest
Arthur M. Pappas, MD
    Section on Orthopaedics

Frederick W. Baker, MD
    Canadian Paediatric Society
Richard Malacrea
    National Athletic Trainers
    Association
Consultants
E. Dennis Lyne, MD, *Chair*
    Section on Orthopaedics
Gerald Erenberg, MD *Chair*
    Section on Neurology
Bruce R. Parker, MD *Chair*
    Section on Radiology
Albert C. Fremont, *Chair*
    Committee on Children with
    Disabilities

REFERENCES

1. Tishler JM, Martel W. Dislocation of the atlas in mongolism: Preliminary report. Radiology 1965;84:904–906.

2. Martel W, Tishler JM. Observations on the spine in mongolism. AJR 1966; 97:630–638.

3. Dzentis AJ. Spontaneous atlanto-axial dislocation in a mongoloid with spinal cord compression: Case report. J Neurosurg 1966;25:458–460.

4. Sherk HH, Nicholson JT. Rotary atlanto-axial dislocation associated with ossiculum terminale and mongolism. J Bone Joint Surg 1969;51-A:957–963.

5. Martel W, Ulyham R, Stimson CW. Subluxation of the atlas causing spinal cord compression in a case of Down's syndrome with a "manifestation of an occipital vertebra." Radiology 1969;93:839–840.

6. Gerard Y, Segal P, Bedoucha JS. L'instabilite de l'atlas sure l'axis dans le mongolisme. Presse Med 1971;79:573–575.

7. Aung MH. Atlanto-axial dislocation in Down's syndrome: Report of a case with spinal cord compression and review of the literature. Bull Los Angeles Neurol Soc 1973;39:197–201.

8. Finerman GAM, Sakai D, Weingarten S. Atlanto-axial dislocation with spinal cord compression in a mongoloid child: A case report. J Bone Joint Surg 1978; 58-A:408–409.

9. Semine AA, Ertel AN, Goldberg MJ, et al. Cervical spine instability in children with Down syndrome (trisomy 21). J Bone Joint Surg 1978;60-A:649–652.

10. Whaley WJ, Gray WD. Atlantoaxial dislocation and Down's syndrome. Can Med Assoc J 1980;123:35–37.

11. Shield LK, Dickens DRV, Jensen F. Atlanto-axial dislocation with spinal cord compression in Down syndrome. Aust Paedriatr J 1981;17:114–116.

12. Hungerford GD, Akkaraju V, Rawe SE, et al. Atlanto-occipital and atlanto-axial dislocations with spinal cord compression in Down's syndrome: A case report and review of the literature. Br J Radiol 1981;54:758–761.

13. Hreidarsson S, Magram G, Singer H. Symptomatic atlantoaxial dislocation in Down syndrome. Pediatrics 1982;69:568–571.

14. Coria F, Quintana F, Villalba M, et al. Craniocervical abnormalities in Down's syndrome. Dev Med Child Neurol 1983;25:252–255.

15. Pueschel SM, Scola FH, Perry CD. Atlanto-axial instability in children with Down syndrome. Pediatr Radiol 1981;10:129–132.

16. Stevens JC, Cartlidge NEF, Saunders M, et al. Atlanto-axial subluxation and cervical myelopathy in rheumatoid arthritis. Q J Med 1971;40:391–408.

17. Herring JA. Cervical instability in Down's syndrome and juvenile rheumatoid arthritis. J Pediatr Orthop 1982;2:205–207.

18. Kopits SE, Perovic MN, McKusick V, et al. Congenital atlanto-axial dislocations in various forms of dwarfism. J Bone Joint Surg 1972;54:1349–1350.

19. Special Olympics Bulletin. Participation by individuals with Down syndrome who suffer from atlantoaxial dislocation condition. Washington, DC, Special Olympics Inc., March 31, 1983.

20. Locke GR, Gardner JI, Van Epps EF. Atlas-dens interval (ADI) in children: A survey based on 200 normal cervical spines. AJR 1966;135–140.

21. Giblin PE, Michell LJ. Management of atlanto-axial subluxation with neurologic involvement in Down syndrome: A report of two cases and review of the literature. Clin Orthop 1979;140:66–71.

22.   Spierings ELH, Braakman R. The management of os odontoideum: Analysis of 37
       cases. J Bone Joint Surg 1982;64-B:422–428.
23.   Diamond LS, Lynne D, Sigman B. Orthopedic disorders in patients with Down's
       syndrome. Orthop Clin North Am 1981;12:57–71.

This statement from the American Academy of Pediatrics has been approved
by the Council on Child and Adolescent Health. Reprinted from *Pediatrics*
74:152–154, 1984.

(See Chapter 11 for a discussion of this recommendation.)

Appendix C

Books About Down Syndrome for Professionals and Parents

References for Physicians

Dmietriev, Valentine and Olwein, Patricia, Editors. *Advances in Down Syndrome*, 1988 (324 pp.), softcover. Special Child Publications, Box 33548, Seattle, WA 98133. A fine general resource book with a wide scope that includes medical and educational strategies; gross motor activities; nutrition; behavior management; living skills for adolescents and adults; and the impact on the family of a child with Down syndrome.

Lane, David and Stratford, Brian, Editors. *Current Approaches to Down's Syndrome*, 1985 (345 pp.), prepaid. Greenwood Press, 88 Post Road W., Box 5007, Westport, CT 06881-9990. An exploration of current initiatives relating to Down syndrome in the medical, educational, and social fields. Written for multidisciplinary audience.

Patterson, David and Epstein, Charles J., Editors. *Molecular Genetics of Chromosome 21 and Down Syndrome*, 1990 (294 pp.). Wiley-Liss, New York. This is based on a 1989 symposium held by the National Down Syndrome Congress. The title speaks for itself.

Pueschel, Siegfried and Rynders, John. *Down Syndrome: Advances in Biomedicine and the Behavioral Sciences*, 1982 (524 pp.), Academic Guild Publishers, Box 397, Cambridge, MA 02138. A useful reference for researchers, physicians, educators, psychologists, and sociologists. This textbook attempts to view research findings in a manner emphasizing scientific advances that have been made or could have been made given adequate attention.

Pueschel, Siegfried. *The Young Child with Down Syndrome*, 1984 (371 pp.), Human Sciences Press, 72 Fifth Avenue, New York, NY 10011-8004. A group of reports that resulted from a special study by Dr. Pueschel and 20 other professionals knowledgeable in the field of Down syndrome. This book is of special interest to medical and educational professionals, but most of it is quite readable by non-physicians.

Pueschel, Siegfried, Tingey, Carol, Rynders, John, Crocker, Allen, and Crutcher, Diane, Editors. *New Perspectives on Down Syndrome*, 1987 (393 pp.), Paul H. Brookes Publishing, Box 10624, Baltimore, MD 21285-0624. The proceedings of the State-of-the-Art conference on Down syndrome held in Boston, April 1985. This book contains current information in the areas of biomedicine, education, community living, and psychosocial aspects with emphasis on future goals. Necessary reference book for professionals and parents alike regarding all facets of Down syndrome. Also available from the National Down Syndrome Congress, 1800 Dempster, Park Ridge, IL 60068-1146.

Trisomy 21 (Down Syndrome). American Journal of Medical Genetics, Supplement 7, 1990 (330 pp.). Sixty papers presented at the International Congress in Rome in 1989 cover a wide range of new and future research work in Down syndrome.

Van Dyke, D.C., Lang, D.J., Heide, F., van Duyne, S., Soucek, M.J. *Clinical Perspectives in the Management of Down Syndrome*, 1990. Springer-Verlag, New York. A description of many different investigations of 190 children, aged 1 to 20 years. Useful to the physician.

Especially for New Parents

Cunningham, Cliff. *Down's Syndrome: An Introduction for Parents*, 2nd edition, 1988 (187 pp.). Distributed exclusively in the United States by Brookline Books, Box 1046, Cambridge, MA 02238. Cunningham modestly describes this newest book as "an attempt to provide some answers to the immediate questions parents ask." Excellent basic book.

Dmitriev, Valentine. *Time to Begin*, 1984 (248 pp.), hardback; softcover. Caring, Box 400, Milton, WA 98354. A current and complete volume, in workbook style, on early intervention for infants and toddlers with Down syndrome. Based on model early childhood programs for children with Down syndrome.

Hanson, Marci. *Teaching the Infant with Down Syndrome: A Guide for Parents and Professionals*, 2nd edition, 1987 (268 pp.), Pro-Ed, 8700 Shoal Creek Blvd., Austin, TX 78758-6897. A manual for parents with step-by-step instructions for teaching skills to infants with Down syndrome.

Horrobin, Margaret and Rynders, John E. *To Give an Edge: A Guide for New Parents of Children with Down's Syndrome*, revised edition, 1984 (103 pp.), Margaret Colwell, %Colwell Industries, 123 N. Third Street, Minneapolis, MN 55401. Make checks payable to To Give An Edge. Contains a wealth of information for new parents of children with Down syndrome as well as parents of older individuals with Down syndrome.

Pueschel, Siegfried, Editor. *Down Syndrome: Growing and Learning*, 1978 (173 pp.), Andrews & McMeel, 4900 Main Street, Kansas City, MO 64112. An excellent overview of Down syndrome, starting with diagnosis and outlining developmental expectations from infancy to adulthood.

Pueschel, Siegfried, M., Editor. *A Parent's Guide to Down Syndrome: Toward a Brighter Future*, 1990. Brookes Publishing, Box 10624, Baltimore, MD 211285. A comprehensive reference book especially for new parents but useful and informative to "seasoned" parents as well. Range of topics include: history of Down syndrome, physical characteristics, developmental expectations, early intervention, feeding the young child, the school years, recreation, adolescence and adulthood, vocational training and employment.

Stray-Gundersen, Karen, Editor. *Babies with Down Syndrome: A New Parent's Guide*, 1986 (237 pp.), Woodbine House, 5615 Fishers Lane, Rockville, MD 20852. A comprehensive guide for new parents and interested others on how to help a child with Down syndrome reach his or her potential.

Simons, Robin. *After the Tears*, 1987 (88 pp.), hardcover, paperback, Harcourt, Brace & Jovanovich, Attn: Trade Dept., 1250 Sixth Avenue, San Diego, CA 92101-4311. This book is subtitled, "parents talk about raising a child with a disability" and is beautifully edited, illustrated, and designed. Parental experiences are integrated into short, readable chapters. Suggestions of simple, constructive things to do follow each chapter.

Turnbull, H.R. III, and Turnbull, Ann P. *Parents Speak Out (Then and Now)*, 2nd edition, 1984, Charles E. Merrill Publishing, 1300 Alum Creek Drive, Box 508, Columbus, OH 43216. This book contains the then and now reflection of parents, who are also professionals in the field of developmental disabilities.

Schiff, Harriet Sarnoff. *The Bereaved Parent*, 1977 (146 pp.), paperback, Viking/Penguin, 120 Woodbine Street, Bergenfield, NJ 07621. Very understanding, commonsense book, especially useful to parents who may not have a strong particular religious faith.

Books About Playing With Your Child

Adcock, Don and Marilyn Segal. *Noval University Play and Learn Program* (College Ave., Ft. Lauderdale, FL 33314). Four volumes: *From Birth to One*

Year. One Year to Two Years. Two-Years-Old, Playing and Learning. Social Competence, Two Years. Paperback. Rolling Hills Estates, CA: B.L. Winch and Associates, 1979. Available from: B.L. Winch and Associates, 45 Hitching Post Drive, Building 2, Rolling Hills Estates, CA 90274. (213) 547-1240.

Gordon, Ira J. *Baby Learning Through Baby Play: A Parent's Guide for the First Two Years.* 1970, paperback. St. Martin's Press, 175 Fifth Ave., New York, NY 10010.

Gordon, Ira J. *Baby to Parent, Parent to Baby: A Guide to Loving and Learning in a Child's First Year.* 1977, paperback. St. Martin's Press, 175 Fifth Ave., New York, NY 10010.

Sinker, Mary. *The Lekotek Guide to Good Toys.* 1983, paperback. Lekotek, 613 Dempster St., Evanston, IL 60201. (312) 328-0001.

Stein, Sara Bonnett. *Learn at Home the Sesame Street Way.* 1979, hardback. Simon & Schuster Building, Rockefeller Center, 1230 Avenue of the Americas, New York, NY 10020. Excellent, creative collection of play activities. A great rainy day (and every day) reference.

Other Developmental Books

Lehane, Stephen. *Help Your Baby Learn: 100 Piaget-Based Activities for the First Two Years of Life.* 1976, paperback. Englewood Cliffs, NJ: Prentice-Hall, 1976.

Levy, Janine. *The Baby Exercise Book: For the First Fifteen Months.* 1973, paperback. New York, NY: Pantheon Books, a division of Random House.

Obtaining Services (Advocacy and Practical Problems)

Anderson, Chitwood and Hayden. *Negotiating the Special Education Maze: A Guide for Parents and Teachers,* 2nd edition, 1989 (250 pp.), paperback. Woodbine House, 5615 Fishers Lane, Rockville, MD 20852. This book was designed to help parents become effective educational advocates for children with disabilities.

How to Get Services by Being Assertive, 1980, revised 1985 (100 pp.), Coordinating Council for Handicapped Children, 20 East Jackson, Room 900, Chicago, IL 60604. A manual that will quickly bring out of the shadows of being "only a parent" into the ranks of being a mover for your child and all children with handicaps.

How to Organize an Effective Parent Group and Move Bureaucracies, 1980 (131 pp.), Coordinating Council for Handicapped Children, 20 E. Jackson,

Room 900, Chicago, IL 60604. Details and common sense suggestions about what new groups encounter and how to handle these situations.

Perske, Robert and Perske, Martha. *New Life in the Neighborhood*, 1980 (78 pp.), Abingdon Press, 201 Eighth Avenue, S., Box 801, Nashville, TN 37202. A timely upbeat book developed from 158 interviews with people living close to 87 family-like residences, each containing six or fewer persons with disabilities. Warm beautiful illustrations.

Russel, L. Mark. *Alternatives, A Family Guide to Legal and Financial Planning for the Disabled*, 1983 (194 pp.), paperback, postpaid. First Publications, Box 1832, Evanston, IL 60204. This book gives a general overview of the subject and is comprehensive and readable. It is written by an attorney who has a brother with a mental disability. It would be good reading for attorneys as an introduction to the special considerations; also good for laypersons.

Wernz, Ann Hart. *Planning for the Disabled Child*, 1980, revised 1984 (32 pp.), Northwestern Mutual Life Insurance, 720 E. Wisconsin Ave., Milwaukee, WI 53202. Request Order #22-3033 and mark "Attention: Field Orders." This study was prepared for Northwestern Mutual. It is an excellent reference to hand to your attorney for his or her perusal. It is thorough yet concise and speaks an attorney's language.

Appendix D

Parent Support Organizations

Argentina

Asociacion Sindrome de Down de la Republica Argentina
Charcas 4649-Cap. Fed. 1425
Tel: 773-5771

Australia

Australian Down Syndrome Assoc., Inc.
91 Hutt Street
Adelaide 5000
Australia
Tel: 08-365-1577

Brazil

Projeto Down
Centro de Informacao & Pesquisa da Sindrome de Down
Ave Briz. Faria Lima 1698 4
Andar Cep. 01452
Sao Paulo, Brazil
Tel: (55) 11-813-4688

Centro Da Dinamica De Ensino
Nancy Derwood Mills Costa
Executive Director
Rua Tenente Negrao, 188
Itaim CEP 04530

Canada

Jeanne Sheldon Robertson
Speech-Language Pathologist
Nova Scotia Hearing
%St. Rita Hospital
409 Kings Road
Sydney, Nova Scotia
Canada B2S 1B4
Tel: 564-5414

Losi Paterson RN
Hereditary Disease Nurse
Red Deer Health Unit
Provincial Building
4920 51st Street
Red Deer, Alberta
Canada T4N 6K8
Tel: 408-343-5340

Sheila Achkewich
EIP Program Worker
Alberta East Central Health
Unit #10, 4703-53 Street
Camrose, Alberta
Canada T4V 1Y8
Tel: 672-3161

Community Health Nursing
5th Floor
Seventh Street Plaza
10030 107th Street
Edmonton, Alberta
Canada T5J 3E4

Mrs. Fran Flanagan
Coordinator
Infant Stimulation Program
Peterborough County City Health Unit
835 Weller Street
Peterborough, Ontario
Canada K9J 4Y1
Tel: 705-743-1160

Joan Devoe
Secretary
Infant Development Program
477 Queen Street East
Suite 104
Sault Ste. Marie, Ontario
Canada P6A 1Z5
Tel: 705-942-3103

Early Education Program
10950-159 Street
Edmonton, Alberta
Canada T5P 3C1
Tel: 403-484-5770

Ms. Katy Cox
Box 69
Peach River Health Unit
Peach River, Alberta
Canada T0H 2X0
Tel: 624-3611

Physio Therapy Dept.
Dr. George-L Dumont Hospital
Moncton, New Brunswick
Canada E1C 2Z3

Holy Cross Hospital
2210 2nd Street, SW
%Allan & Johnston
Calgary, Alberta
Canada T2S 1S6

Rob Danson
Special Needs
Jewish Family and Child Service of Metropolitan Toronto
4600 Bathurst Street
Willowdale, Ontario
Canada M2R 3V3

Burnaby Infant Development Program
6161 Jilpui Street
Burnaby, British Columbia
Canada V5G 4A3
Julia Hart
Tel: 294-7260

The Canadian Down Syndrome Society
#303 501 18th Avenue, S.W.
Calgary, Alberta
Canada T2S 0C7
Tel: 403-235-0746

Judith Pepler
Family Education Center
Calgary Association for the Mentally Handicapped
303, 1147 17th Avenue SW
Calgary, Alberta
Canada T2T 0B7
Tel: 403-244-9335

Ft. McMurray & District Health Unit
Early Intervention Program
9921 Main Street
Ft. McMurray, Alberta
Canada T9H 4B4
Tel: 403-743-3232

Margaret Dediluke
Program Director
Terrace Child Development Centre
2510 South Eby Street
Terrace, British Columbia
Canada V8G 2X3

Ms. Armour
Book Editor
National Institute on Mental Retardation
Kinsmen NIMR Building
York University Campus
4700 Keele Street
Downview, Ontario
Canada M3J 1P3
Tel: 416-661-9611

Betty M. Youson, RN
Nurse Coordinator
Department of Genetics
The Hospital for Sick Children
555 University Avenue
Toronto, Ontario
Canada M5G 1X8
Tel: 416-597-1500

Donna Dawkins
Executive Director
Planned Parenthood New Brunswick
65 Rue Brunswick
Fredericton, New Brunswick
Canada E3B 1G5
Tel: 506-454-1808

The Dr. Charles A. Janeway
Child Health Care Centre
Receiving Department
Newfoundland Drive
Pleasantville, St. John's
Newfoundland, Canada A1A 1R8

Colombia

Corporacion Sindrome de Down
Apartado Aereo 91925
Bogota
Colombia
Tel: (571) 266-7090, 253-0131

Chile

Walter Sanches
Instituto de Estudios Internacionales
Universidad de Chile
Casilla 14187 Suc. 21
Santiago, Chile

France

A.P.E.M.
4 Rue de la Maison Communale
B-4802 Heusy, France
Tel: (087) 22-88-44

Section Charleroi
Entre Sambre et Meuse
76, Rue du corby
6110 Montigny-Le Tilleul, France
Tel: (071) 51-24-67

Section Hesbaye Condroz
102, Rue de Leumont
5250 Antheit/Wanzw, France
Tel: (085) 21-50-01

Section Liege
12, Rue de la Forge
4030 Grivegnee, France
Tel: (041) 42-35-81

Hong Kong/Japan

Ms. Adeline Sybesma
Hokkaido International School
41-8 Jukuzum
Sapporo, Hokkaido, 062
Japan

Shirley B. Cheyfitz
The Matilda Child Development Center
41 Mount Kellett Road
Hong Kong
Tel: 5-8496138

Lee Guild, Director
Educational Services Exchange with China, Inc.
1641 West Main Street, #401
Alhambra, CA, USA 91801
Tel: 818-570-9721

Ireland

Down Syndrome Association of Munster
Ireland

Down Syndrome Association of Ireland
27 South William Street
Dublin 2
Tel: (01) 6793322

Israel/Saudi Arabia

HELP
Guidance and Counseling Center
PO Box 1049
Jeddah, Saudi Arabia 21431
Tel: 660-0013, Ext. 70
Telex: 601130 SJ

Israel Association for Rehabilitation of the Mentally Handicapped
Branch: 16, Bialik St.
Tel Aviv 65241
Israel

Ms. Dahlia Nissim
National Guidance Center for Special Education and Rehabilitation in Israel
Beit "SHEMS"
30 Plitei Hasfar Street
Tel Aviv 67948
Israel

Italy

Associazione Banmbini Down
Viale Delle Milzie 106
00192 Roma, Italy
Tel: 384949, 317976

Associazione Bambini Down
Via Zianotte 25
Roma, Italy

Associazione Bambini Down
Via Pietro Ciaunoue 25
Roma
Maure Cova %HERNEMAU
407 West 54th Street
New York, NY
Tel: 212-586-2466

Mexico

Centro De Terapia
Educativa De Morelia, Mich AC
Lic. Bucio 63 Fracc,
Ocolusen, Morelia, Mich.
Mexico
Tel: 2-73-41

Asociacion Mexicana de Sindrome de Down, A.C.
Boulevard de la Luz 232
Jardines del Pedregal
01900 Mexico, D.F.
Tel: (525) 652-42-00

Down Association of Monterrey AC
20 De Noviembre Sur 846
Monterrey, N.L., Mexico

Fundacion Down de la Laguna
Avenida Morelos, No. 43 Ote.
Torreon, Coah. 27000
Mexico
Tel: 18-58-05

The Netherlands

STICHTING
"DOWN'S SYNDROOM"
Bovenboerseweg 41
NL-7946 Al Venneperveen
Tel: 05228-1337

Puerto Rico

Dulce Delirro
Asociacion de Padres
Pro-Bienestar de Ninos Impedidos
PO Box 21301
Rio Piedras, Puerto Rico 00928

University of Puerto Rico
School of Medicine
Myriam Castro de Castaneda
GPO Box 5067
San Juan, Puerto Rico 00936

Ms. Eva Lopez
Founder & Director
Fundacion Para Servicios a Ninos Mentalmente Retardados
de Puerto Rico, Inc.
Americo Salas No. 1422
Santurce, Puerto Rico 00910
Tel: 725-5571

Singapore

Head
Disabled Persons Section
Development Division
Ministry 06 Social Affairs
Pearl's Hill
Singapore 0316

Spain

Fundacio Catalana por a la Sindrome de Down
Carrer Valencia, 229, 3.er, 2.a
08007 Barcelona
Spain
Tel: (93) 215-1988

Fundacion Sindrome de Down de Cantabria
Avda. de General Davila, 24-A, 1.0,C
39005 Santander
Spain
Tel: (942) 278028

Escola Municipal
"Vil-la Joana"
Carretera De Les Planes, S/N
Vallvidrera-Barcelona-17, Spain

Asociacion Sindrome de Down de Baleares
Carretera Palma-Alcudia, Km. 7,5
07141 Marratxi, Baleares
Spain
Tel: 600857

United States

Association for Children with Down Syndrome
2616 Martin Ave.
Bellmore, NY 11710
Tel: 516-221-4700

National Down Syndrome Society
666 Broadway
New York, NY 10012
Tel: 212-460-9330 (800-221-4602)

National Down Syndrome Congress
1800 Dempster St.
Park Ridge, Ill 60068-1146
Tel: 312-823-7550 (800-232-6372)

Special Resource

Down Syndrome Adoption Exchange
56 Midchester Ave.
White Plains, NY 10606
Tel: 914-428-1236

Appendix E

Preventive Medicine Checklist: Neonatal Through Adult

I. Neonatal period (birth–2 months)
   A. History
      1. Parental concerns
      2. Feeding pattern
      3. Stooling pattern
   B. Physical examination
      1. Complete general physical and neurological examination.
      2. Plot height and weight on Down syndrome growth chart.
      3. Look for signs of congenital heart disease such as cyanosis, irregular heart rate, or heart murmur.
      4. Careful examination for otitis media and cataracts.
      5. Screen hearing.
   C. Lab
      1. Karyotype
      2. Thyroid function
      3. Echocardiogram
   D. Consults
      1. Cardiology
      2. Genetic
   E. Recommendations
      1. A follow-up appointment at a Down syndrome center
      2. Parent and education support
      3. Referral to infant education program

II.   Infancy (2 months–12 months)
    A.   History
        1.   Review parental concerns.
        2.   Review medical history, especially in relation to otitis media and constipation.
    B.   Physical examination
        1.   General physical and neurological examination.
        2.   Plot parameters on Down syndrome growth chart.
    C.   Lab
        1.   Audiology assessment
        2.   Thyroid screening that includes T4 and TSH at one year of age
    D.   Consultation
        1.   Cardiology
        2.   Infant developmental specialist or team of occupational therapist, physical therapist, and speech and language therapist
        3.   Ophthalmology
        4.   Nutritional where indicated
    E.   Recommendations
        1.   A follow-up appointment at the Down syndrome center
        2.   Continue infant education program
        3.   Continue family education support
III. Childhood (1–12 years)
    A.   History
        1.   Review parental concerns
        2.   Review educational program
        3.   Inquire about behavioral problems
        4.   Inquire about hearing or vision problems
    B.   Physical examination
        1.   General physical and careful neurological examination.
        2.   Plot height and weight on Down syndrome growth chart.
    C.   Lab
        1.   Annual thyroid screening with T4 and TSH
        2.   Hearing screening
        3.   X-ray cervical spine
    D.   Consults
        1.   Ophthalmology annually
        2.   Ears nose and throat when indicated
        3.   Dental annually after the age of one
    E.   Recommendations
        1.   A follow-up appointment at the Down syndrome center

       2. Infant and child education program
       3. Regular exercise and recreational programs
       4. Continue parent education support
       5. Discuss respite care with family

IV. Adolescence (12–18 years)

    A. History

       1. Review parent concerns.
       2. Inquire about symptoms of hypothyroidism.
       3. Inquire about vision and hearing problems.

    B. Physical examination

       1. Good general physical as well as neurological examination.
       2. Plot growth parameters on Down syndrome growth chart.

    C. Lab

       1. Annual thyroid screening with T4 and TSH.
       2. Hearing screening annually.
       3. Echocardiogram where indicated for mitral valve prolapse.
       4. Repeat cervical spine film at 18 years of age.

    D. Consultations

       1. Pelvic exam and pap smear for teenage girls
       2. Ophthalmology consult yearly
       3. Dental

    E. Recommendations

       1. Continue appointments at the Down syndrome center.
       2. Review educational and transitional vocational plans.
       3. Continue parent education support.
       4. Regular exercise recreational program.
       5. Sexuality education.

V. Adulthood (over 18 years)

    A. History

       1. Review for symptoms of dementia, such as decreased memory or care skills.
       2. Screen for hearing and vision problems.

    B. Physical examination

       1. General physical/neurological examination.
       2. Gynecology examination/pap smear.
       3. Monitor weight closely for obesity.

    C. Lab

       1. Annual thyroid screening with TSH and T4
       2. Hearing screening
       3. X-ray cervical spine at the age of 30

4. Echocardiogram for mitral valve prolapse where indicated
5. Pap smear annually
6. Baseline mammogram at 35 years of age
7. Follow up where indicated by physical examination and family history thereafter

D. Consultations
    1. Ophthalmology
    2. Dental

E. Recommendations
    1. Continue appointments at the Down syndrome center
    2. Vocational training
    3. Continue adult education where indicated
    4. Sexuality education
    5. Continue family and education support
    6. Regular exercise and recreation program

Appendix F

Financial Checklist for Families

1. Establish family budget.
2. Document all medical-related expenses. Include all out-of-pocket expenses, such as health insurance premiums, physical and occupational therapy, prescribed medical equipment, mileage for transportation costs to and from medical care, and home adaptations necessary because of a child's condition.
3. Negotiate a realistic repayment schedule with hospitals and physicians.
4. Assess closely associated fringe benefits when seeking a new employment opportunity.
5. Make sure you are receiving all of the appropriate government services and tax benefits allowed.
6. Make a long-term financial plan that includes a testamentory trust, low cost life insurance, and a savings account.

This list was adapted from the following article: Worley G, Rosenfeld L, and Lipscomb J. Financial counselling for families of children with chronic disabilities. Developmental Medicine Child Neurology: 1991; 33:679–689.

Appendix G

Using Computers to Stimulate Developmental Skills

Many parents wonder what they can do at home to improve their child's development. Microcomputers can help children gain developmental skills. A home computer may benefit a child in several ways [1]:

1. Improve communication skills. Newer programs provide a synthesized voice in response to a child's selections of objects on the screen.
2. Increase motivation. Children's interaction with a computer can be entertaining and engaging.
3. Enhance self-esteem. As a child learns how to control a computer, it can provide a sense of accomplishment.

Parents should determine whether their child is ready developmentally for a computer. A child needs to have visual motor skills at about a 2- to 2½-year level to profit from having a home computer. If the child can use a remote control for television, he or she is ready to operate a computer.

The next step is to select the specific skills that the parents wish to develop in their child, for example, improving articulation or specific prereading skills. By talking to the child's therapists or teachers, parents can learn what skills need the most improvement. It is important to decide on goals so that a computer can be selected with appropriate equipment to meet an individual child's needs.

The next step is the selection of the hardware (the actual computer unit). The two major types of computers for education are manufactured by Apple Computer and IBM. Apple makes several computers, including the Macintosh, that have been used extensively in schools. The Apple computers offer many advantages for educational use over the IBM and IBM-compatible computers. Macintoshs are easy to use and easy to learn. They have a high quality of output, a graphic interface (that is, the use of a hand directed mouse to manipulate icons on the screen instead of using specific key sequences), and a high rate of user satisfaction [2]. Disadvantages include their initial cost and less acceptance in the business world. The IBM and IBM-compatible computers have an initial lower cost and have general acceptance in the business world. However, they require a longer time to learn how to use. A recently introduced software package provides a graphical interface for the IBM computers and may change the traditional differences between the two computers.

Both companies can provide information that will help in choosing hardware. The following are the addresses to write to obtain more information about each companies' computers for educational programs.

Apple Computer
Office of Special Education
20525 Mariani Avenue
Cupertino, CA 95014
408-973-4475

IBM
National Support Center for Persons with Disabilities
P.O. Box 2150
Atlanta, GA 30055

Other computer users can also provide helpful information with deciding on a computer. User groups are clubs of people using computers and often are divided into smaller special interest groups, such as those persons interested in educational use of computers. Contacting several persons in a user group can help provide information not only about which computer to buy, but also where to buy it. It is helpful to buy from a dealer that provides support (that is, technicians or knowledgeable salespeople who would be available to answer questions about operation of the computer) and education in computer use after the sale. Computer magazines such as *MacUser* and *PC* are available on the newsstand and print informative articles about computer models. Two other noncommercial resources to consult are:

Trace Research & Development Center
S-151 Waisman Center
1500 Highland Avenue
Madison, WI 53705
608-262-6966

Closing the gap
P.O. Box 68
Henderson, MN 56044
612-248-3294

Once a computer is purchased, the next decisions concern the purchase of software. Software refers to the actual program that runs the computer. Software is packaged in a small, flexible mylar disk that is 3½ inches or 5¼ inches in size.

There are several ways to find software that fits your child's learning needs. The Menu, available from the International Software Database Corporation (1-800-The Menu), is one source that lists (with brief descriptions) all of the software available for Apple or IBM computers. The Special Education Software Center (1-800-327-5892) is a federally supported clearinghouse that provides information about software for educational needs.

The following are a few additional suggestions for selecting software for children [3]:

1. Always try a program before buying it.
2. Written instructions should be very simple and never more than one or two words.
3. Words in the program should be in large type.
4. Start-up should be very simple. The game or program selection should be easy for the child to do.
5. When appropriate, programs should have some form of built-in speech synthesizer so that a child receives both visual and oral clues.
6. A program also should have the capability to produce a printed product that a child can see and show to others.

A home computer can be a helpful tool in stimulating a child's developmental skills. Proper selection of hardware and software guarantees that a child will use the equipment purchased. If, after some effort, a parent is still not sure which computer or software to buy, a final word of advice is to try renting a computer and see which works best for their child.

REFERENCES

1. Willner J. Using computers to help children with Down syndrome. New York: The National Down Syndrome Society,* 1989.

---

*The address for the National Down Syndrome Society is 666 Broadway, New York, New York, 10012.

2. Malone G. Issues of hardware acquisition for K–12 education. Technol Horizons in Educ J 1989;April(suppl):59–63.
3. Wellington A. Educating Mac. MacGuide Magazine 1989;2:42–45.

Index

About the Authors

PAUL T. ROGERS is Director of the Rehabilitation of Chronic Illness program at Mt. Washington Pediatric Hospital and Instructor in the Department of Pediatrics at the Johns Hopkins School of Medicine, Baltimore, Maryland. The author of numerous book chapters and articles, Dr. Rogers is a Fellow of the American Board of Pediatrics and the American Academy of Pediatrics, as well as a member of the Society for Developmental Pediatrics and the American Academy of Cerebral Palsy and Developmental Medicine. Dr. Rogers received the B.S. degree (1967) in microbiology from the Ohio State University, Columbus, and the M.D. degree (1971) from the University of Maryland School of Medicine, Baltimore.

MARY COLEMAN is an emeritus member of the Department of Pediatrics, Georgetown University School of Medicine, Washington, D.C. The author of numerous books and papers, Dr. Coleman has directed much of her research and writing toward enhancing the quality of life of individuals with Down syndrome and their families. She is a member of the Child Neurology Society, the American Academy of Neurology, the American Epilepsy Society, and the American Society of Neurochemistry, among others. Dr. Coleman received the B.A. degree in general studies from the University of Chicago, Illinois, and the M.D. degree from the George Washington University School of Medicine, Washington, D.C.

Printed in the United States
by Baker & Taylor Publisher Services